P. E. Ochsner (Ed.) • **Total Hip Replacement**

Springer-Verlag Berlin Heidelberg GmbH

Peter E. Ochsner (Ed.)

Total Hip Replacement

Implantation Technique and Local Complications

Presentation based on the system according to M.E. Müller with long-term follow-up

With Contributions by
M. Brunazzi • P. Ferrat • S. Häfliger • M. Klein
G. Kohler • M. Lüem • T. Maurer • T. Münch • B. Nachbur
P. E. Ochsner • A.S. Pirwitz • U. Riede • M. Sarungi
M. Schafroth • A. Schweizer • R. Sommacal • H.R. Stöckli
Y. Thomann • D. Toia • J. Vaeckenstedt • W. Zimmerli

Foreword by M. E. Müller

With 169 Figures in 361 Separate Illustrations, 84 in colour, and 24 Tables

Springer

Professor Dr. med. PETER EMIL OCHSNER
Chefarzt der Orthopädischen Klinik
Kantonsspital

CH-4410 Liestal
Switzerland

Translator:

Robert Hinchliffe
2 The Gully
Winterbourne

Bristol BS36 1QW
United Kingdom

The German Edition appeared under the title
Peter Ochsner (Hrsg.): Die Hüfttotalprothese

ISBN 978-3-642-62868-9 ISBN 978-3-642-55679-1 (eBook)
DOI 10.1007/978-3-642-55679-1

Cataloging-in-Publication Data applied for

A catalog record for this book is available from the Library 9f Congress.

Bibliographic information published by Die Deutsche Bibliothek
Die Deutsche Bibliothek lists this publication in the Deutsche Nationalbibliografie;
detailed bibliographic data is available in the Internet at http://dnb.ddb.de

http://www.springer.de

Originally published by Springer-Verlag Berlin Heidelberg New York in 2003
Softcover reprint of the hardcover 1st edition 2003

Medical illustrations: J. Kühn, Heidelberg
Graphics: G. Hippmann, Nürnberg
Cover design: deblik Berlin
Typesetting and reproduction of the figures: AM-productions GmbH, Wiesloch

Printed on acid-free paper SPIN 10718477 24/3150PF 5 4 3 2 1 0

THIS BOOK IS DEDICATED
TO MAURICE E. MÜLLER
AND HANS WILLENEGGER †
AND TO OUR PATIENTS

Foreword

"Total Hip Replacement" by Peter Ochsner and his colleagues is a unique, exemplary, instructive and valuable addition to the world of surgery.

Shortly after taking charge of the newly established department for orthopaedic surgery in Liestal in June 1984, the new medical director, Peter E. Ochsner, decided to document all total hip replacement operations prospectively and then follow these up regularly over a minimum period of 10 years.

The former director of the surgical clinic, Professor Hans Willenegger, had previously established a documentation secretariat. The documentation system selected by Peter Ochsner was based on the code forms A (first hospital stay), B (revision procedure) and C (follow-up), which were developed in 1984 by the MEM Institute for Documentation in Berne, each form incorporating over 400 check boxes. The forms are supplemented by the radiograph card, with affixed copies of the most important images, and the preoperative plans. New forms revised by IDES ("International Documentation and Evaluation System") and accepted by SICOT were used from 1991.

With the application of a little discipline, consistent completion of the A form did not prove to be a problem, provided that every operator was prepared to write the surgical report immediately after the procedure. This task took up little more than 5 minutes of the surgeon's time. Follow-up planning, however, proved rather more difficult according to Peter Ochsner, although it still proved possible to invite and follow-up over 96 % of operated patients who were still living.

Once the code forms have been correctly marked and imported into the database, either by the optical scanner or by hand, the surgeon then has at his disposal an incredibly valuable information resource. At the press of a button, the computer can provide not only the complete medical histories, but any desired statistical compilation or lists with data summaries. By 2000, data were available from over 1500 primary hip replacements and 478 revisions. In order to ensure the inclusion of a sufficient follow-up period for patients with complications, it was decided that the statistical analysis should only take into consideration those patients undergoing surgery prior to 1997. Excluding deceased patients, this resulted in 1081 primary cases and 330 revision procedures. Each group of complications was analysed according to all possible criteria, which meant that not only could number, cause, treatment and outcome, previous procedures, age and weight be determined, but also the precise diagnoses, per- or post-operative sources of error and complications of a local and general nature.

The various chapters, including those on surgical technique and planning, postoperative haematomas and dislocations, fractures and other perioperative complications, trochanteric problems, leg length discrepancies, limping, periarticular ossification, pain, revision rates, are objectively and comprehensively discussed by various collaborators. In the difficult chapters on infections, nerve lesions and vascular injuries, Peter Ochsner sought the assistance of well-known specialists. Special emphasis has been placed on preoperative patient briefing. Additionally, the literature, including the last five years of the principal orthopaedic journals, has been reviewed and compared with the authors' own results. The data were collated from all the patients undergoing surgery at the clinic, i.e. roughly one third were operated on by the medical director himself, one third by senior registrars and experienced assistants and the last third by more junior registrars.

Over the course of the last five years, medical documentation technology has advanced in leaps and bounds. Electronic medical histories coupled with digital archiving of radiographs and integrated quality control, regardless of the specialist field, have now become commonplace. All of the information that is important for the clinic director, surgeon, theatre nurse, patient, administration, clinical researcher, health insurance scheme, healthcare policy-maker, medical technologist, not forgetting the lawyer, can be collated in one and the same database. At the same time, these systems represent a substantial saving on paperwork for the surgical assistant. The main question nowadays is whether the information should be saved via an Internet platform or via optical scanners.

While no-one can say how soon this trend will become a reality in Swiss hospitals, one thing is certain: systematic, prospective, seamless, patient-oriented documentation is here to stay, and should become a quality benchmark for procedures performed by any conscientious orthopaedic surgeon.

To sum up: the work of Peter Ochsner and his colleagues is unique because all total hip replacements undertaken between 1984 and 1997 at the Liestal Cantonal Hospital have been documented almost seamlessly (> 96%). The book shows, in an exemplary manner, how to publish in book form data for a whole clinic that have been prospectively collated and stored over many years.

The book is instructive in several respects, since it shows how the quality of a surgical team can be discerned through seamless documentation and provides senior surgeons and assistants with a wealth of data for presentations and scientific papers. These individuals can then draw on the experience thereby gained throughout their career.

The book is particularly valuable for those who seek to perform total hip replacements correctly and avoid complications, yet manage them competently when they occur. It will help the junior orthopaedic surgeon acquire a solid grounding in these areas. But thanks to the wealth of detailed information, it also enables the experienced orthopaedic surgeon, in particular, to deal in depth with the problems associated with complications and the options for systematic documentation.

The book is recommended to all those who deal with problems relating to hip surgery and statistics in medicine, and is also of particular interest to general practitioners.

Maurice E. Müller

Preface

Our aim in writing this book is to convey as much practical information as possible on the surgical technique of total hip replacement and the prevention and treatment of complications. Chapter 3, "Surgical Technique", deals with special design features of the implants used, operation planning and the detailed sequence of surgical steps in primary and revision procedures. The uniformly structured chapters on complications focus on definitions, frequency, prophylaxis, treatment and literature references. Numerous examples and sketches, some described and illustrated in considerable detail, are intended to stimulate a rational debate. Many cross-references are included for further enlightenment. Separate chapters are devoted to the subjects of documentation, patient population and preoperative briefing. The comprehensive survival curves for the implants used constitute a key scientific element of the book and cover all the implants developed by M.E. Müller and currently on the market, as well as the Wagner SL revision stem. By way of a reminder, it was in 1977 – exactly 25 years ago – that M.E. Müller introduced two of his most important implants, the straight-stem prosthesis and the acetabular reinforcement ring.

The book aims to encourage both recently qualified and experienced orthopaedic surgeons to compare their own experiences and problems with those of a hospital that has been monitoring its own patient population in a regular follow-up programme for 18 years. The idea of a standardised surgical technique and systematic documentation for total hip replacements was suggested to the editor of this book on his arrival at Liestal in 1984 by Maurice E. Müller, who also provided financial support to initiate the scientific research work at the newly formed Orthopaedic Hospital. Since 1989, the editor has also regularly been invited by the company Protek to attend the meetings of its technical committee. This committee was made up of engineers, marketing specialists and orthopaedic surgeons, including H.-B. Burch, R. Ganz, N. Gschwend, E. Morscher, R. Schneider, H. Vasey and H. Wagner. Working with this committee, M.E. Müller successfully developed a number of hip and knee implants with specific features. Unfortunately, these activities were scaled down when the company was transferred to Sulzer Orthopaedics. A similarly composed, albeit smaller, group remained for the sole purpose of managing the products developed by M.E. Müller, who transferred his chairmanship of this committee to the editor some time ago. The enthusiasm for his subject conveyed by M.E. Müller and the commitment of our hospital to the scientific monitoring of these products were the driving forces behind this book.

The first paper by M.E. Müller on arthroplasty of the hip appeared in 1950. The objective of the study was to analyse the results obtained by his host at that time, Cornelis Pieter van Nes, in the Annaspital in Leiden following the implantation of Smith–Petersen shells and femoral head prostheses according to Judet [2]. The two themes of surgical technique and management of complications appear like a central thread running through the principal works of Müller on total hip replacement [3–5]. Three other publications dealing primarily with the management of complications deserve to be mentioned: a congress report by Postel in 1970 [6] and two books, one edited by Ling in 1984 [1] and the other by Steinberg and Garino in 1999 [7].

In this book we have adopted the approach of M.E. Müller by combining surgical technique with the management of complications. In addition to a literature analysis, the scientific basis of the book is provided by a comprehensive evaluation of our own patient population. The data analysis was made possible by the MEM hip documentation system, which has been in operation since 1984. The tradition of complete, seamless documentation was developed in Liestal by Hans Willenegger, at that time the head of surgery, who, with M.E. Müller, was one of the four co-founders of the *Arbeitsgemeinschaft für Osteosynthesefragen* (Association for the Study of Internal Fixation). Hans Willenegger established a documentation secretariat for organising the scrupulous follow-up of all internal fixations and for recording the resulting data. This facility remains at our disposal to this day. Willenegger's constant willingness to accept patients with complications for treatment has resulted in a growing influx of such patients into our hospital. A considerable proportion of our wealth of practical experience in the management of complications derives from these patients.

All orthopaedic collaborators working on this book are indebted to our orthopaedic department. They have written their chapters with considerable energy and initiative and, together with the editor, have made many revisions. As regards the non-orthopaedic subjects, we have been able to count on the cooperation of a number of acknowledged experts in their field, specifically the vascular surgeon Bernhard Nachbur, the neurologist Hansruedi Stöckli, the infectious diseases specialist Werner Zimmerli and our own engineer Martin Lüem. A proper statistical analysis of our patient population was made possible thanks only to the collaboration with the Institute for Medical Biometrics and Medical Informatics in Freiburg in Breisgau, under the direction of Martin Schuhmacher. Documentation played a key role in this study. As documentation secretary, Susanne Häfliger ensured that patient data were meticulously recorded. We also received excellent support in perfecting our database from our partnership with the M.E. Müller Institute in Berne, particularly from Mrs. Thomet and Mrs. Rösli. In the Pathology Institute of the Canton of Basel-Land (Prof. Gieri Cathomas) we were able to use the anatomical preparations as a basis for the corresponding drawings in Chaps. 11 and 13. The histological investigations were conducted by the laboratory jointly operated by the Orthopaedic Department and Stratec AG Oberdorf under the leadership of Peter Zimmermann. Ursula von Allmen provided skilful photographic input, while Anna Berchtold helped with the literature acquisition. The company Centerpulse has supported our scientific work financially, with the explicit proviso that this funding would not influence the results. The company Stratec placed their laboratory, directed by Peter Zimmermann, at our disposal for the histological investigations. The two hospital directors Hans Bider and Heinz Schneider have supported the scientific projects conducted at the Orthopaedic Hospital and generously provided us with the necessary facilities. I should like to offer my sincere thanks to all the aforementioned individuals. But I should also particularly like to thank all those numerous colleagues who, without being named, conducted thousands of follow-up evaluations and who gave the book's authors the time to produce this work.

I should like to thank Springer-Verlag for the helpful multi-coloured layout of the book, which I find very appealing. Mr. Kühn has taken on the task of reworking my original drawings and the anatomical photographs into printer's copy. Mrs. Schröder, Mr. Schmidt, Mrs. Hofmann and Mrs. Pfaff, together with many others, have worked on the book with considerable care and sensitivity. They have repeatedly surprised me with impressive design details.

We should like to dedicate this book to our patients, to Maurice E. Müller and to the late Hans Willenegger. Our hope for our patients is that they should not have to endure avoidable suffering. We are grateful to M.E. Müller for his continuing and generous support for our work. We thank Hans Willenegger for encouraging us to work for the benefit of those patients who suffer complications, and for the portrayal of our hospital as a contributor to scientific research.

Liestal, April 2002 PETER E. OCHSNER

References

1. Ling RSM (Hrsg) (1984) Complications of total hip replacement. Churchill Livingstone, Edinburgh
2. Müller M, Sibay R (1950) Zur Arthroplastik des Hüftgelenkes. Z Orthop 80: 8–16
3. Müller ME (1966) Proceedings, SICOT Congress Paris, pp 323–333
4. Müller ME (1970) Total hip prosthesis. Clin Orthop 72: 46–68
5. Müller ME, Jaberg H (1990)Total hip reconstruction. In: McCollister E (ed) Surgery of the musculoskeletal system, 2nd edn. Churchill Livingstone, New York, pp 2979–3017
6. Postel M (1970) Les complications des prothèses totales de hanche. Revue Chir Orthop 56: 27–120
7. Steinberg ME, Garino JP (eds) (1999) Revision total hip arthroplasty. Lippincott Williams & Wilkins, Philadelphia

Table of Contents

List of Contributors

BRUNAZZI, MARCO, Dr. med.
Chefarzt
Orthopädie/Traumatologie
des Bewegungsapparates
Thurgauisches Kantonsspital
CH-8500 Frauenfeld
Switzerland
e-mail: marco.brunazzi@kttg.ch

FERRAT, PIA, Dr. med.
Oberärztin
Universitätskinderklinik beider Basel
Kantonsspital
CH-4101 Bruderholz
Switzerland
e-mail: pia.ferrat@ksli.ch

HÄFLIGER, SUSANNA
Dokumentationsmitarbeiterin
Wissenschaftliche Abteilung
der Orthopädischen Klinik
Kantonsspital
CH-4410 Liestal
Switzerland
e-mail: susanna.haefliger@ksli.ch

KLEIN, MATTHIAS, Dr. med.
Oberarzt
Orthopädische Klinik
Kantonsspital
CH-4101 Bruderholz
Switzerland
e-mail: matthias.klein@ksbh.ch

KOHLER, GREGOR, Dr. med.
Leitender Arzt
Orthopädie/Traumatologie
des Bewegungsapparates
Thurgauisches Kantonsspital
CH-8500 Frauenfeld
Switzerland
e-mail: gregor.kohler.@kttg.ch

LÜEM, MARTIN, Dipl. Ing. HTL
Wissenschaftliche Abteilung
der Orthopädischen Klinik
Kantonsspital
CH-4410 Liestal
Switzerland
e-mail: martin.lueem@ksli.ch

MAURER, THOMAS, Dr. med.
Oberarzt
Orthopädische Klinik
CH-4410 Liestal
Switzerland
e-mail: thomas.maurer@ksli.ch

MÜNCH, THIERRY, Dr. med.
Praxis im Kurzentrum
Roberstenstr. 31
CH-4310 Rheinfelden
Switzerland
e-mail: twhmuench@bluewin.ch

NACHBUR, BERNHARD, Prof. Dr. med.
Talmoosstr. 48
CH-3063 Ittigen
Switzerland
e-mail: nachbur@bluewin.ch

OCHSNER, PETER EMIL, Prof. Dr. med.
Chefarzt
Orthopädische Klinik
Kantonsspital
CH-4410 Liestal
Switzerland
e-mail: peter.ochsner@ksli.ch

PIRWITZ, ANJA-S., Dr. med.
Hôpitaux de la ville
CH-2000 Neuchâtel
Switzerland
e-mail: pir-bie@bluewin.ch

Riede Ulf, Dr. med.
Orthopädische Klinik
Kantonsspital
CH-4410 Liestal
Switzerland
e-mail: ulf.riede@ksli.ch

Sarungi, Martin, MD
Department of Orthopaedic
and Trauma Surgery
MAV Hospital
H-1062 Budapest
Hungary
e-mail: sarungi@dpg.hu

Schafroth, Mathias, Dr. med.
Oberarzt
Academisch Medisch Centrum
NL-1107 WR Amsterdam
The Netherlands
e-mail:
m.u.schafroth@amc.uva.nl

Switzerlander, Andreas, Dr. med.
Orthopädische Klinik
Kantonsspital
CH-4410 Liestal
Switzerland
e-mail: andreas.Switzerlander@ksli.ch

Sommacal, Renato, Dr. med.
Werner Kälin-Str. 16
CH-8840 Einsiedeln
Switzerland
e-mail:
orthopaedie.einsiedeln@bluewin.ch

Stöckli, Hans Rudolf, Dr. med.
Konsiliararzt für Neurologie
Kantonsspital
CH-4410 Liestal
Switzerland
e-mail: hrstoeckli@datacomm.ch

Thomann, Yves, Dr. med.
Praxis im Kurzentrum
Roberstenstr. 31
CH-4310 Rheinfelden
Switzerland
e-mail: yrthomann@bluewin.ch

Toia, Damien, Dr. med.
Chefarzt Radiologie
Institut für Radiologie
Kantonsspital
CH-4410 Liestal
Switzerland
e-mail: damien.toia@ksli.ch

Vaeckenstedt, Joachim, Dr. med.
SUVA Basel
St. Jakobsstr. 24
CH-4002 Basel
Switzerland
e-mail: vaeckenstedt@web.de

Zimmerli, Werner, Prof. Dr. med.
Ordinarius für Innere Medizin
Medizinische Universitätsklinik
Kantonsspital
CH-4410 Liestal
Switzerland
e-mail: werner.zimmerli@ksli.ch

Chapter 1

Documentation

Susanna Häfliger, Peter E. Ochsner

The data in this book originate from various documentation sources, some of which are prospective and others retrospective in character.

1.1 Prospectively Recorded Data

Since Autumn 1984, all primary and revision hip implants have been registered in the MEM documentation system and followed up after 4 months and 1 year respectively. To provide a better basis for the analysis of test series, follow-up evaluations were initially conducted every 2 years. During preparations for the EBRA migration analysis, which investigated the migration of acetabular implants in relation to the bony pelvis, it emerged that an accurate assessment was only possible after making measurements on 4 radiographs. This led to the recording of postoperative pelvic radiographs after 4 months and 1 and 2 years. Additional evaluations after 5, 10 and 15 years enable the existing situation to be compared against the prevailing standard. If a routine check-up reveals findings that need to be monitored, interim checks are arranged and likewise fully documented. Patients are thus followed up at comparable postoperative points (Fig. 1.1), allowing the progress of the results to be analysed in relation to the time after operation.

The patient data are recorded on three different case report forms. Separate forms (A, B) are provided for primary and revision operations and include multiple-choice questions about the preoperative status, the operation and postoperative progress. A third form (C) is used for follow-up purposes. The questionnaire concept was first employed in its 1984 version. In 1992, the questions were extended and internationalised to become known as the IDES (International Documentation and Evaluation System). This step also enabled us to standardise the definition of terms and questions [1]. A significant advantage of the system is that it asks not just about joint function, but also about patients' abilities, thereby managing to remain up-to-date over the years. A disadvantage is that the internationally widespread "Harris hip score" [1] can only be determined approximately and is only intended for the postoperative phase. The Merle d' Aubigné score, on the other hand, is included in full [2].

Also recorded prospectively were any changes made to implants and the materials used. If, for example, a straight stem made from a chromium-cobalt alloy was replaced by a stem made from a

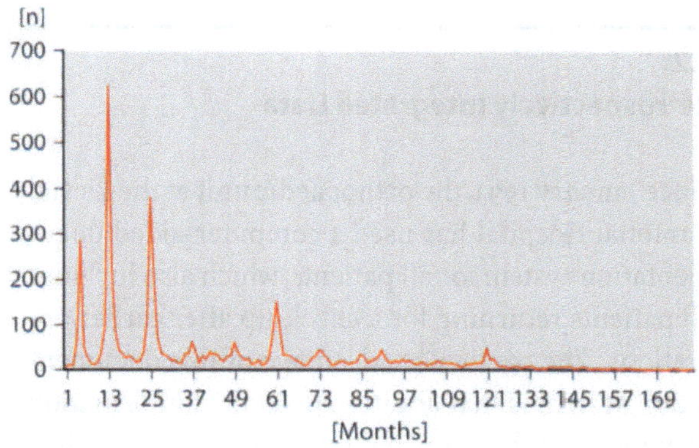

Fig. 1.1. Total number of follow-ups of our patients undergoing primary and revision total hip replacement, based on the postoperative month in which they were seen. The figure clearly shows that the great majority of follow-up evaluations took place almost exactly after 1, 2, 5, 10 and 15 years

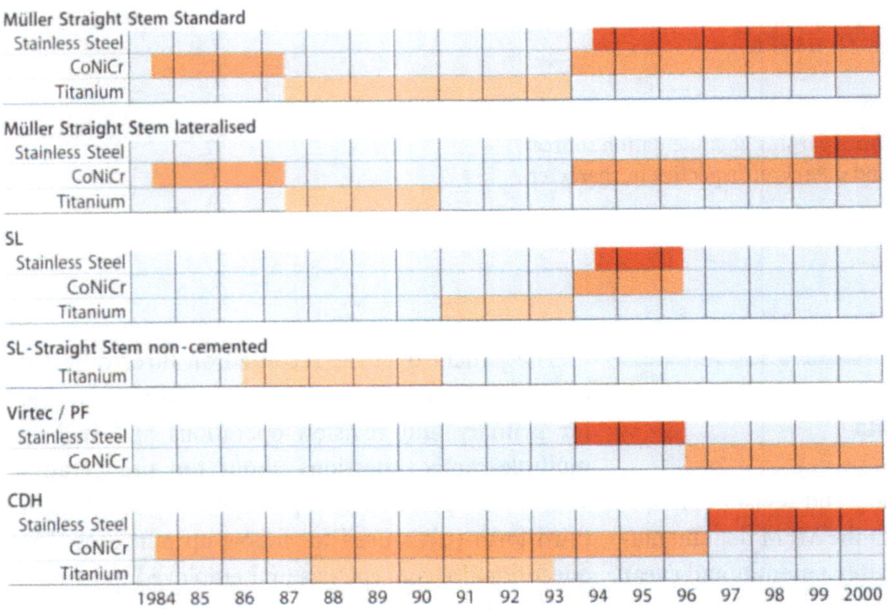

Fig. 1.2. Change in prosthesis types during the period 1984–2000, taking the example of femoral components. With few exceptions, the change from one type to the next occurred on a fixed date, i.e. with no overlap

titanium alloy, then all prostheses in all sizes were changed on a specified date (Fig. 1.2). This was of prime importance especially for the scientific management of problems encountered by us with the cemented titanium stem, although we had no idea of the significance of this change at the time. Only by making this clear separation between the use of both products were we able to assign the cases unambiguously to the corresponding groups. We adopted a similar procedure when changing the bone cement employed. No such sharp demarcation was made, however, in the application of new implantation methods, e.g. the introduction of the motorised femoral rasp. Such changes were tried out for a fairly prolonged period in each case.

1.2 Retrospectively Integrated Data

Since January 1993, the orthopaedic unit at the Liestal Cantonal Hospital has used a computer-aided documentation system for all patients, which also includes all patients returning for a check-up after earlier operations. The particular advantage of this documentation system is that additional detailed information on patients with an unfavourable course can be called up from any workstation without having to search for the corresponding medical file. However, a statistical analysis of the corresponding data is not possible with this system.

In February 2001, the scientific and clinical documentation systems were combined in the "Qualicare" system. All data can now be accessed from a single system. Simple statistical analyses are also possible, for example with Kaplan-Meier survival curves. The system is currently being networked so as to allow access to radiographic images, clinical photographs and any existing transparencies.

1.3 Data Entry

At the end of every year, during preparation of the annual statistics, our documentation secretary is responsible for checking whether any patient has failed to be entered in the scientific MEM documentation system. As a result, individual patients are occasionally entered at a later date in order to ensure that the follow-up details remain complete. The corrected lists serve as a basis for arranging prospective follow-up appointments for patients. Those who fail to turn up are contacted personally. Where patients cannot be reached, the documentation secretary conducts a separate search via the local authorities. Any dates of death are registered. Patients who are not fit for transportation are asked to complete a questionnaire. If the patient is unable to complete the questionnaire himself, we ask his carer to enter the replies.

The data for the basic documentation (forms A and B) are entered jointly by the operator and the relevant assistant surgeon. During follow-up, the subjective data have, since 1995, been entered with the aid of a questionnaire issued to the patient for completion before the actual examination. The clinical data are recorded by the examining doctor. Since the training status of the doctors involved varies considerably (students, specialist assistant surgeons in training, specialist surgeons, head of department), errors also inevitably creep in, as became apparent particularly in the analysis of leg length discrepancies for example (Chap. 9). The documentation secretary checks the data. When the sheets have been read into the system using a special scanning device, the data undergo a simple, automated plausibility check incorporated in the MEM documentation software. Impossible combinations of answers are highlighted for subsequent correction. All checked data are periodically forwarded to the MEM Institute in Bern and the Institute for Biometrics and Medical Informatics at the University of Freiburg in Breisgau for checking and joint evaluation.

1.4 Data Correction

If only part of the patient population is to be scientifically analysed, a sub-group of the whole is formed. At the same time, the data are checked specifically in respect of the planned analysis. Numerous errors are regularly discovered during this process, e.g. incorrect designation of prosthesis size, metal alloy used, etc. A particularly important basis for our data checks is the fact that all new implants, in all sizes, are introduced on a specific date and the superseded implants are completely withdrawn on the same day (Fig. 1.4). This allows us to check detailed information concerning the implants recorded in the questionnaires by the operators and the assistant surgeons responsible for follow-up. During an analysis, we also frequently note missing entries, e.g. for patients' weights and heights. The documentation secretary – supported by the research assistant – is responsible for correcting such mistakes, always entering the corrections in the primary data record as well. The corrected data are periodically exchanged with the scientific partners. This data correction is an extremely important, albeit very time-consuming, process. It is also clear that these scientific, prospectively recorded data cannot be included as a fully integrated part of the regular medical file which, by law, may not be altered at a later date.

1.5 Data Basis for this Book

For the statistical analysis of complications described in this book we relied on data from all our patients undergoing surgery up to the end of 1996. Basic documentation was available in every case. Clinical follow-up was not possible in just 4.3 % of patients. The annual check-ups served as the basis for recording complications. The advantage of our documentation system is that the questions before and after operation are always identically formulated and therefore comparable. We also noted corresponding headings for the commonest complications, although a few genuine problems did come to light:

- Under the heading "preoperative details", no information was provided about the degree of limping observed preoperatively, thus preventing any subsequent comparison with the preoperative status.
- During recording of functional leg length difference, no precise details of the recording method were provided. Nor was any distinction made between correctable and non-correctable leg length discrepancies.
- Neurological complications have been recorded since 1984. However, in view of the great importance attached to these complications, we decided, in 1988, to start looking for these systematically from the immediate postoperative period onward and to refer affected patients to the neurologist H. R. Stöckli, who treated these patients with especially meticulous care.

In all the analysed cases of complications, the medical files were also included, usually via the "Emil" system, in addition to the data recorded in the MEM documentation system up to the end of 2000.

References

1. Harris WH (1969) Traumatic arthritis of the hip after dislocation and acetabular fractures: treatment by mold arthroplasty. An end-result study using a new method of result evaluation. J Bone Joint Surg Am 51: 737–755
2. Merle d'Aubigné R, Cauchoix J, Ramadier JV (1949) Evaluation chiffrée de la fonction de la hanche. Application à l'étude des résultats des opérations mobilisatrices de la hanche. Rev Chir Orthop 35: 541–548
3. SICOT Presidential Commission on Documentation and Evaluation (1990) Report of the SICOT Presidential Commission on Documentation and Evaluation. Int Orthop 14: 221–229

CHAPTER 2

Patient Population

MARTIN LÜEM

Between June 1984 and the end of 2000 we recorded 1570 primary and 479 revision operations (Fig. 2.1). Men were overrepresented in the primary operations, at 55%, and to an even greater extent in the revision procedures, at 63%.

For the acetabular components we predominantly used Müller original products. In the primary operations we tended to insert the cemented polyethylene cup (PE), the acetabular reinforcement ring (ARR) and the uncemented SL cup (Figs. 2.5–2.7). The ARR with cemented PE cup and the Burch–Schneider (BS) antiprotrusio cage were predominantly used as revision implants.

On the femoral side (Figs. 2.8–2.10), original Müller products were used in 95% of primary implantations and 48% of revision procedures. During the period 1984–1990, a straight stem was inserted in nine out of ten operations. A newly developed product made from titanium alloy, and known as the cemented SL stem, almost completely replaced the straight stem between 1990 and 1996. A randomised study (straight stem vs. Virtec stem) was initiated in the summer of 1996. The stem was cemented in 95% of primary implantations. A similar trend was also apparent between 1984 and 1990 for the revision procedures. Additionally, the uncemented Wagner stem was used for revisions from the start of 1988, while the PF prosthesis was introduced in 1994. Overall, we inserted a cemented stem in 76% of all revision operations.

2.1 Introduction

Thanks to the introduction of the systematic documentation and recording of all implantations and hip prostheses in June 1984, when the orthopaedic department was opened, statistical analyses have become routine and can now be performed easily and quickly for addressing specific questions (see Chap. 1). All figures are taken from this database. Radiographs, surgical reports and – where available – removed implants, served as verification sources for the figures.

2.2 General Analysis of the Patient Population

2.2.1 Recorded Cases

Between the start of electronic recording in mid 1984 and the end of 2000, we registered 2049 total hip prostheses (1570 primary implantations, 479 revisions) at the Liestal Cantonal Hospital. To ensure an adequate follow-up period, we have used the data for those cases recorded only up to the end of 1996 for the statistical analysis in this book (Table 2.1).

■ **Primary Operations.** 1098 patients received a primary prosthesis: 606 men (55%) and 492 women (45%). Of these 1098 patients, 17 died before the 1-year follow-up evaluation. Of the remaining 1081 patients, 96.7% were clinically and radiologically assessed after 1 year.

■ **Revision Operations.** A revision procedure was performed on 330 patients (209 or 63% men, and 121

Table 2.1. Overview of patient follow-up after 1 year, 1984–1996

	Primary THR		Revision THR	
	[n]	[%]	[n]	[%]
Patients registered	1098		330	
Died before the 1-year-follow-up	17	1.5	11	3.3
Examinable patients	1081	100	319	100
Examined after 1 year	1046	96.7	292	91.5
No follow-up	35	3.3	27	8.5
Living too far away	10 out of 35	29	8 out of 27	30
Poor general health	11 out of 35	31	13 out of 27	48
Other reasons	14 out of 35	40	6 out of 27	22

or 37% women). The total implant was replaced in 153 cases, the cup in 81 cases and the stem in 96 cases. Of the 330 patients, 11 died before the 1-year follow-up evaluation. Of the remaining 319, 91.5% returned for the check-up after 1 year (Table 2.1).

Patients were asked about the reason for their failure to attend the 1-year check-up. The long journey was given as the reason by one third of those patients not followed up after a primary implantation. The other patients stated a variety of reasons. After revision operations, half of the patients not followed up failed to attend because of poor general health, one third because of the long journey and only a sixth gave a variety of other reasons.

2.2.2 Characteristics of the Patient Population

■ **Overview of Patient Data.** 61% (674) of the primary operations were performed by senior registrars and registrars. The remaining 39 % (424) were operated on by the head of department. Two-thirds (69%) of the revision operations were performed by the head of department, while the remaining third (31%) were carried out by senior registrars. The number of implanted hip prostheses shows a rising linear trend over the years, from 70 in 1985 to over 150 in 1996 (Fig. 2.1).

■ **Age at Operation and Average Stay in Hospital.** The average age of the patients at operation remained very constant, with a figure of 68.2±1.5 years (Fig. 2.2) for primary operations and 75.6±2.25 years (Fig. 2.3) for the revisions. The average stay in hospital for the

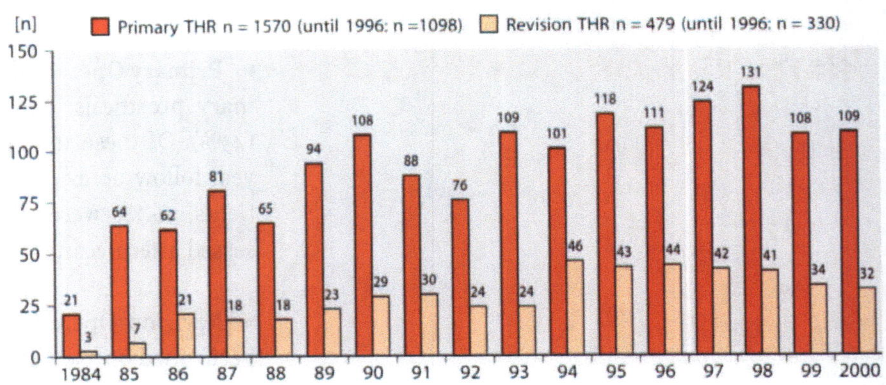

Fig. 2.1. Overview of total hip replacements implanted each year between the start of electronic recording in June 1984 and the end of 2000 (1996)

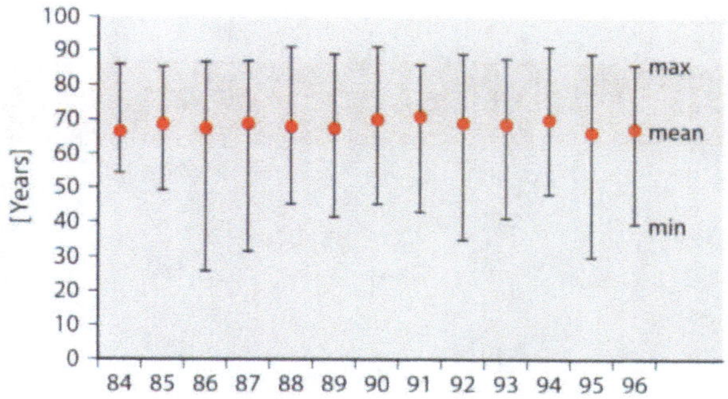

Fig. 2.2. Average age of patients undergoing a primary operation

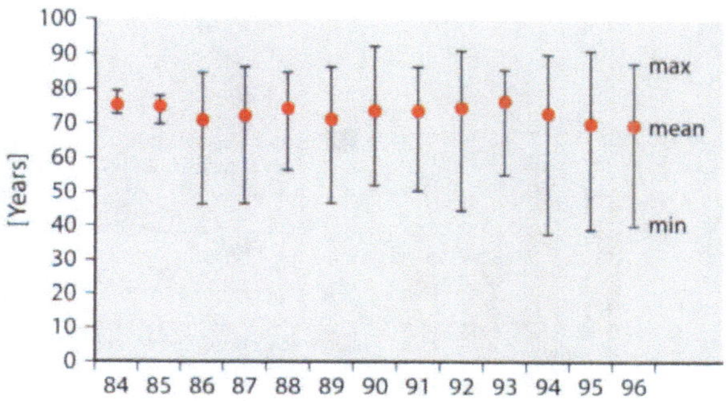

Fig. 2.3. Average age of patients undergoing a revision operation

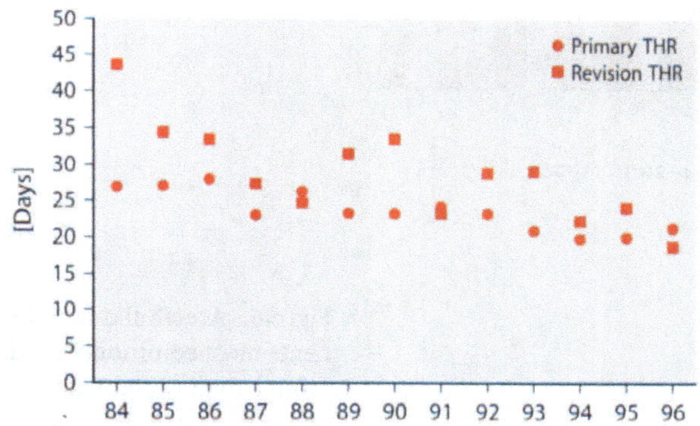

Fig. 2.4. Average stay in hospital for patients undergoing primary and revision operations

primary procedures (Fig. 2.4) declined during the period under review from 27±6.7 to 21±5.5 days. For revision procedures, the hospital stay dropped over the same period from over 40 to 21 days.

■ **Diagnoses.** The most common diagnosis for the primary procedures was primary arthrosis (71%). This group also included patients with minor deviations in the shape of the head. Special abnormalities noted included dysplasia (19%), femoral head necrosis (4%), fractures (3.5 %) and miscellaneous (2.5%). Among the revisions, aseptic loosening was the main reason for revision in 82% of cases. Other conditions observed included a post-Girdlestone scenario (4%), trochanteric pathologies (3%), infections (2%), fractures (2%) and various other diagnoses (7%).

2.3 Prostheses Used

The overview of the operations performed between mid-1984 and the end of 1996 shows certain fluctuations (Fig. 2.1). The temporary drop in the figures after 1990 is probably attributable to the departure of two senior surgeons who then set up a two-person practice in the same town as our hospital. The increased percentage of patients undergoing a primary procedure elsewhere and the higher number of cases of early loosening of cemented titanium stems explain the increase in revision operations since 1994.

2.3.1 Primary Operations on the Acetabulum

(Figs. 2.5 and 2.6; Table 2.2)

Cemented polyethylene (PE) cups were implanted in over 90% of cases between 1984 and 1986. From 1987 onward, cemented PE cups combined with armament screws predominated. The proportions in 1987 and 1988 were as follows: 40% PE cups with armament screws, 40% ARR and 20% cemented PE cups without armament screws. The proportions of the two types of cemented PE cups subsequently declined, eventually disappearing completely in 1990. Since the cemented PE cup without armament screws produced positive results at least over a 10-year period (see also Chap. 15), it was occasionally used again from 1996 for patients with a shorter life expectancy.

The introduction of the titanium hemispherical SL cup in March 1988 led to a decline in the number of ARR and PE cups, and the proportion of primarily implanted ARRs only rose back to the 25% level from 1995. Since their introduction, the percentage of SL cups has always exceeded 70%. Overall, SL cups were employed in 661 of 1098 primary implantations. Of

Table 2.2. Overview of acetabular components used, 1984–1996

Acetabular side	Primary	Revision	Total
SL cup	661	40	701
Müller acetabular reinforcement ring	203	144	347
PE cup – cemented	117	6	123
PE cup with armament screws	110	3	113
Burch-Schneider antiprotrusio cage	7	40	47
Burch-Schneider antiprotrusio cage	0	1	1
Total	1098	234	1332

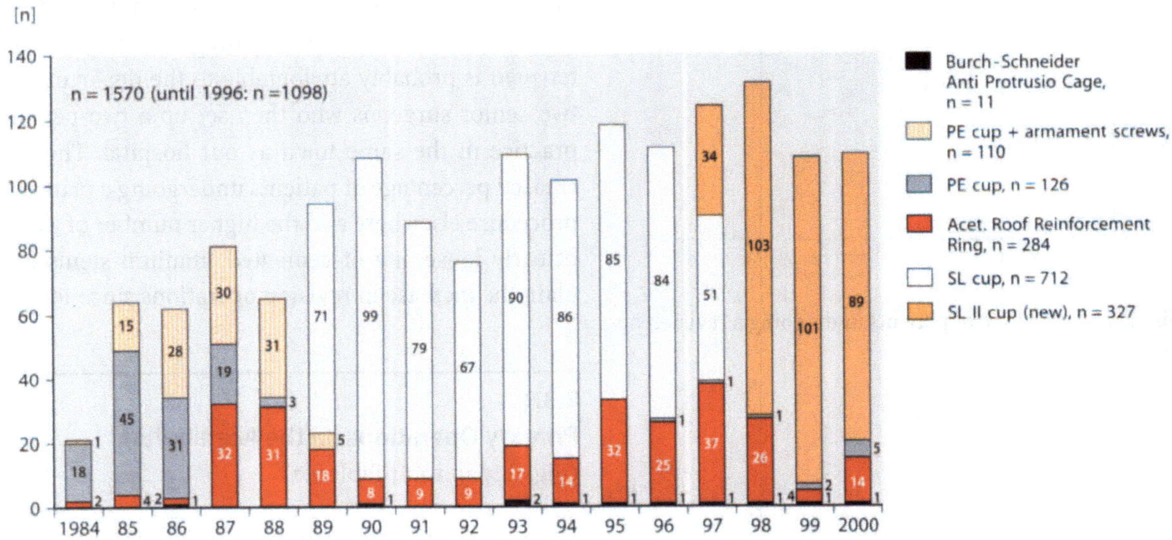

Fig. 2.5. Primary acetabular implantations per year from 1984–2000 (1996)

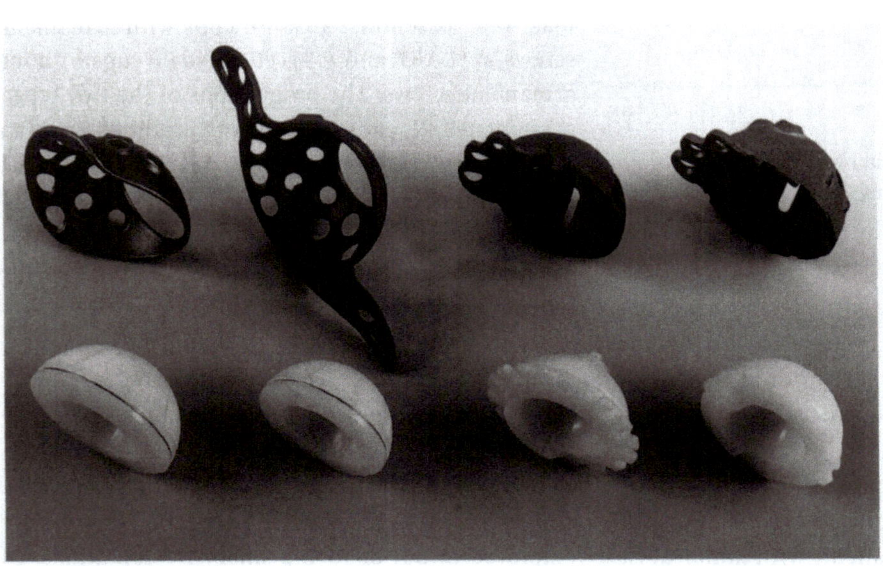

Fig. 2.6. Acetabular components most commonly used: From l. to r.: Acetabular reinforcement ring according to M.E. Müller, Burch-Schneider antiprotrusio cage, SL cup according to M.E. Müller, SL shell according to Müller/Ochsner

the total patient population, 17% received an ARR. In seven cases, a Burch-Schneider antiprotrusio cage was implanted (see also Sect. 3.3.1).

As bearing couples we used polyethylene-metal in 21% of cases and PE-ceramic in 68% of cases. The metal-metal articulation (trade name: Metasul) has been used 124 times (11%) since its introduction in March 1992.

2.3.2 Revision Operations on the Acetabulum

(Figs. 2.6, 2.7; Table 2.2)

The acetabular reinforcement ring (ARR) was used in 61% (144 out of 234) of all acetabular revision procedures. Since 1992 it has been by far the most frequently used revision implant, invariably accounting for 50%–60% of cases.

The SL cup was used in 17% (40 out of 234) of cases. Since we view it principally as a primary acetabular component, we have used the SL cup as a revision implant only rarely in recent years.

The Burch-Schneider antiprotrusio cage was also introduced to deal with the growing number of second and third revision operations and complex situations involving excessive destruction of the acetabular bone stock. Its increased use from 1994 is attributable partly to the referral of problem cases and partly to the introduction of a new trial shell for simplifying the implantation procedure (Fig. 3.10). As with the ARR, the antiprotrusio cage was also manufactured from titanium instead of steel from 1987. This refinement resulted in improved intraoperative malleability and better integration with the bone postoperatively. This latter property was further improved in 1995 with the introduction of rough-blasting.

As a bearing couple in our revision operations we used polyethylene-metal in 36% of cases, PE-ceramic in 61% of cases and metal-metal in 3% of cases.

2.3.3 Primary Operations on the Femoral Shaft

(Figs. 2.8, 2.9, Table 2.3)

The original M.E. Müller straight stem (with a cement abutment collar) was used as a cemented primary implant in over 90% of all primary operations during the years 1984–1990. Uncemented SL straight stems with attached collars were used between 1986 and 1989 in 31 cases.

At the beginning of July 1987, production of the straight-stem Müller prostheses switched from the rigid cobalt-nickel-chromium alloy (trade name PROTASUL-10) to the more elastic titanium-aluminium-niobium alloy (trade name PROTASUL-100). No changes were made either to the shape or to the surface design.

In 1990, the traditional straight stem was replaced by the SL straight stem, which has no cement abutment collar or ventral/dorsal groove and which is slightly thicker, more angular and rough-blasted at the proximal end. This stem was subsequently used in over 90% of primary operations. The stem material was changed yet again at the end of 1993. Because of the increasing

Table 2.3. Overview of femoral components used, 1984–1996

Femoral side	Femoral side	Revision	Total
Müller straight stem	459	63	522
SL stem	488	35	523
Virtec/PF stem	50	62	112
CDH-stem	55	8	63
Wagner SL revision stem	3	54	57
Müller curved stem 180 mm	55	15	20
SL stem uncemented with collar	31	4	35
CLS stem	5	3	8
Other	2	5	7
Total	1098	249	1347

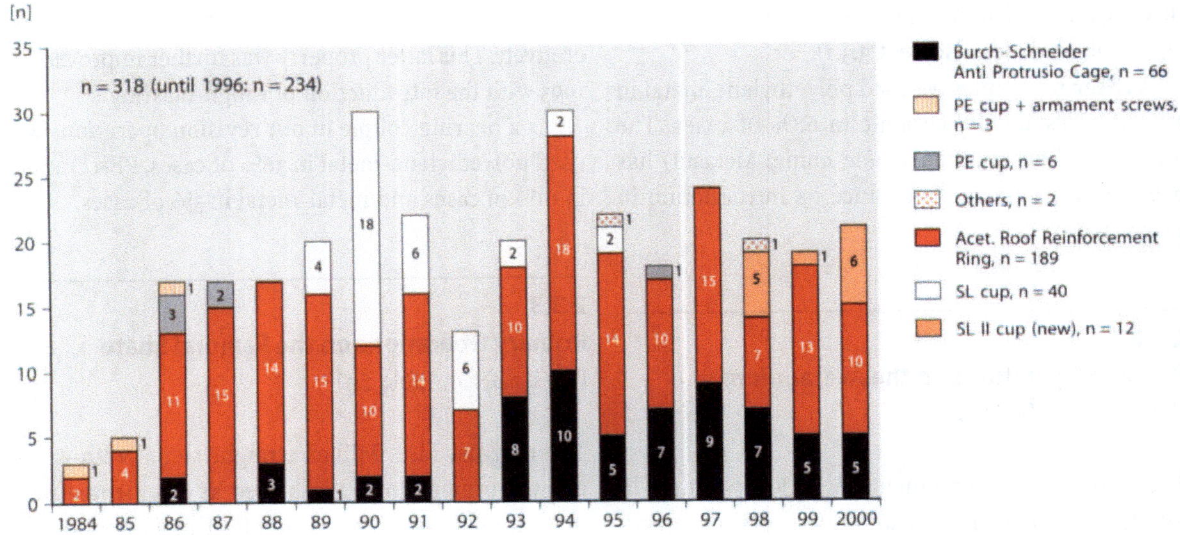

Fig. 2.7. Cup revisions per year, 1984–2000 (1996)

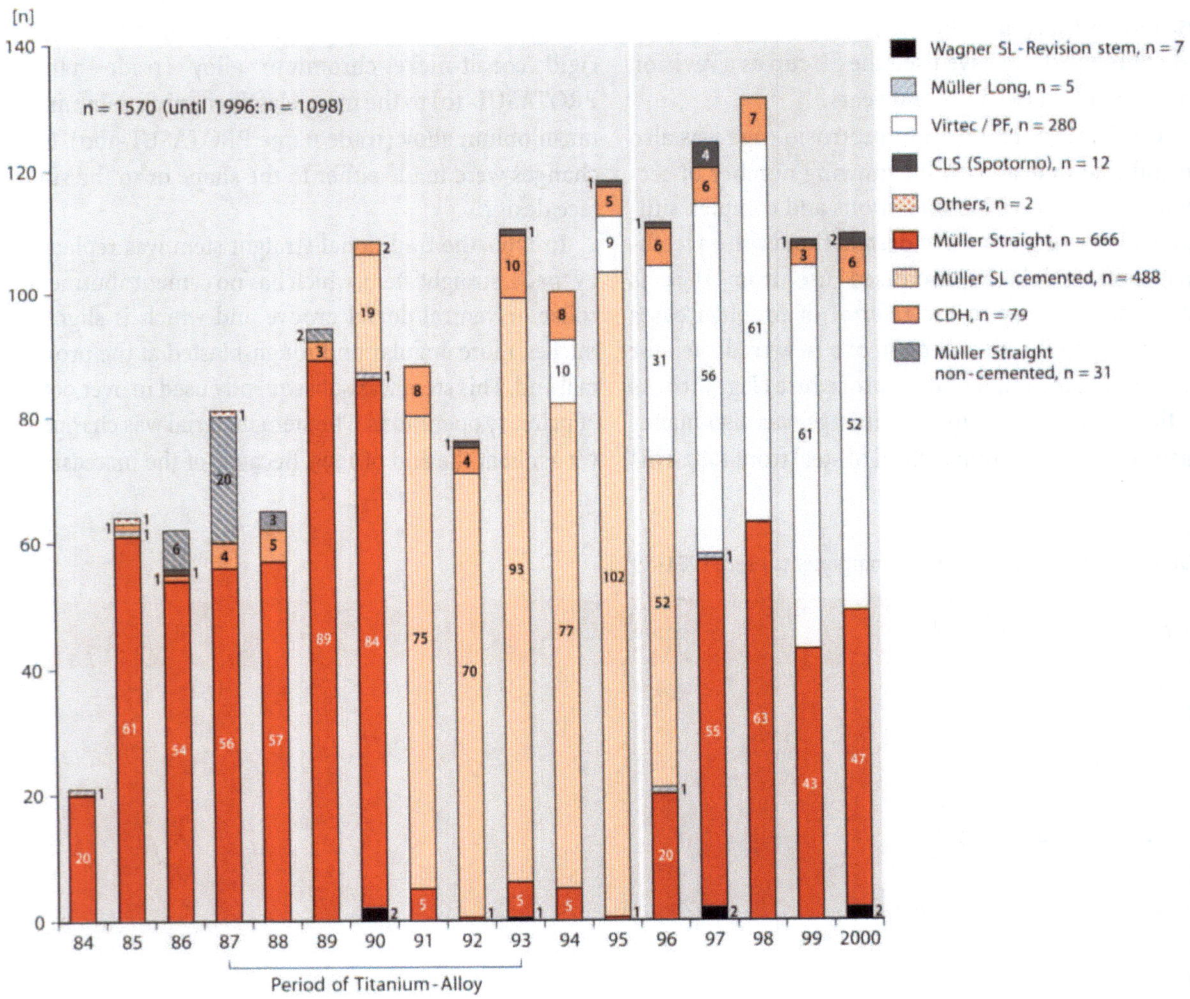

Fig. 2.8. Primary stem implantations per year, 1984–1996

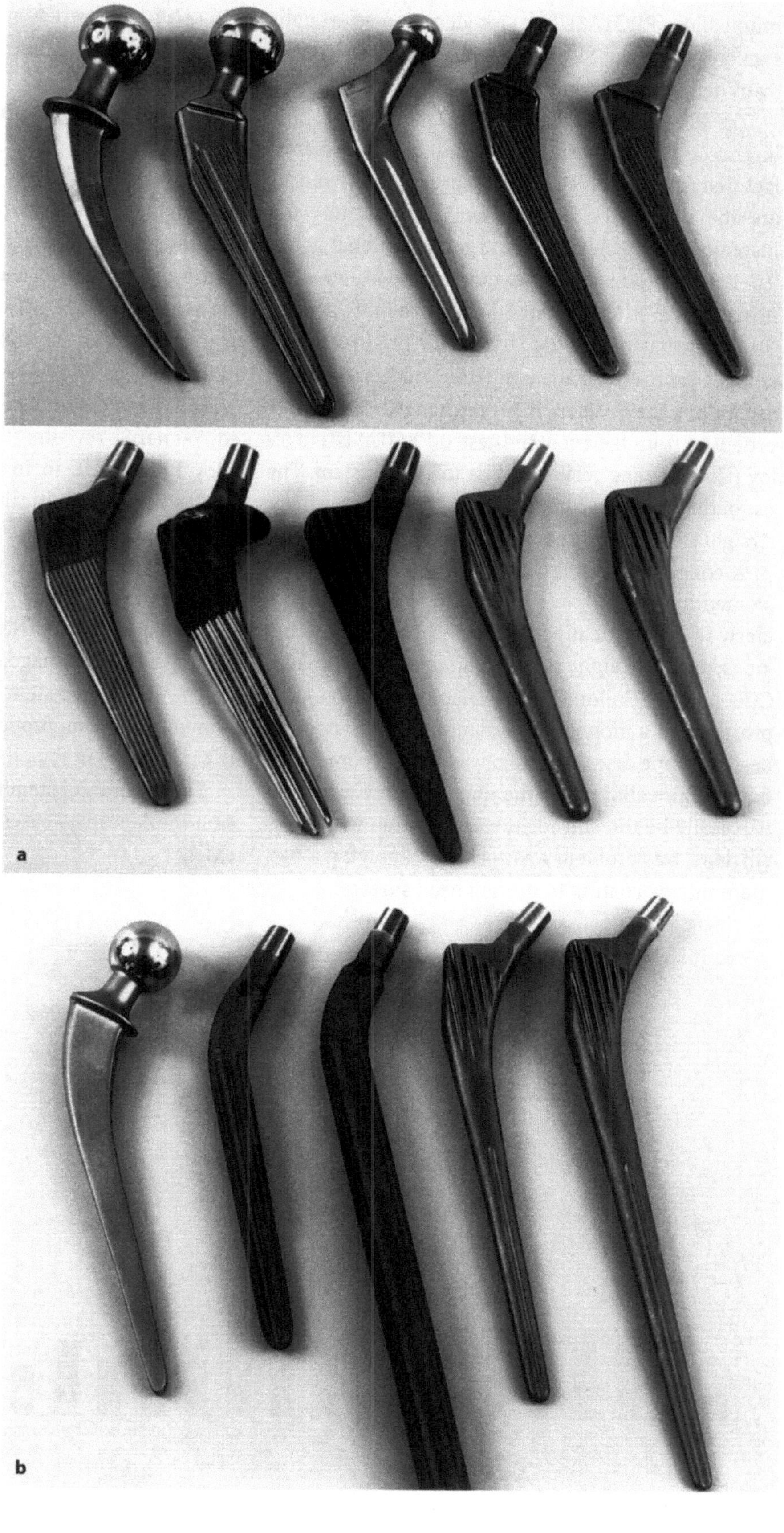

Fig. 2.9. a Stems used for primary implantation (from left to right); *top:* curved stem, straight stem Monoblock 32mm, CDH stem, standard straight stem, lateralising straight stem; *bottom:* SL stem, SL uncemented stem with collar, CLS stem, Virtec standard, Virtec lateralising. **b** Stem implants used for revision operations (from left to right) MEM long stem, Wagner SL revision stem (l = 385 mm), Virtec long stem (sizes 8/225 and 10/265)

number of stem revisions [1], the titanium alloy was changed back to the tried-and-tested cobalt-chromium alloy (PROTASUL 10) for all cemented straight stem systems. The SL stem system was discontinued by us definitively in mid-July 1996.

The PF stem was introduced in January 1994. This is also a straight stem prosthesis, but one manufactured from steel (FeCrNi). The principal differences are the oval shape of the stem cross-section, the increased proximal stiffness and good rotational stability. Between January 1994 and July 1996, 29 (3%) primary operations employed this system. Following the discontinuation of the SL stem, the original Müller straight stem was again used from mid-1996. At the same time, the PF stem, in an unchanged design, was produced from the tried-and-tested PROTASUL 10 alloy (CoNiCr) and relaunched as the Virtec stem. The use of this stem was compared with the original Müller straight stem in a prospective randomised study.

A congenital dysplastic hip (CDH) stem was implanted in approx. 5% of primary operations, particularly in dysplastic hips. This prosthesis likewise belongs to the straight stem group, but has a smaller CCD angle (Collum-Centre-Diaphysis). The CDH prosthesis is a monoblock system without a modular head. In some cases, this stem was also prepared from the titanium alloy. Since the titanium alloy would intrinsically be too soft for the articulation with polyethylene, this problem was solved by applying a titanium nitride coating to the ball head surface.

An uncemented Spotorno stem (CLS) was used in only five cases (0.5%).

2.3.4 Revision Operations on the Femoral Shaft

(Figs. 2.9 and 2.10; Table 2.3)

As with the primary operations, the straight stem was also the prosthesis most commonly implanted in revision procedures, at least until 1990. In four cases, the uncemented SL straight stem (with collar) was used as the revision implant. The CLS stem was used in three cases.

Following the implantation of the first uncemented Wagner SL revision stems made from the titanium alloy PROTASUL 10 in 1988, their use in revisions grew steadily. As with the Burch-Schneider antiprotrusio cage, the increased use is explained less by the failure of a procedure with the cemented straight stem and more by the growth in the referrals of patients requiring a further revision or a revision involving a badly damaged femoral shaft.

The PF / Virtec stem has proved very suitable for cemented revision procedures, and its use grew from 12 cases (34%) in 1994 to 29 (70%) in 1996.

The SL straight stem was used as a cemented revision implant in 35 cases and the CDH stem in eight cases.

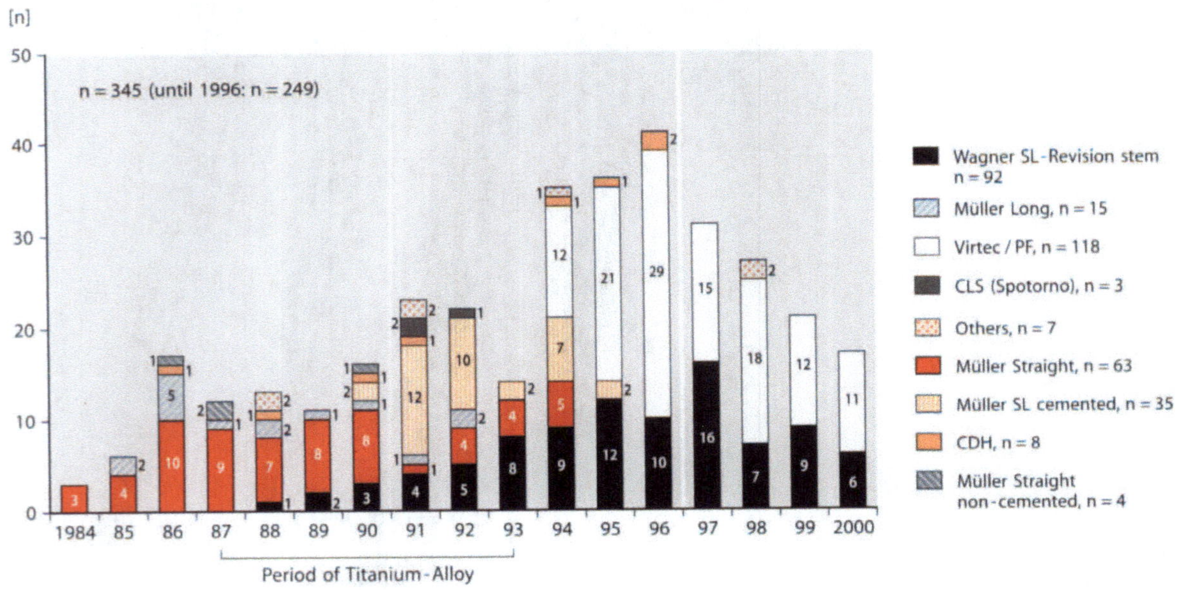

Fig. 2.10. Stem revisions per year, 1984–2000 (1996)

2.4 Frequency of Complications

Limping and leg length discrepancies are the most commonly observed complications, occurring understandably to a greater extent in patients after revision operations (Fig. 2.11). As regards the other complications (Fig. 2.12), haematomas and infections occur more frequently after revisions, whereas dislocations, fractures and neurological complications are, surprisingly, rarer after revisions than after primary operations.

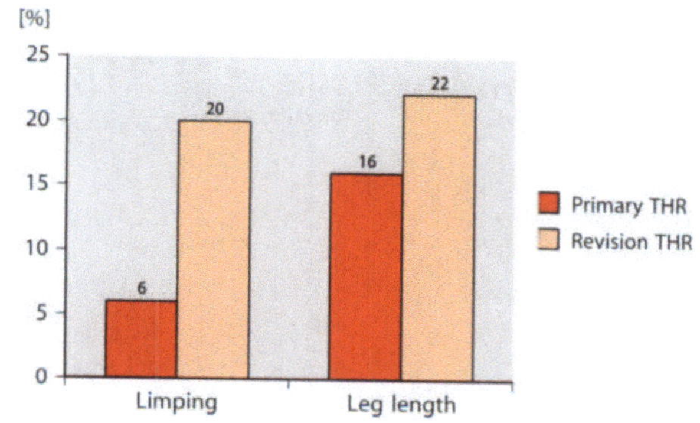

Fig. 2.11. The most common local complications: limping and leg length discrepancy

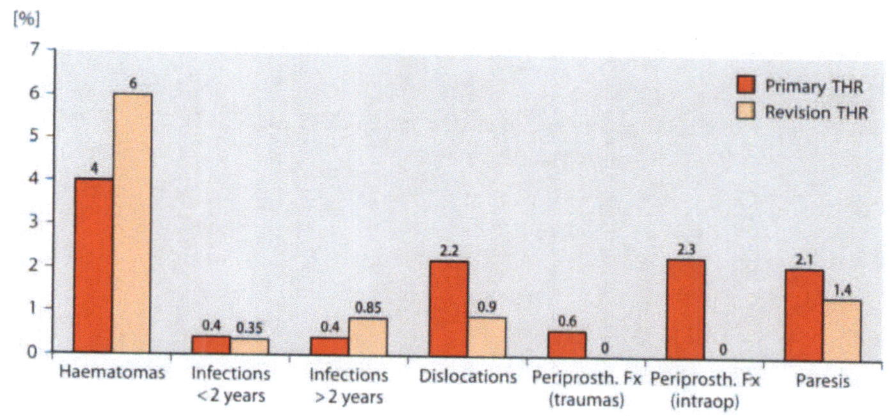

Fig. 2.12. The rarer local complications

Reference

1. Maurer TB, Ochsner P, Schwarzer G, Schumacher M (2001) Increased loosening of cemented straight stem prostheses made from titanium alloys. An analysis and comparison with prostheses made of cobalt-chromium-nickel alloy. Int Orthop (SICOT) 25: 77–80

Surgical Technique

3

PETER E. OCHSNER, ANDREAS SCHWEIZER

This chapter assesses the prosthesis system according to M.E. Müller and provides instruction in its use. The reader of the chapter on complications should be able to determine, through careful study, the reasons underlying the onset of any complications.

The concept of total hip replacement according to M.E. Müller is based on six factors: simple operation planning, reliable instruments, a standardised surgical procedure, prepared solutions for dealing with any complications, retrievability of implants and the documentation of results. The detailed planning of the procedures is illustrated with examples of typical primary operations and revisions and is designed to enable operators to address the prevailing problems preoperatively and then compare the outcome with the original plan. The surgical technique for primary operations is described in detail, together with corresponding variants. Reference is also made to the particularly important instruments and their use. Special hazards are highlighted. The presentation of revision procedures is restricted to the technical aspects of surgical approach and prosthesis retrieval, while a few remarks on implantation are included in the section on planning.

3.1 Introduction

The orthopaedic department at the Liestal Cantonal Hospital is a teaching facility. Each year - partly in rotation with other teaching hospitals attached to the University of Basel – two to four future orthopaedic surgeons visit the unit to familiarise themselves with our surgical technique. In order to ensure consistency of instruction, all supervisory staff use the same surgical method. Changes are discussed in advance and definitively introduced on specific dates (see also Table 2.1). This chapter performs a double function in this book:

- To furnish the reader of the chapters on complications with details of the surgical technique used, enabling him, in the light of his own technique, to better evaluate the extent to which high complication rates are attributable to our or his own surgical technique. We would be very grateful to any readers if they would notify us of any unrecognised errors in our technique.
- To present a clearly structured description of the system for the implantation and revision of total hip replacements as elaborated by M.E. Müller, so that those interested in this surgical technique are in a position, if they so wish, to appropriate the system for themselves. This system remains one of the most complete of its kind in the world. Although it has already been extensively described in 1989 by Schneider [16] in book form and in 1992 by M.E. Müller himself [14], the system has since undergone numerous modifications, hence the need for a new description.

3.2 Concept of Total Hip Replacement According to M.E. Müller

Based on an analysis of the works of M.E. Müller on total hip replacement, his guidelines can broadly be summarised in a concept incorporating six factors:

- Simple operation planning
- Reliable instruments
- Standardised surgical procedure
- Prepared solutions for dealing with complications
- Retrievability of implants
- Documentation of results

■ **Simple Operation Planning.** The operator should have at his disposal readily understandable resources for the detailed planning of the forthcoming operation. The planning should be sufficiently detailed to ensure that, together with the appropriate surgical technique, the outcome of the operation is in line with the original plan, or alternatively that, in the event of any difficulties at operation, any incorrect assessments made during planning are disclosed.

■ **Reliable Instrumentation.** Over a period of several decades, M.E. Müller has personally sought to develop high-quality, easy-to-use precision instruments for the implantation of prostheses. The details of instrument design were discussed with the instrument manufacturer directly at the operating table. His first technical partner was Robert Mathys senior (†), who had to make countless modifications to the instruments, or else manufacture them from scratch, until M.E. Müller was satisfied with the result. His last technical assistant in instrument development was Jürg Küfer. It is easy to understand why M.E. Müller is not particularly pleased when he hears his bone or soft tissue levers sweepingly referred to as "Hohmann" retractors. In fact, Hohmann merely described a retractor with a wide front end to be placed in pairs around the bone during an osteotomy to protect the soft tissues.

■ **Standardised Surgical Procedure.** To ensure a consistent standard, M.E. Müller strongly believes that an operation should, as a rule, follow a standardised procedure. This has proved particularly effective in the training of young surgeons and in serving as a guide to a large team in achieving consistency of quality. Putting these beliefs into practice, M.E. Müller has written surgical instructions for all his implants [14].

■ **Prepared Solutions for Dealing with Complications.** As early as 1966, M.E. Müller [13] was describing complications after total hip replacements, and he realised that early complications, in particular, posed the greatest threat to good results in the long term. Accordingly, the prosthesis system that he developed incorporates implants and instruments designed to eliminate early and late complications. The acetabular reinforcement ring, the Burch-Schneider antiprotrusio cage, long-stem prosthesis and numerous special instruments are the results of these efforts.

■ **Retrievability of Implants.** Before being introduced, every implant in this system was tested for its retrievability. The patient needs to be protected from the particular risks associated with implant retrieval, for example those observed with the Sulmesh cup according to Morscher, or the porous metal stems according to Lord.

■ **Documentation of Results.** In 1958, M.E. Müller introduced a detailed and prospectively structured documentation system for fracture management. This system enabled him to identify and eliminate any mistakes in the internal fixation technique at an early stage. Building on this experience, he then managed to develop a far more efficient documentation system with the aim of improving the total hip replacement procedure. Regular checks in the system not only benefited the individual patient, through the early detection of impending problems, but also the developer through the identification of systematic errors. The elimination of such errors ultimately leads to better implants and instruments. All total hip replacement operations undertaken at the Liestal Cantonal Hospital since 1984 have been documented and followed up (see also Chap. 1).

3.3 Implants and Corresponding Indications

In this section, the various implants used in our hospital are analysed and certain fundamental aspects of implantation explained. The survival curves are grouped together in Chap. 15.

3.3.1 Acetabular Implants

General Information on Implantation

■ The Normal Acetabulum. In the normal acetabulum, the bone contour of the femoral head approaches Köhler's radiographic teardrop to within about 5–8 mm (Fig. 3.1a). Forces are transmitted from the hip to the pelvis – emanating from the centre of the femoral head – via a strong, hourglass-shaped pillar of bone – in the direction of the iliosacral joint.

In order to maintain a high degree of mechanical resistance cranially, the well-perfused subchondral sclerosis should, if possible, be preserved (Figs. 3.1b,c).

■ Acetabular Wear and Restoring the Acetabulum. An acetabulum subjected to wear is usually shifted in the cranial direction and eroded to form a transverse oval, with an increased transverse diameter (Figs. 3.1b,c, Fig. 3.6a), and a slightly decreased sagittal diameter (Fig. 3.6b).

A number of options are available for matching an implant to the bone stock:

- The implant is adapted to the bony bed. This results in numerous different implants.
- The existing bone stock is adapted to an optimally preshaped implant. A spherical shape will involve less bone loss than a conical design. A slightly oversized implant (by a maximum of 2 mm) will produce good wedging.
- Since the acetabulum is usually worn to a transverse oval, circular reaming out to the transverse diameter will cause an unnecessarily large amount of bone to be sacrificed ventrally and dorsally. As an alternative to increased reaming, the implant can be wedged ventrally and dorsally, while the gaps remaining on the lateral side, and exceptionally on the medial side, can be filled with cement (Fig. 3.1b) or cancellous bone from the femoral head (Fig. 3.1c).
- In the case of acetabular defects, e.g. those occurring in severe congenital hip dysplasia or a pronounced defect with cup loosening, a solid autologous bone block (Fig. 3.8) or cancellous graft, protected by robust acetabular reinforcement (Fig. 3.1d,e), serves as structural material that is subsequently remodelled into a strong bone stock.

■ Selection of Head Centre and Cup Position. As a general rule, we try to restore the original head centre (Figs. 3.6, 3.8). In cases of advanced coxarthrosis, this usually moves increasingly in the lateral, cranial and ventral directions (Figs. 3.6a–c, 3.8a). In other words, the centre has to be moved back to a more medial, dorsal and distal position. Only in protrusion coxarthrosis is the head centre shifted ventrally and laterally (Fig. 3.7). There is important evidence to suggest that a correct head centre, combined with a cup inclination of 35–40° will prolong the life of the implant [5]. An anteversion of 14–18° is an important precondition for preventing ventral impingement and dislocations (Chap. 6). In acetabular revisions, meticulous investigation of the pathological cup position is essential for a successful outcome (Fig. 3.9).

Primary Stability and Prevention of Migration Through Screw Fixation

The aim in an acetabular replacement procedure is to achieve a primary stability that allows immediate full weight-bearing, and one that respects the rules of stable osteosynthesis, affording protection until permanent secondary stability is achieved as a result of bone remodelling and osteointegration. This secondary stability is absolutely essential for any prosthesis. Restoring and preserving the natural head centre is one of the objectives of primary osteosynthesis, and secondary migration also needs to be excluded at the same time. Screw fixation is one of the basic principles of osteosynthesis. Given the wide variety of acetabular defects, the complexity of screw fixation and the reinforcements needed to achieve stability differ from case to case, although the basic technique and the objective of screw fixation remain the same.

■ Principle of Screw Fixation. The strongest anchoring zone is the conical pillar of supporting bone proximal to the acetabulum in the direction of the iliosacral joint (Figs. 3.1a–e, 3.2). Screws can almost always gain purchase in this zone. If pronounced os-

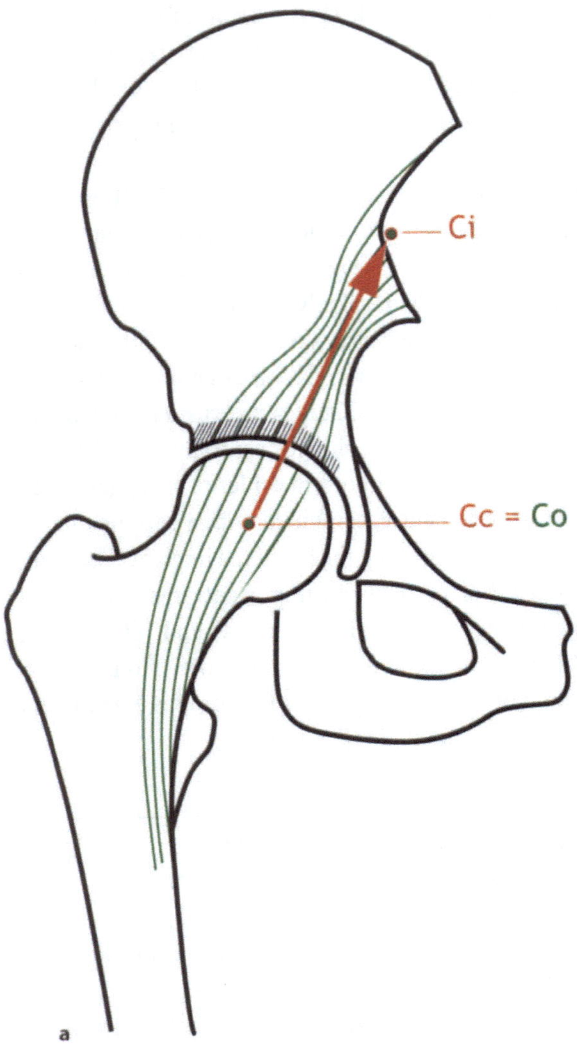

Fig. 3.1a–e. Cup implants and their anchorage; **b, c** cut-away views through the pelvis with view of the implant as shown in Fig. 3.6. Allogeneic bone (*allo*)

a Normal acetabulum. The average resultant of the transmission of forces runs roughly from the centre of the hip (*Cc*) to the centre of the iliosacral joint (*Ci*). This line thus runs through the middle of the hourglass-shaped pillar of bone that links the acetabulum to the iliosacral joint and offers good screw anchorage. Screws are able to gain a secure purchase in this area, and no soft tissue structures are injured by the resulting intraosseous screw positions
b Anchorage of a polyethylene cup with bone cement: The acetabulum is reamed so as to shift the head centre (*Ch*), which is in an excessively lateral position preoperatively, back to a more correct medial position, so that the centre of the acetabular component will match the natural head centre on the opposite, healthy side (*Co*) and so that the subchondral sclerosis zone (*Sc*) is preserved. Anchoring holes approx. 6 mm in diameter along the cup rim allow the cement to dovetail with the bone. The thickness of the bone cement (*ce*) cranially should be at least 2–4 mm
c Anchorage of an uncemented SL-II cup: The acetabulum is prepared as for **a**. Since the arthritic acetabulum generally has a transverse oval shape, small gaps remain on the medial and lateral sides, while the shell is firmly wedged ventrally and dorsally. The gaps are filled with autologous cancellous bone from the femoral head (*auto*). The cup is then tapped home, and primary stable anchorage is achieved with two to three screws directed towards the centre of the iliosacral joint. See Fig. 13.8 for the risks associated with screw fixation
d Anchorage of an acetabular reinforcement ring: Irregular gaps are preferably filled with autologous (*auto*) bone. The acetabular reinforcement ring is screwed firmly in the direction of the iliosacral joint. In revision cases, the projecting screw heads provide welcome distalisation of the polyethylene cup and head centre, although not quite as far as the natural centre on our drawing. A smaller cup will produce additional medialisation of the head centre. See Fig. 13.9 for the risks associated with screw fixation
e Anchorage of a Burch-Schneider antiprotrusio cage: The antiprotrusio cage allows primary stability to be achieved even in the absence of any cranial abutment. The flange bent onto the iliac bone is anchored by horizontal screws, or by screws pointing slightly distally and dorsally. The distal tip in the ischium prevents protrusion. The cranial defects are filled with autologous cancellous bone. Medial cavities can be filled with allogeneic bone (*allo*). During cementing of the polyethylene cup, primary stability is enhanced by an additional mediocranial pillar of cement (*ce*). The head centre (*Cc*) in the drawing, though still in an excessively cranial position despite distalisation, is on the line joining the iliosacral joint. See Fig. 13.11 for the risks associated with screw fixation

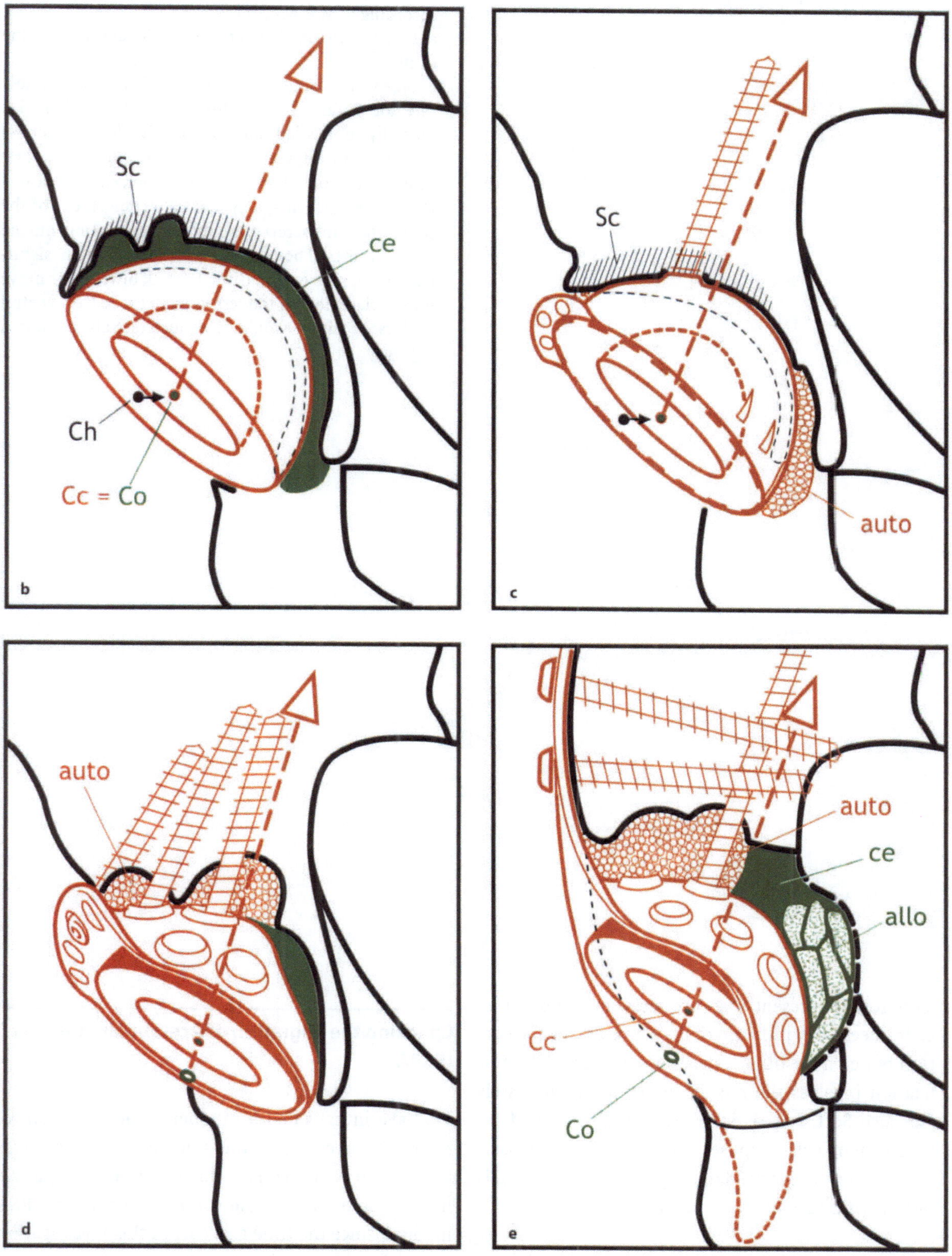

Fig. 3.1 b-e

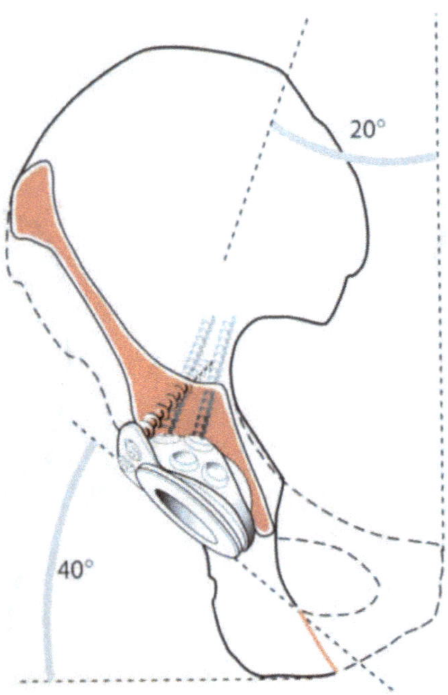

a

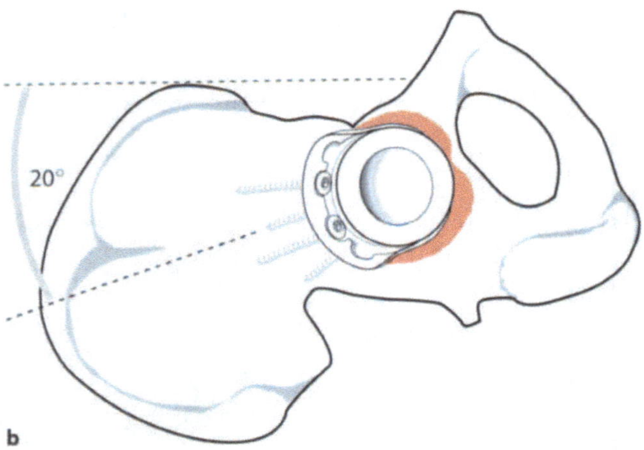

b

Fig. 3.2a, b. Three-dimensional orientation of screw anchorage (example: acetabular reinforcement ring according to M.E. Müller)
a Front view with iliac bone partially cut away at the front
b Side view: The central screw is the first to be inserted. The hole is drilled in the direction of the resultant, i.e. cranially, 20° medially and 20° dorsally. The other screws are screwed in at a conical angle in relation to the first screw. If the bone structure is very poor, e.g. in a case of rheumatoid arthritis, a cylindrical arrangement of the screws, with the screw tips only just penetrating into the adjacent cortical bone, is recommended. This can significantly improve cup fit. Given the risk of vessel or nerve injury, placement of the screws in an excessively ventral or dorsal position should be avoided (see also Sect. 13.4, Fig. 13.9)

teoporosis is present, a secure screw fit can often be guaranteed only if the tip of the screw grasps the cortical bone on the other side. A less than careful screw fixation involves the risk of injury to blood vessels (see also Sect. 13.4.2). Excessively ventral screw fixation in particular exposes the external iliac vessels (Figs. 13.3–13.7). Nerve damage, on the other hand, is only described in exceptional cases.

■ **Screw Fractures.** If, despite the presumed existence of primary stability, migration occurs in a weakly supporting bone stock, fatigue fractures of the screws can occur as a result of excessive loading.

Checking the Migration of Acetabular Implants (EBRA)

We have investigated a number of possible control methods for checking the suitability of techniques for providing immediate stable cup anchorage. We made a conscious decision not to opt for the RSA method, since the time and cost of this investigation per patient is excessive, even though it does offer an impressive degree of accuracy. For the purposes of comparison, we investigated four measuring techniques that were much less time-consuming [7, 8].

The expenditure:accuracy ratio proved to be particularly favourable for the EBRA (*Einbildröntgenanalyse* = single X-ray image analysis) method developed by the Innsbruck study group [9]. A precondition for this measuring method are consistently recorded ap pelvic X-rays (Fig. 3.5.a). Although the regular preparation of usable images requires a certain amount of training on the part of the radiographic personnel, the images can be used both for clinical evaluation and for making measurements – in contrast with the RSA method, in which the radiostereometric images are largely worthless in clinical respects.

The EBRA measuring method is accurate to within ±1 mm and increases with the number of evaluable radiographic images. Since our experience to date suggests that the maximum permitted movement of a cup that still allows secure integration is 1.6 mm, this level of accuracy can be considered adequate, though not outstanding. We have supplemented the traditional presentation of migration with curves with a pseudo three-dimensional presentation [3].

As a rule we are able to achieve a permanently stable anchorage with the surgical techniques presented in this chapter, even in situations involving major defects (Figs. 5.11f, 5.13e). Even if large bone grafts are used to overcome acetabular defects, the cups remain stable provided the direct transmission of forces after operation is absorbed by the existing undisturbed bone stock (Figs. 3.8, 9.1). A slight migration tendency is occasionally observed, and gradual deformation of the acetabulum is also a possibility in exceptional cases (Fig. 3.11d).

Acetabular Implants Used

During the period under review we used four different groups of acetabular implants with a spherical design. We continue to use all these types today:

▪ **Cemented Polyethylene Cup** (Figs. 2.6, 3.1b). With the cemented cup, the gap between the cup and acetabulum is filled with bone cement. Our long-term results have been good where the thickness of the cement layer cranially was at least 2–4 mm. The cement prevents contact between polyethylene and bone, including in cases of gradual loosening with consequent dissemination of granulation tissue between implant and bone. Restoring the natural head centre and inclining the cup at 35–40° also appears to have a positive impact on implant durability [5]. Because of positive results over a period of 5–15 years we have recently reintroduced this solution for occasional primary procedures in elderly patients (Fig. 2.5). The attempt by Schneider [16] to reinforce the bony acetabulum with "armament" screws and thereby redistribute the pressure over a larger bone surface area has produced fairly poor long-term results (Figs. 15.7, 15.8).

▪ **Uncemented SL Cup** (Figs. 2.6, 3.1c). An uncemented spherical cup must fit as accurately as possible in the reamed acetabulum. If the acetabulum has deformed into an oval shape, any cavities present in the frontal plane after centring of the cup centre are filled with autologous bone. The original SL cup according to M.E. Müller was replaced in 1997 by an improved design with a thinner wall, rougher surface and wedge-shaped teeth on the outer surface (Figs. 2.5, 2.6).

▪ **Acetabular Reinforcement Ring** (Figs. 2.6, 3.1d) If the supporting bone stock of the acetabulum is irregular or discontinuous as a result of subchondral cysts in the case of primary prostheses, or defects filled with granulation tissue in the case of revisions, the acetabular reinforcement ring according to M.E. Müller offers a suitable solution. After the cavities are cleaned, the acetabulum is levelled out a little with the acetabular reamer. The remaining gaps are filled with autologous cancellous bone. The acetabular reinforcement ring is wedged in place such that its cranial end abuts securely against the remaining bone stock and its medial ring is located directly on the medial wall of the acetabulum (Fig. 3.12).

Three or four screws are then screwed firmly in place in the direction of the iliosacral joint with the aim of achieving a primary stability that allows weight bearing. Any exposed autologous cancellous bone is covered with a reabsorbable net, e.g. made from Vicryl, to prevent any cement from penetrating between the cancellous chips. The polyethylene cup can now be cemented in place in the desired inclination of 35–40° and anteversion of 14–18°. If a large cup is selected, the head centre is shifted in the distal direction, while a small cup will move the head centre medially. We do not recommend the Ganz ring with hook because its flat hollow does not allow the head centre to be shifted sufficiently in the medial direction and because the shell does not butt against the bone on the craniomedial side if the hook tab is too short. The acetabular reinforcement ring is widely used as a primary and revision implant (Figs. 2.5, 2.7).

■ **Burch-Schneider Antiprotrusio Cage** (Figs. 2.6, 3.1e) The antiprotrusio cage is used in patients with major bone defects and a lack of proximal support or bone discontinuity. Its increasing use (Fig. 2.7) is attributable partly to the simplified implantation technique as a result of introduction of the trial antiprotrusio cage (Fig. 3.10) and partly to the growing number of large acetabular defects to be managed in our patient population. The cranial flange can be anchored, together with a medial pillar of cement, sufficiently strongly to allow this antiprotrusio cage to effect powerful distalisation of the cup centre (Fig. 3.11). The cranial defect is filled with autologous or, in the event of elderly patients, allogeneic bone material (Fig. 3.11e). We have discontinued the practice of filling with cement alone (Fig. 6.6) because of the risk of overheating and consequent damage to the adjacent bone.

3.3.2 Selection of Femoral Implants

The internal shape of the proximal femur is highly irregular and subject to considerable interindividual variation (Fig. 3.4a). As a rule, the metaphysis is characterised by antetorsion and recurvation, while the diaphysis shows a conical tapering of widely varying degree (Fig. 3.4a) and antecurvation. The narrowest point of the femur, the femoral isthmus, is located approximately 220–240 mm below the head centre. Since off-the-shelf prosthesis systems are unable to match this internal shape precisely, uncemented systems resolve the dilemma by adopting a bulky, wedging design. Depending on the individual case, conical (CLS) or cylindrical implants (Zweymüller) are the appropriate shapes of choice. In the cemented systems, the residual cavities are filled with cement.

A proper evaluation of a prosthetic system must take account of the interrelationships between the shape, the microscopic and macroscopic surface structure, the implant material and its elasticity (see also Chap. 15).

Femoral Implants Used
(Figs. 2.9a,b)

Cemented Straight-Stem Systems

Common features of all systems: The straight-stem systems used (straight stem 77 standard and lateralising, SL 88 and CDH, Virtec standard and lateralising) are characterised by a whole range of common components:

- The following common properties of the six prosthesis ranges mean that just one individual planning template (Fig. 3.3) needs to be produced per range:
  - Constant lateralisation of the prosthesis contouring on the medial side in relation to the head centre. Accordingly, total lateralisation in the larger prostheses, compared to the smaller prostheses, is increased by 50% of the additional prosthesis width.
  - Constant neck angle.
  - Constant wedge angle.
- Wedge shape: The wedge shape is more pronounced in the frontal plane compared with the sagittal plane, resulting in self-centring and three-point contact (Fig. 3.4c).
- Rotational stability, thanks to a flat or oval cross-section, resulting in a more or less pronounced demarcation between ventral and dorsal cement halves (Figs. 3.4c,e).
- Standard-lateralising prosthesis: The difference in the lateralisation of the corresponding sizes is 6 mm, but increases to 12 mm if the standard prosthesis has a short head and the lateralising stem is fitted with a long head. This classification into two prosthesis types permits more accurate imitation of the preoperative situation. In men, the lateralising prosthesis tends to produce a better fit, while the standard prosthesis is more likely to match the anatomical contouring of women. There is evidence to suggest that wear is reduced and the quality of the clinical outcome is superior with greater lateralisation [15], although other authors argue that this can result in slightly earlier loosening.
- Cementing: A highly secure bond with the cement requires fine-blasted prosthesis surfaces. In combination with ventral and dorsal cement abutment collars, this results in a highly stable bond. In this context, additional cement projecting beyond the

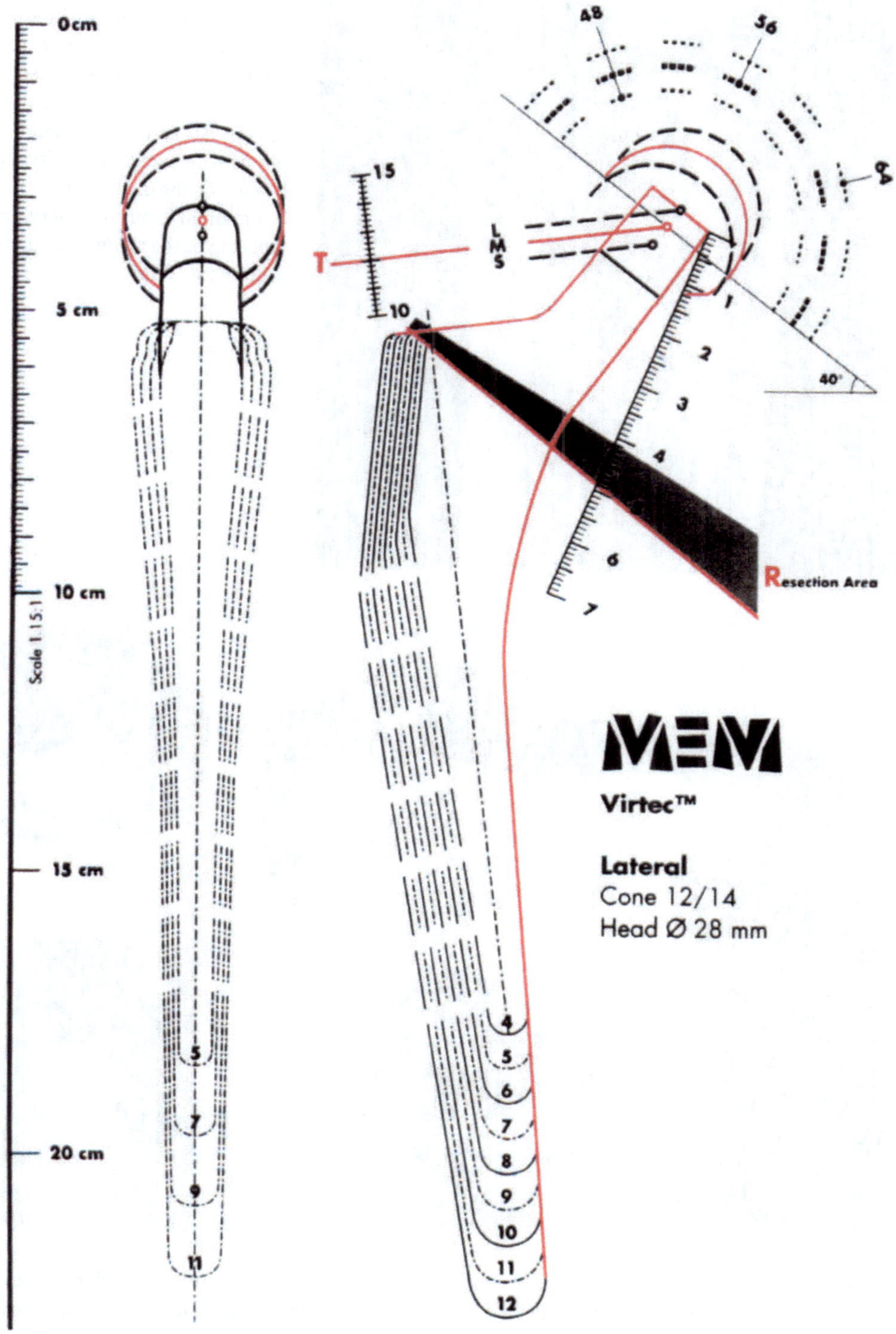

Fig. 3.3. Example of a drawing template for a prosthesis from the straight stem system: Virtec lateralising. The outlines marked in red are common to all sizes. The trochanter line T is used to prepare for, and establish, the distalisation/proximalisation of the head centre in relation to the tip of the greater trochanter. The location of the head neck resection is shown as an area in which the distance from the edge of the cone can be measured. With ascending prosthesis size, the lateralisation increases by half the amount of prosthesis widening. The acetabular opening angle is shown with 40° inclination. An inclination of 35–40° combined with an anteversion of 14–18° is considered ideal for preventing dislocations and impingement (Chap. 6). By way of illustration, three spherical cup outlines with differing diameter are shown. The lateral prosthesis projection is also shown on the left

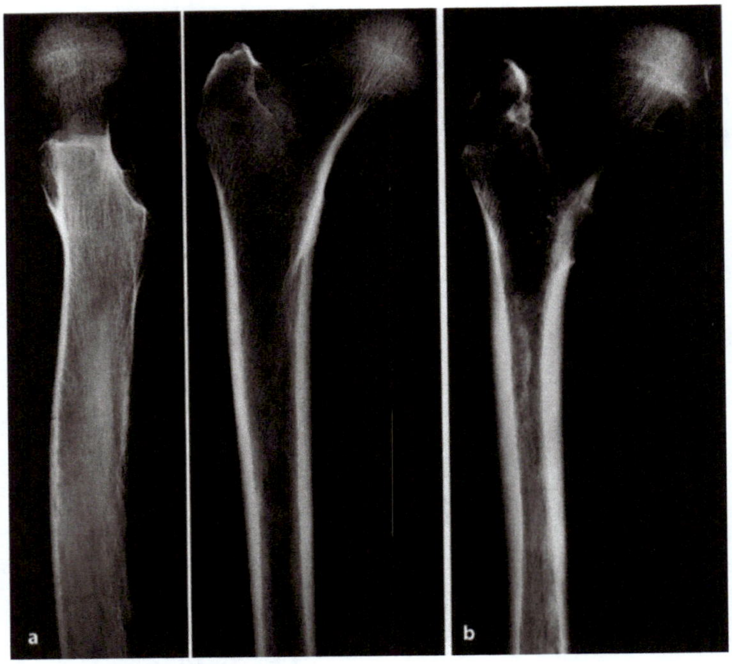

Fig. 3.4a–e. Three-dimensional view of the proximal femur and anchorage of the straight stem/Virtec prosthesis
a Proximal femur, ap and axial views – Radiographs of a femur in isolation. Antetorsion and recurvation are present at the metaphysis and antecurvation at the diaphysis. The medullary cavity tapers slightly towards the distal end
b Proximal femur with very pronounced tapering of the medullary cavity and prominent isthmus

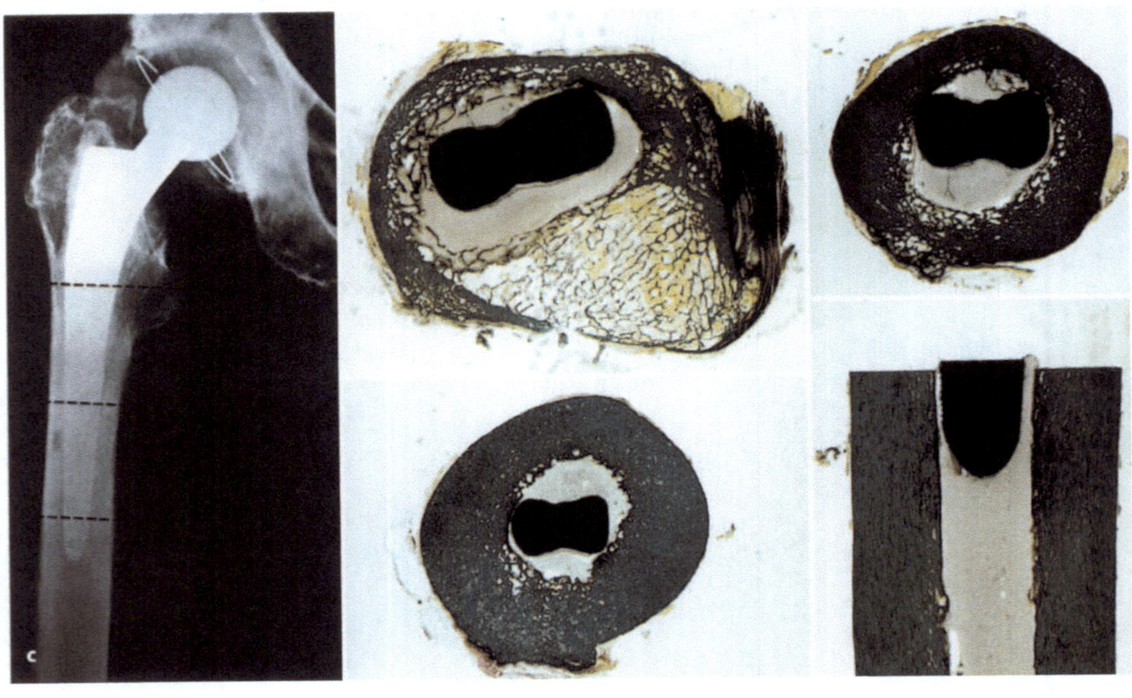

c Anchorage of a straight-stem prosthesis in the proximal femur. Post mortem examination with non-decalcified histology technique. S.E., male, 80 years (O. 8990). No pain at clinical follow-up after 11 years. Died 12 years after implantation. The three transverse sawn sections correspond with Grun's zones, the distal tip has been sawn in the frontal plane. Section thickness of approximately 100 µm. Mounted on opaque Plexiglas, stained with toluidine blue. Specially detailed areas were cut to a thickness of 6 µm using a special microtome. The lateral cortical bone shows a small patch of brightness as the first sign of granulation tissue. No evidence of stress protection in terms of cortical thickening distally on the very rigid implant. No seam formation between cement and bone. The cutaway views show individual localised points of contact between prosthesis and bone. The prosthesis is typically positioned more ventrally at the proximal end and more dorsally at the distal end. The cement mantle is wholly intact and remains integrated with the honeycomb structure of the bone. The cortical bone remains almost unchanged. No intermediate tissue has entered between the cement and the bone. The cement plug distal to the prosthesis tip is too long, and the limiting intramedullary plug made from bone from the femoral head is largely resorbed

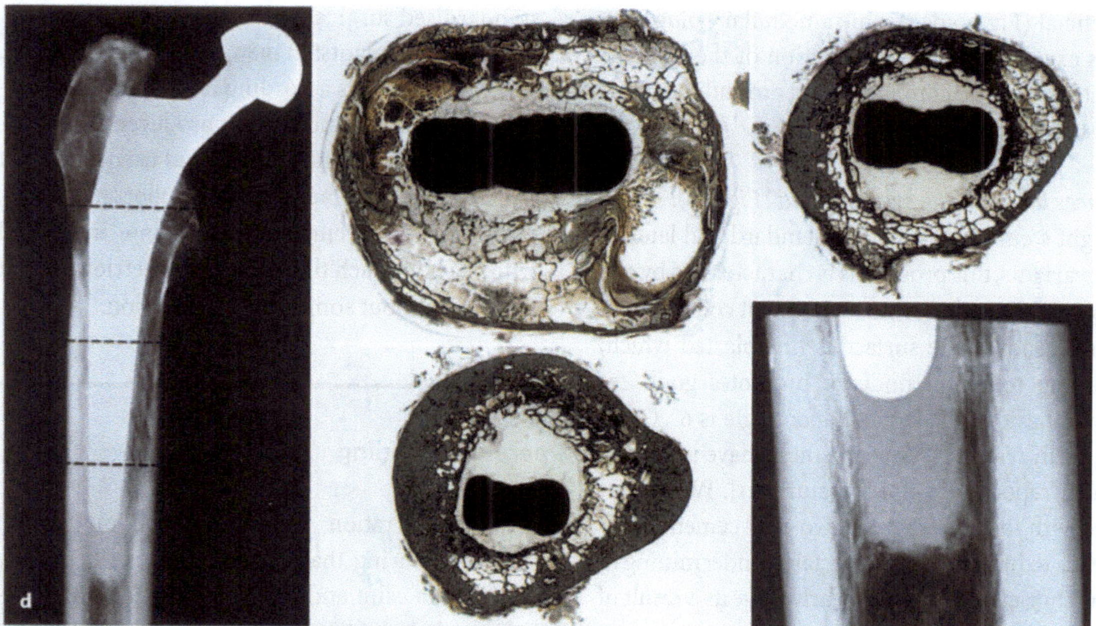

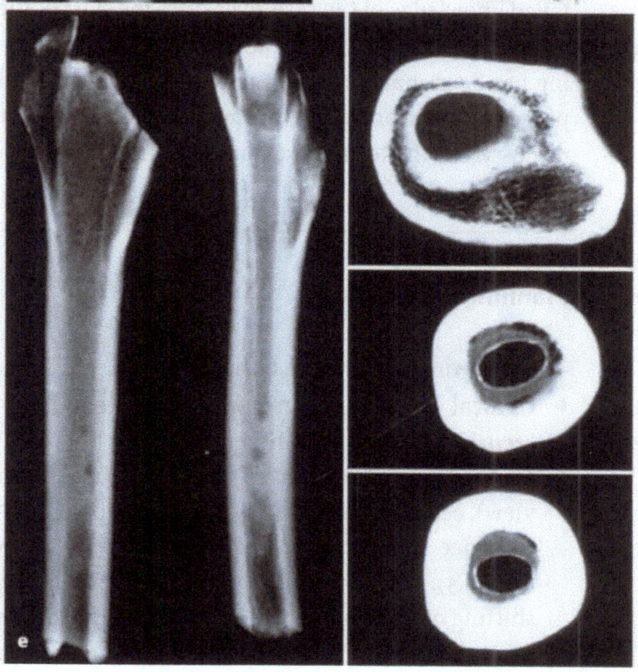

Fig. 3.4.d Second example: S.I., female, 84 years (O. 7884). After 5 years the patient assessed the result as very good, reported no pain, was able to walk for more than an hour and flex the hip through 90°, after 10 years she had already become very frail. She died 13 years after implantation. Same preparation as for Fig. 3.4c. Severe osteoporosis with loosened cortical bone, particularly on the proximal and medial sides. Two spreading cavities filled with granulation tissue are apparent in Grun's zones 1 and 7, i.e. proximally where the stem enters the femur. This is a manifestation of polyethylene wear from the joint. Beyond this point distally, the cement mantle remains completely undisturbed. Adjacent to the cement, however, substantial cancellisation of the cortical bone has occurred, particularly medially and dorsally. This is clearly apparent especially distal-medial to the cement tip projecting beyond the prosthesis. Almost nothing remains of the autologous intramedullary plug
e Experimental implantation with a Virtec prosthesis made from a radiolucent plastic: The general ap and axial views on the left show very central positioning of the prosthesis even though a centraliser was not used. Three sectional views show a largely regular cement mantle, with contact points between the stem and cortical bone limited to small areas

tip of the prosthesis distally by 5–10 mm can prove beneficial (Fig. 3.4d). An intramedullary plug prevents excessively deep penetration of the cement, resulting in more compact filling around the prosthesis.

Differences between the systems used (Fig. 2.9):

- Straight stem 77: Available in standard and lateralising variants, this prosthesis is characterised by anterior and posterior cement abutment collars and a central groove. The surface is fine-blasted which, according to recent findings, promotes good cement adhesion. The frontal taper angle is 6°. Good long-term results for this prosthesis have repeatedly been reported in the literature [11]. We do not agree with the view that the two-part cement mantle leads to histologically detectable undermining of the anchorage at a relatively early stage as a result of granulation tissue formation [4]. Two of nine prostheses histologically examined by the non-decalcified technique after an average of 11 years in situ are cited by way of example (Figs. 3.4c,d).
- The CDH prosthesis possesses an oval cross-section and a frontal taper angle of 6°.
- The SL 88 prosthesis is rough-blasted and, compared with the GS 77 prosthesis, is slightly more rectangular in cross-section and slightly thicker on the lateral side compared to the medial side. A central groove on the anterior and posterior sides – a familiar feature of the GS 77 prosthesis – is lacking in the SL 88 stem. The frontal taper angle is 6°.
- The Virtec prosthesis is oval in cross-section. Rotational stability is ensured partly by this oval cross-section and partly by additional vertical slits at the proximal end (Fig. 2.9a). In view of the fairly rounded cross-section, care must be taken during insertion of the prosthesis to prevent incorrect antetorsion by using a forked impactor. The cement mantle is more regularly formed than is the case with the straight stem (Fig. 3.4e). The frontal taper angle is 5°.

Uncemented Femoral Components

- As primary implants: The SL collar prosthesis according to M.E. Müller has been tried on an experimental basis. Little use has been made of uncemented components, not on principle, but because of our special teaching hospital status. The systems used need to be simple and allow a standardised surgical technique.
- As revision implants: In 1989, we introduced the SL revision prosthesis according to Wagner for bridging major defects, and this has produced good clinical results. This is the only implant used by us that has not been designed by M.E. Müller, and it can, under certain circumstances, become integrated with the bone such that subsequent retrieval is not possible without some bone destruction.

3.4 Operation Planning

Meticulous operation planning is the method of choice for ensuring that the operator can begin the operation in a calm and collected manner with a detailed knowledge of the case. Ever since the start of the period under review, preparation of a planning drawing has been mandatory for all total hip replacement procedures performed in our hospital. The plans are discussed by the team at each morning report.

3.4.1 Planning Preparations

The following serve as the basis for planning:

- Clinical examination in respect of leg length discrepancy and hip mobility.
- Up-to-date radiographs: Pelvis (anteroposterior view), centred low on the symphysis, supplemented since approx. 1990 by a "faux profil" view (Fig. 3.5). This projection primarily reveals any shifting of the head centre anteriorly (Fig. 3.6b) or posteriorly (Fig. 3.7a). The radiographs should have been taken within the previous 3 months. Any available earlier images plotting the patient's progression are retrieved, or requested, and included in the assessment.
- Planning templates according to M.E. Müller for the prostheses used (Fig. 3.3).

3.4.2 Objectives of Planning

The operation planning should enable the operator to form as accurate a picture as possible of the sequence

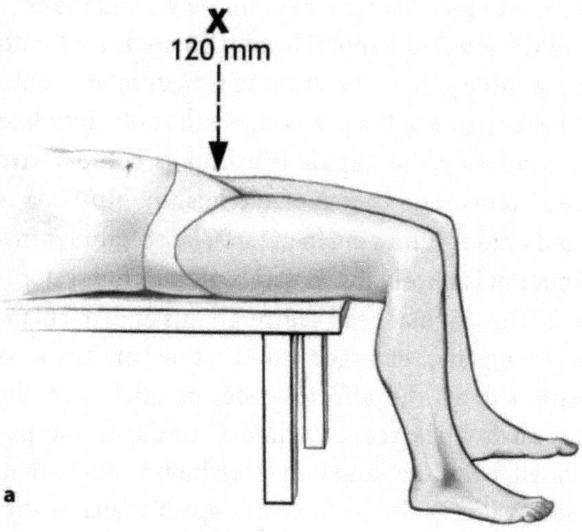

a

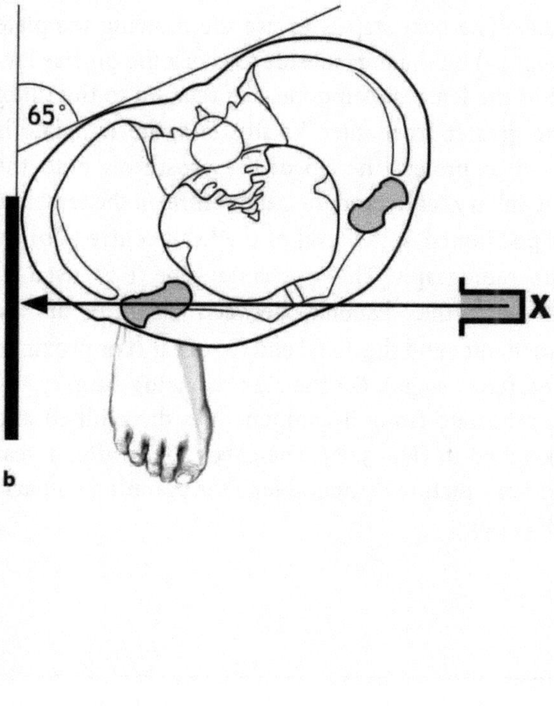

b

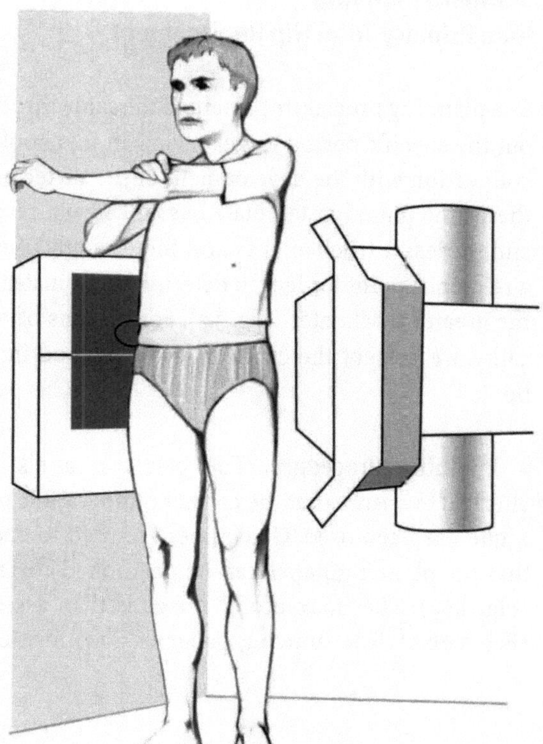

Fig. 3.5a, b. Recording technique for reproducible standard radiographs
a Pelvis antero-posterior, low centred with legs hanging down (Fig. 3.6.a): The knees are touching, the lower legs hang over the edge of the table and are parallel. The central beam is targeted on the upper edge of the symphysis, film focal distance 120 mm. Ensure that the pelvis is not tilted. The postoperative X-ray should therefore be recorded only after several days. For the purposes of better reproducibility grid plates should not be used

b Hip "faux profil" [10]: The pelvis of the standing patient is rotated 25° towards the back, producing an angle of 65° between the radiographic plate and the sacral plane. The foot closest to the plate is aligned parallel with the film. The central beam is targeted on the groin on the side farthest from the plate. The resulting radiograph depicts the hip side next to the plate (Fig. 3.6.b,c) of the operation and any potential problems. The drawing is used to establish the plan and allows certain errors to be identified and corrected before surgery. The surgical team can prepare itself for the procedure, procure the necessary implants and offer their own thoughts during the procedure. If these objectives are to be achieved, there needs to be a clear drawing with large lettering which can easily be viewed by all the team members and which is suspended on the light box next to the preoperative radiographs. The correctness of the operation/drawing can be checked through comparison with the postoperative radiograph.

3.4.3 Standard Planning for a Primary Total Hip Replacement

The planning procedure remained the same throughout the specific period under review in this book. In connection with the development of the Virtec prosthesis, the planning template has since been revised and the lesser trochanter is now increasingly used as a reference point for length determination instead of the greater trochanter (Fig. 3.3). For reasons of topicality, we present the currently used method in this book.

■ **Planning Procedure.** The pelvic x-ray is first checked to ensure that the correct radiographic technique has been used. Guide lines are used to ensure that the planning paper can be positioned correctly (Fig. 3.6a). The "faux profil" image is then assessed (Fig. 3.6b,c). The drawing paper is now positioned correctly on the pelvic radiograph (Fig. 3.6d). The contours of the affected side of the pelvis and the centre of the affected femoral head (Ch) are traced onto the planning paper. The drawing is then rotated onto the healthy side of the pelvis, using the obturator line and Köhler's radiographic teardrop as comparative guide points. The centre of the healthy hip (Co) is traced onto the drawing in green. The acetabular implantation is now planned with a view to the restoration of the original head centre. To this end, the planning template, enlarged to a scale of 1.15:1, is positioned on the affected side, parallel with the body's axis. The circular outline of the cup is now positioned over the diseased acetabulum such that, postoperatively, the head centre again matches that on the healthy side. The operator should select a cup diameter that ensures that the subchondral zone of sclerosis on the affected side is largely preserved (see also Fig. 3.6c). The cup contours are now traced onto the drawing paper placed over the template (Fig. 3.6e). The next step is to use the drawing template (Fig. 3.3) on the normal side to check the precise level of the femoral component in relation to the tip of the greater trochanter. To this end, the template is used to project the tip of the prosthesis onto the medullary cavity, and the head centre on the template is positioned at the level of the head centre (Co) on the radiograph. The trochanter line T is used to measure the distance between the tip of the trochanter and the distal end (coxa vara) or proximal end (coxa valga). On the side requiring surgery, the appropriate femoral component is determined and sketched in (Fig. 3.6f). The check X-ray after 1 year shows a picture comparable to the planning scenario (Fig. 3.6g).

Fig. 3.6a–g. Example of operation plan for a patient with dysplastic coxarthrosis. K.O., female, 83 years (O.14867).
a The two head centres are marked on the pelvic X-ray. Additionally, a line is drawn on the lower edge of the obturator foramen and another line on the lower edge of the iliosacral joint. A vertical line through the symphysis also passes centrally through the coccyx, allowing the viewer to confirm the precise ap projection
b The faux profil radiograph shows that the head centre has clearly shifted ventrally. During operation this is to be relocated to its more dorsal position
c Sketch aid for the faux-profil radiograph: *Ch* head centre, *Cc* centre of the acetabulum, *Fol* obturator foramen left, *Spi* ant. inf. iliac spine, *Sps* ant. sup. iliac spine, *Tmi* lesser trochanter, *Tisch* ischial tuberosity. The spherical acetabular reamer is used to widen the acetabulum in the dorsal-distal direction (*arrows*), while the subchondral sclerosis zone (*Sc*) is preserved cranially
d The upper edge of the transparent paper overlaps the lower end of the iliosacral joint, the medial edge overlaps the symphysis. The contours and the head centre (*Ch*) of the pelvic side undergoing surgery are copied onto the paper

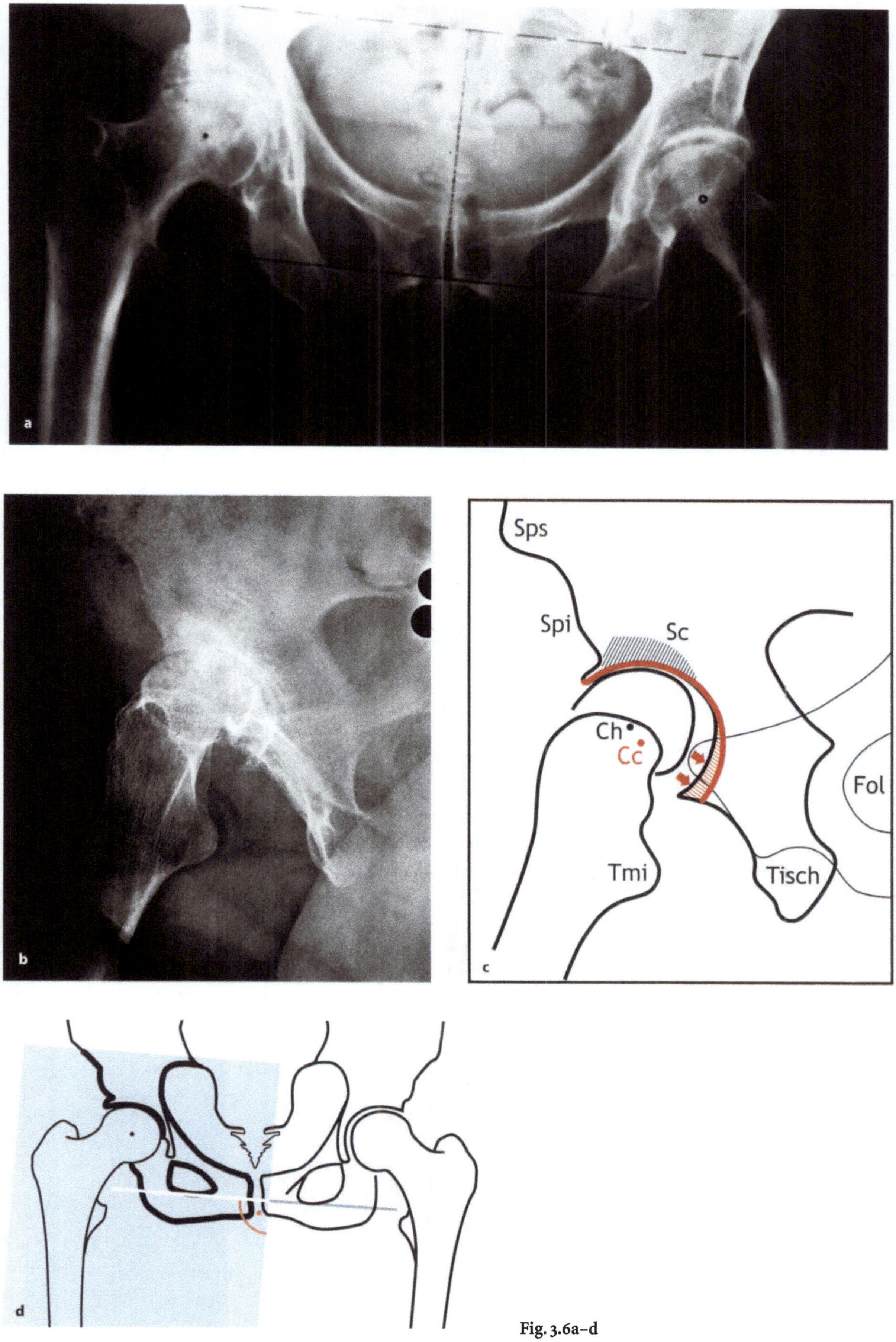

Fig. 3.6a–d

Fig. 3.6e,f

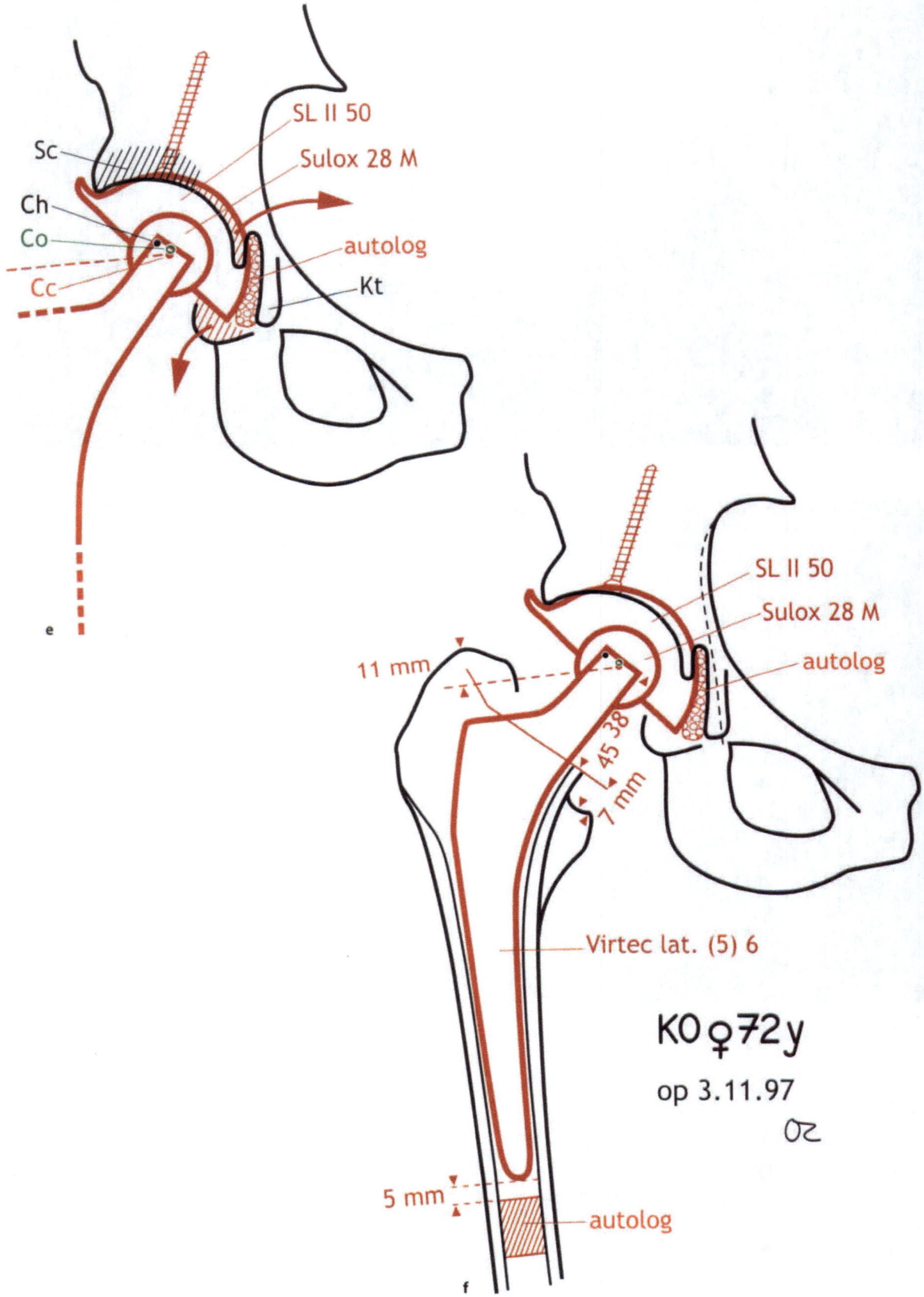
SL II 50
Sulox 28 M
Sc
Ch
Co
Cc
autolog
Kt
e
SL II 50
Sulox 28 M
autolog
11 mm
45 38
7 mm
Virtec lat. (5) 6
KO ♀ 72 y
op 3.11.97
5 mm
autolog
f

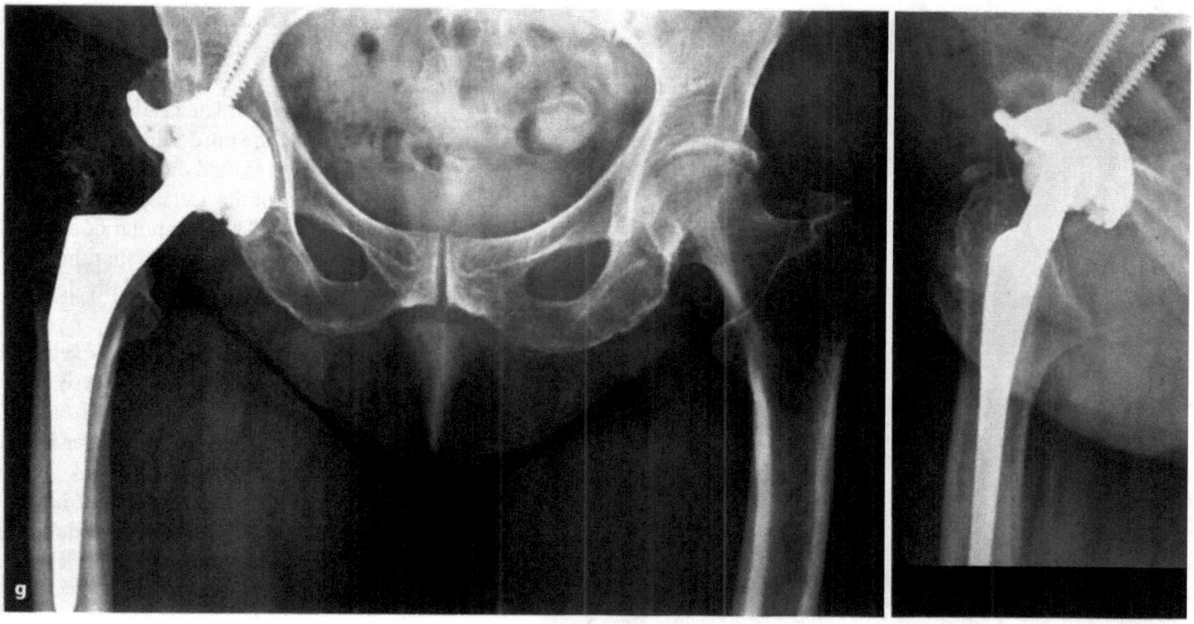

◂ **Fig. 3.6e.** Detail drawing after cup planning and the drawing of the outlines common to all prosthesis sizes. The red-hatched bone sections are removed, while the black-hatched subchondral sclerosis zone (*Sc*) is preserved. *Red* reamed acetabular cavity
f The contours of the femur and the location of the femoral neck osteotomy are determined using the drawing template. The template permits the direct measurement of the distance between the lesser trochanter/planned osteotomy and cone edge. All components are drawn in and the important distances measured. The names of the patient and operator and the date of operation are added
g Check radiograph 2 years postoperatively. The patient was free of symptoms, could walk without sticks for over 1 hour and flex the hip through 100°. She died of other causes shortly thereafter

■ **Specific Points.** Severely worn acetabulum on the cranial side: The new head centre can also be positioned slightly cranially, but not laterally, in relation to the natural centre of the opposite side [5]. By way of compensation, the femoral component can be allowed to protrude in a slightly more proximal direction by the same distance.

Severe dysplastic coxarthrosis: To ensure that the prosthesis head is better centred in the acetabulum by the existing muscle forces we prefer to use a lateralising stem component.

Pronounced protrusion (Fig. 3.7): Lateralising the head centre to its original location also produces distinct lateralisation of the trochanter. We use the narrower standard component to avoid triggering the annoying phenomenon of trochanteric clicking.

Preoperative leg length discrepancies: See Chap: 9.

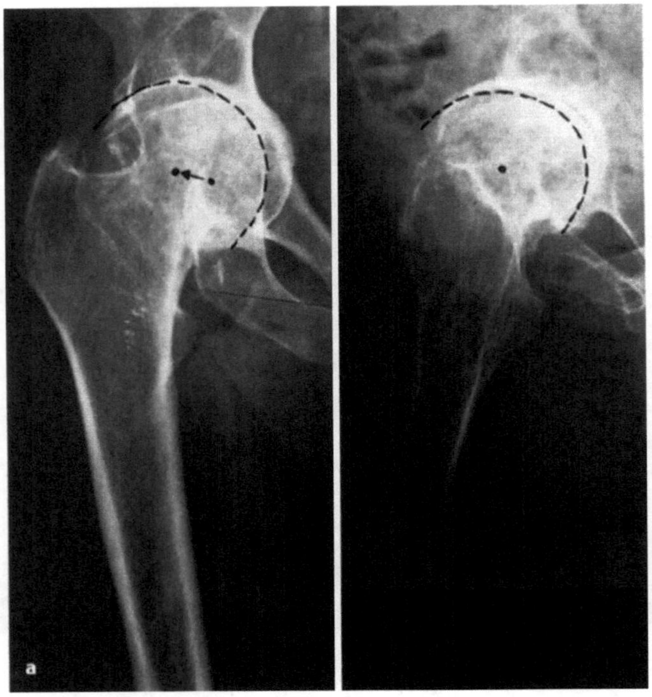

Fig. 3.7a–d. Plan for the primary management of a protrusion coxarthrosis (R.L., female, 80 years (O.11557)) Protrusion coxarthrosis bil., flexion/extension 75 – 15 – 0

a Pelvis ap and "faux profil": The head contour protrudes medially over the borderline of the lesser pelvis. The head centre is shifted dorsally and medially. The dotted outlines of the acetabular component have been drawn on. The acetabular opening is reamed in a single step so as to ensure that the cup wedges in place without subsiding medially deep into the cavity

b On the postoperative view, the hip centre is shifted back to its normal position and the underlying cavity has been filled with cancellous bone from the resected femoral head. The greater trochanter is marked with a tantalum ball

c Two years later, the cup is firmly anchored in the bone in its postoperative position and remodelling of the cancellous bone lining has occurred. Flexion/extension 95 – 0 – 0, no limping, no pain

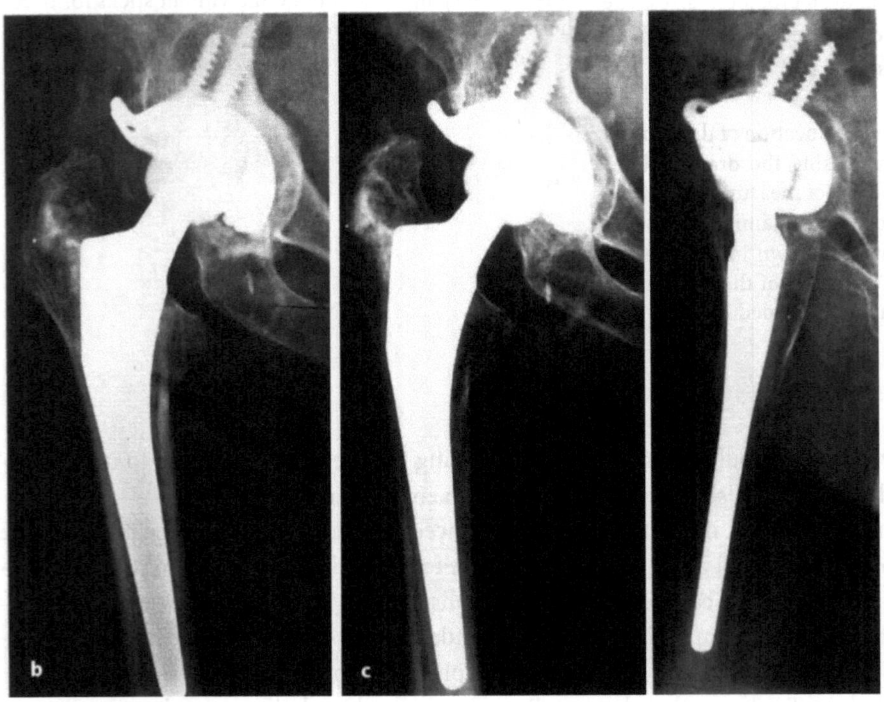

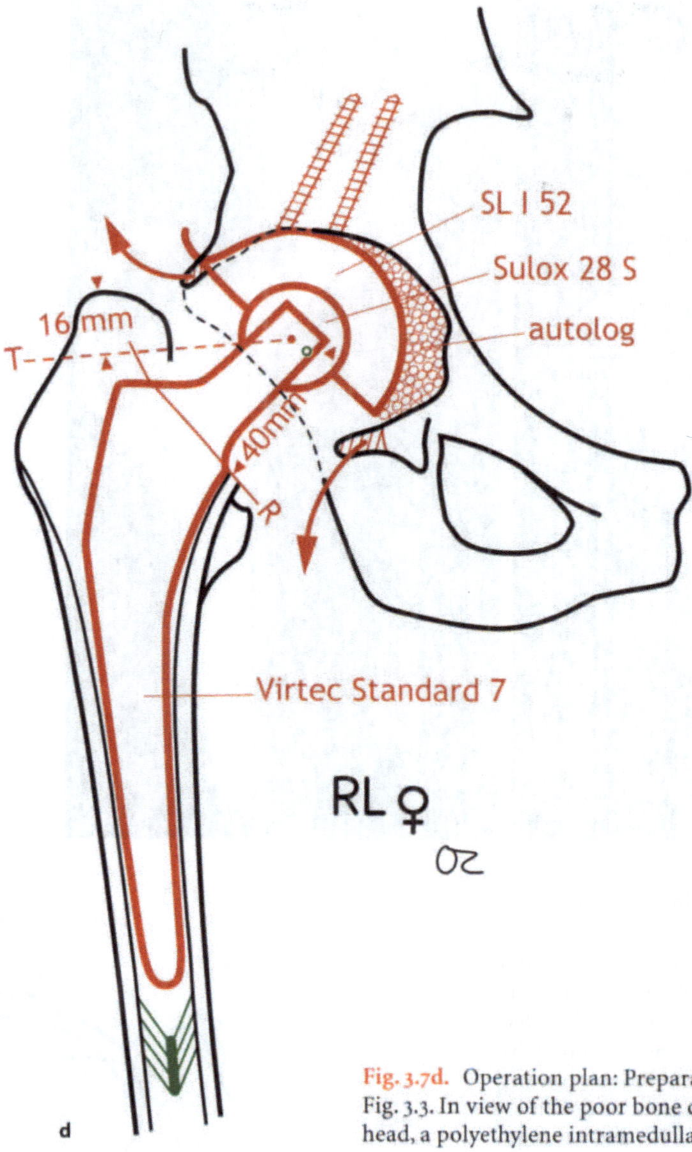

d

Fig. 3.7d. Operation plan: Preparation as described for Fig. 3.3. In view of the poor bone quality of the femoral head, a polyethylene intramedullary plug was used

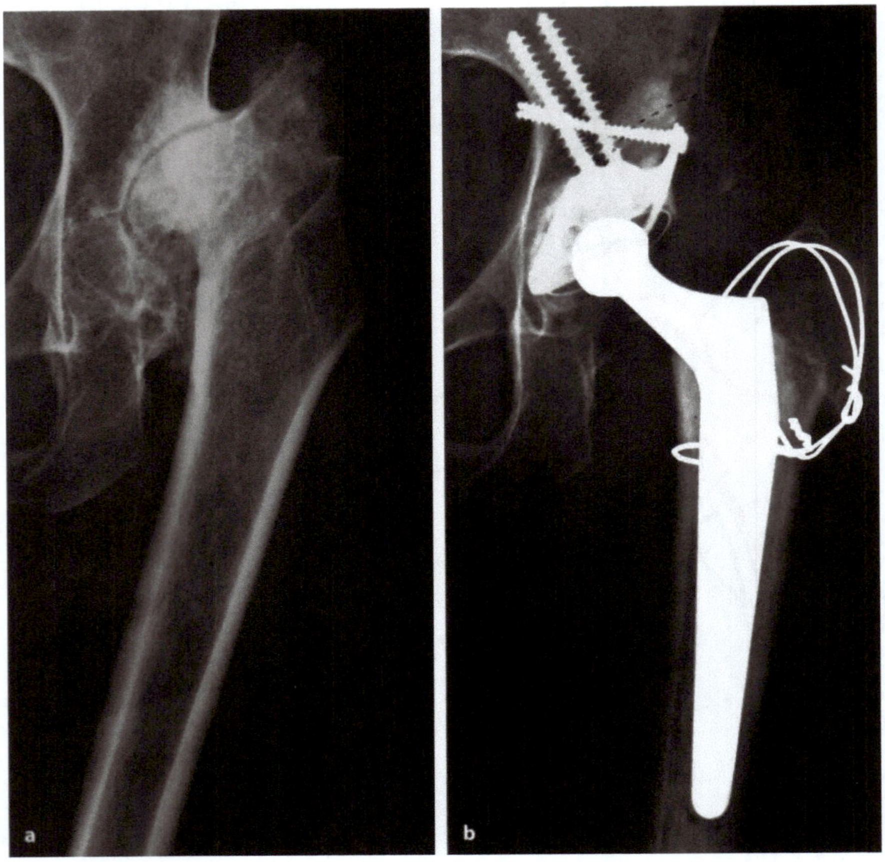

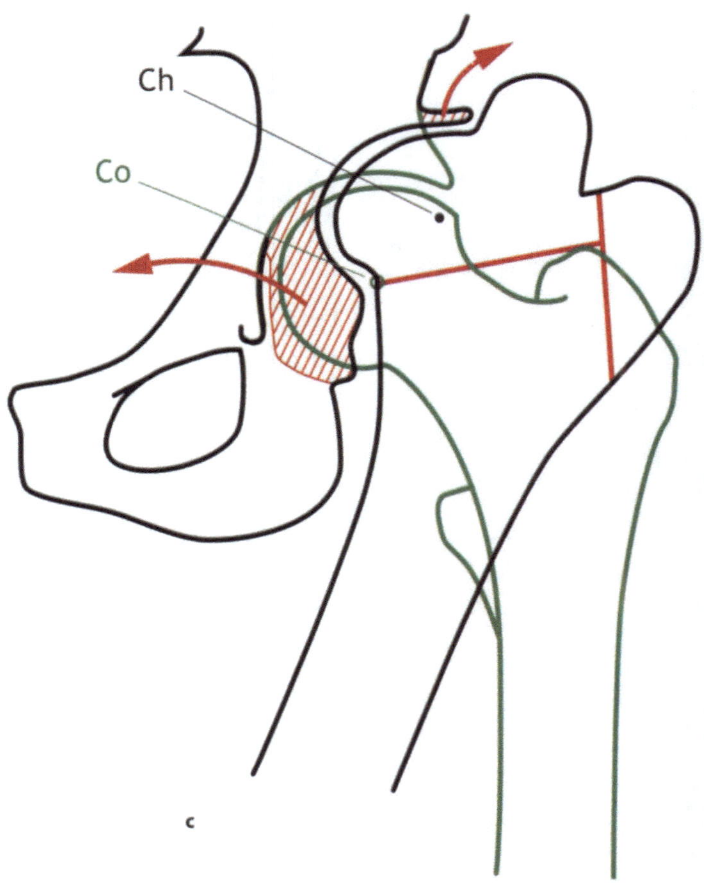

Fig. 3.8a–e. Plan for a primary prosthesis with high subluxation

a G.H., male, 64 years (O.3095). Pinning of a case of femoral head epiphyseolysis at the age of 14 with Steinmann pins, followed by infection and femoral head necrosis. Preoperatively, considerable pain with extreme coxa vara, combined with problems associated with a valgus gonarthrosis on the left and varus gonarthrosis on the right. Preoperatively, a functional leg length discrepancy of 12 cm was noted (see also Fig. 9.1)

b Situation postoperatively. The *dotted line* represents the border with the autologous bone graft (shaped from a section of the resected femoral head). The trochanter is secured with double-wound cerclage wiring, supplemented with cerclage of the femoral shaft (see also Chap. 8)

c If the healthy side (*green*) is compared with the affected (*black*) side on a drawing, it can be seen that approximately half of the acetabular contact surface area is missing from the latter. The floor of the acetabulum is filled in with a large osteophyte and needs to be removed (*red hatching*). The planned osteotomies at the proximal end of the femur are marked in *red*

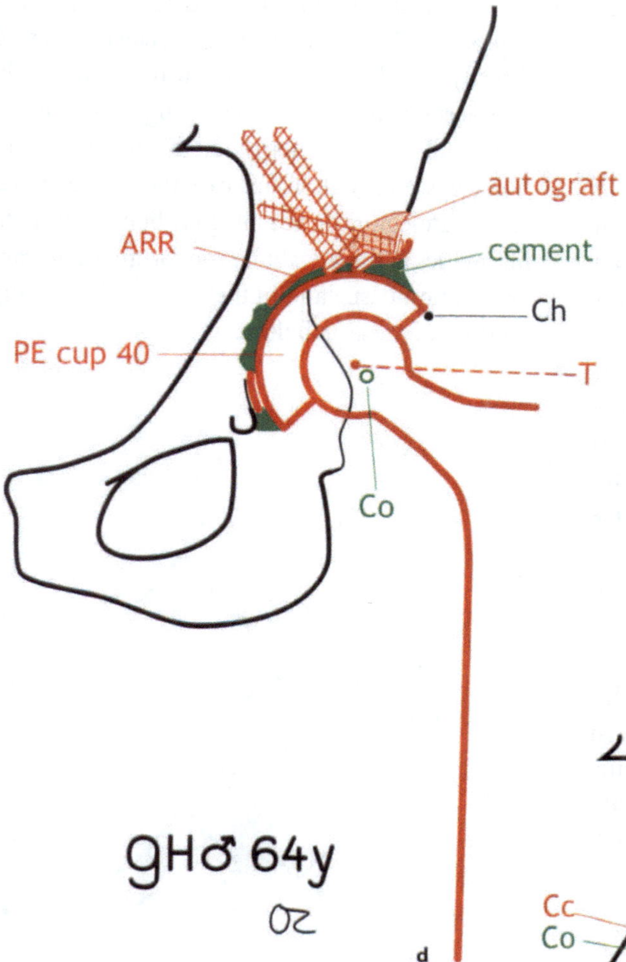

Fig. 3.8.
d The missing section of acetabulum laterally is fashioned from the resected femoral head and screwed onto the freshened acetabular floor. The whole construction is strengthened with an acetabular reinforcement ring (*ARR*). The selected polyethylene cup must be small enough for at least three fifths of its contacting surface to abut against the original bone stock. The use of a 22-mm head is recommended in order to ensure an adequate thickness of polyethylene for such a small cup. The CDH prosthesis combines the features of a small 22-mm head and an especially straight stem, and is particularly suitable for the shaft conditions prevailing in this situation
e The preoperative situation is highlighted by the black dotted area on the completed drawing. While the actual leg lengthening is just 18 mm, the functional leg shortening is reduced from a preoperative 12 cm to 3.5 cm postoperatively, thanks to the concurrent correction of the adduction malposition

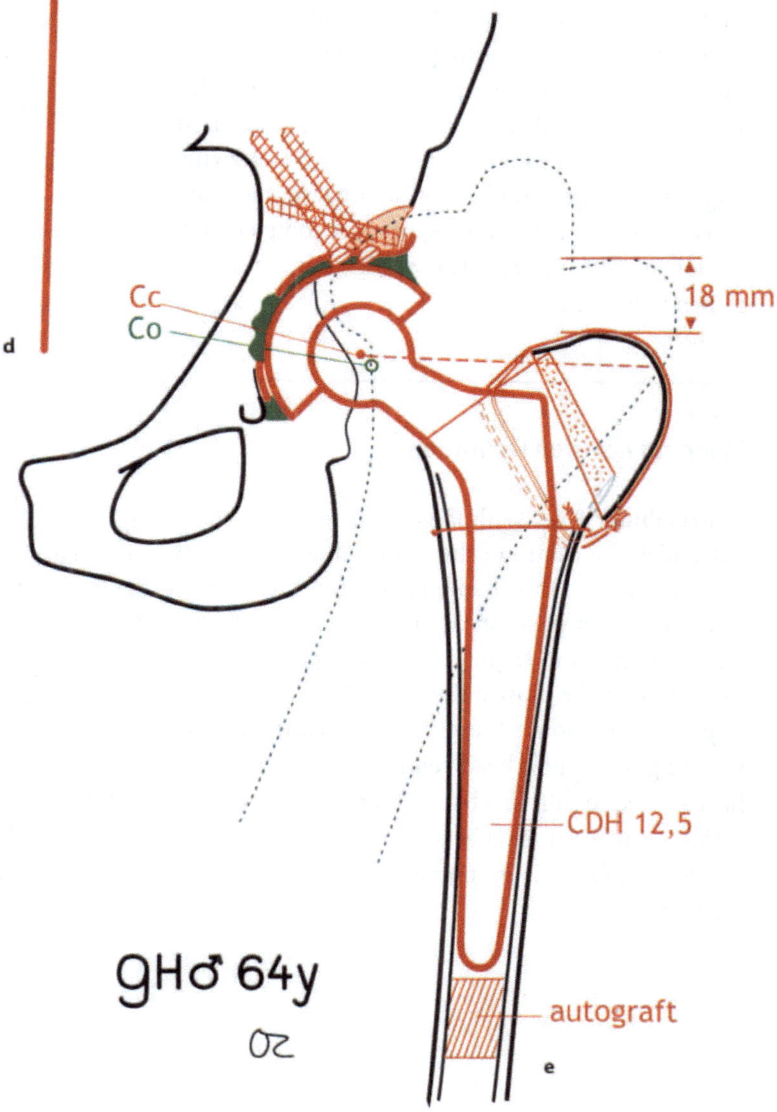

3.4.4
Planning Example for a Complex Primary Prosthesis

As an example we have chosen a high subluxation. In our case (Fig. 3.8), there is a pronounced adduction contracture, lateralisation of the head centre (Ch), an extremely short femoral neck with coxa vara and partial destruction of the acetabular roof. In the first planning step, the situation on the affected side is compared with that on the healthy side and the osteotomies are planned (Fig. 3.8c). The next step is to determine how to reconstruct the acetabulum (Fig. 3.8d), ensuring that the new head centre (Cc) is located under the existing undisturbed bone stock and not under the newly inserted bone block. Even with an acetabular roof reconstruction employing autologous material, full weight-bearing is only possible after a remodelling period of several months. The planned lengthening and trochanteric fixation can be ascertained from the definitive drawing (Fig. 3.8e). In our example an additional supracondylar varisation osteotomy is required for complete correction of the leg axis. The result after 3 years is shown in Fig. 9.1c.

3.4.5
Planning Revision Operations

■ **Acetabular Side.** With large acetabular defects in particular, the centre of the loosened acetabulum is generally shifted to a dysplasia position, more rarely to a protrusion position or along the resultant in a cranial, dorsal and slightly medial direction towards the centre of the iliosacral joint (Fig. 3.9). The most important decision in this planning process is the positioning of the new head centre. From the start, we have strived to shift this back either to its original location or, with large defects, allowed it to migrate a maximum of 1–2 cm in a proximal direction along the resultant.

- Small defects with no need for distalisation of the cup centre: The acetabular implant can be screwed directly into the existing undisturbed bone stock. The acetabular reinforcement ring according to M.E. Müller is particularly suitable for this situation (Figs. 2.6, 13.8). In this case the only purpose of an autologous or homologous bone graft is to fill cavities in the acetabular roof originating from granulation tissue and in the non-weight bearing sections of the acetabulum.

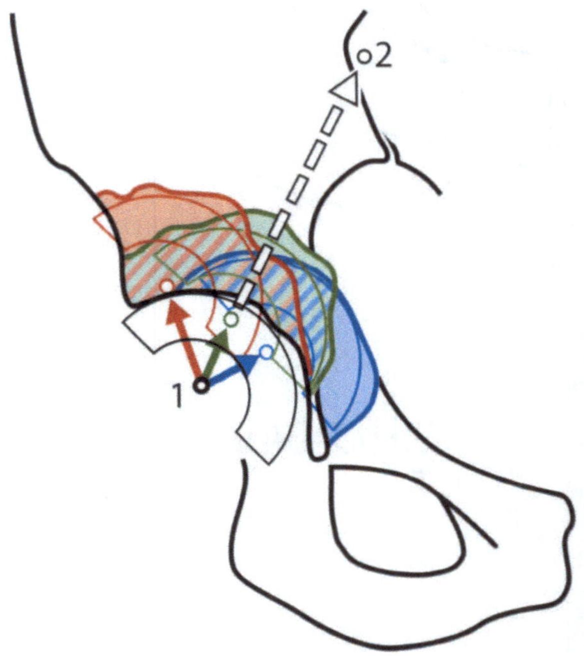

Fig. 3.9. Options for shifting the head centre in the event of substantial cup loosening. The bony border in the various types of defect is marked by a *thick line*, while a *hatched area* of the same colour denotes the corresponding bone loss. The original central cup position with the head centre and the resultant of the forces acting on the cup are drawn in *black*. The resultant passes from the head centre in a cranial, dorsal and medial direction toward the centre of the iliosacral joint (see also Fig. 3.1a). In most cases, a loose cup moves to a laterocranial subluxation position (*red*). Less frequently the centre migrates toward the resultant (*green*) or to a protrusion position (*blue*)

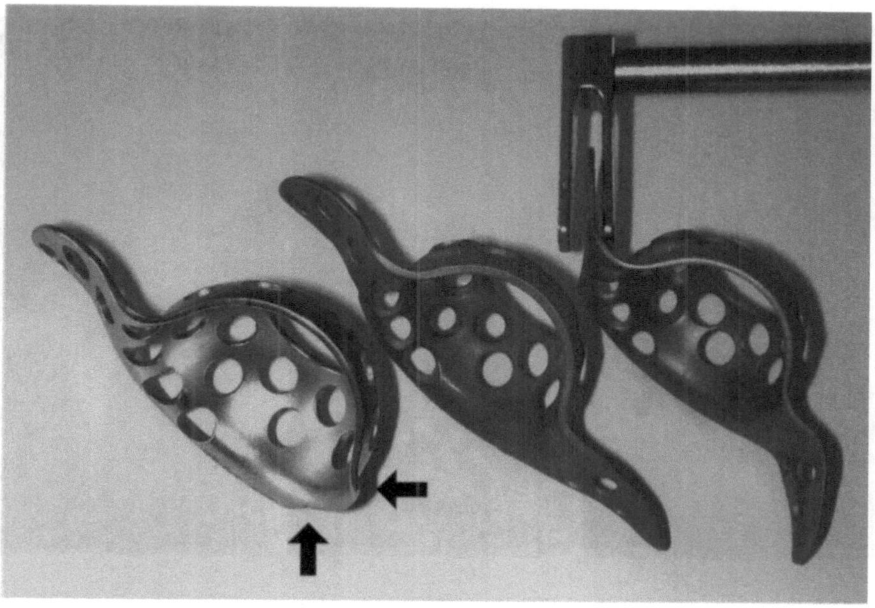

Fig. 3.10. Burch-Schneider antiprotrusio cage. The trial shell (*left*) with marked points just at the distal tip (*arrows*) allows the surgeon to test the position of the shell and flange during operation. The shell can then be bent from its original shape (*centre*) into the appropriate shape to match the specific local situation (*right*)

- Large defects with incomplete bony demarcation: The antiprotrusio cage according to Burch-Schneider can be used to bridge even fairly extensive acetabular defects thanks to the flange, which is screwed onto the side of the iliac bone, and the distal tip, which is anchored in the ischium (Figs. 2.6, 3.10, 3.11). The stability of the whole assembly and the anchorage high on the iliac bone also allows the head centre to be shifted distally and the defect in the acetabular roof to be rectified with an autologous bone graft in such a way that the weight-bearing bone structure again consists of vital bone after the conclusion of remodelling. Caution is indicated when screwing in the antiprotrusio cage to avoid damaging the surrounding vessels and nerves (Fig. 13.10).

■ **Femoral Side: Cemented Revision.** The only options available in the beginning were cemented primary and long-stem prostheses (Fig. 2.9a,b). A cemented primary prosthesis is still used to this day in revision procedures on patients with a well-preserved bone stock. By contrast, cemented long-stem prostheses were envisaged for cases where the proximal anchorage of the implant was compromised by bone defects or shaft perforations that had arisen during cement removal [2].

Although we have not used cemented long-stem prostheses very often, these implants have, contrary to the expectations of many external studies, remained firmly in place in the long term without any loosening. We have therefore resumed their use by introducing the Virtec long-stem prosthesis. Of the various aspects that must be considered during the planning process (Fig. 3.12), the following are particularly important:

- Advantages: Since it is anchored in weight-bearing bone stock over a distance of at least 12 cm, immediate and stable weight-bearing is possible with a minimal subsequent bleeding tendency. If cementation of the fracture is omitted in proximal fractures then bone remodelling takes place, as with non-cemented bridging prostheses (Fig. 3.12h).
- Problems: If the prosthesis is longer than 225 mm, the intramedullary plug is located on the other side of the femoral isthmus (Fig. 3.12), with the consequent risk that the cement filling is unsatisfactory due to inadequate purchase or compactness of the plug. In this case a temporary transosseous fixation of the plug with a Kirschner wire is recommended (Figs. 3.12g,i). With extensive defects, the available long-stem prosthesis is occasionally too thin. In such cases M.E. Müller inserted a bent semi-tubular plate medially and laterally before applying the cement. The cement filling is then pressed through the plate screw holes at certain points by the subsequently inserted prosthe-

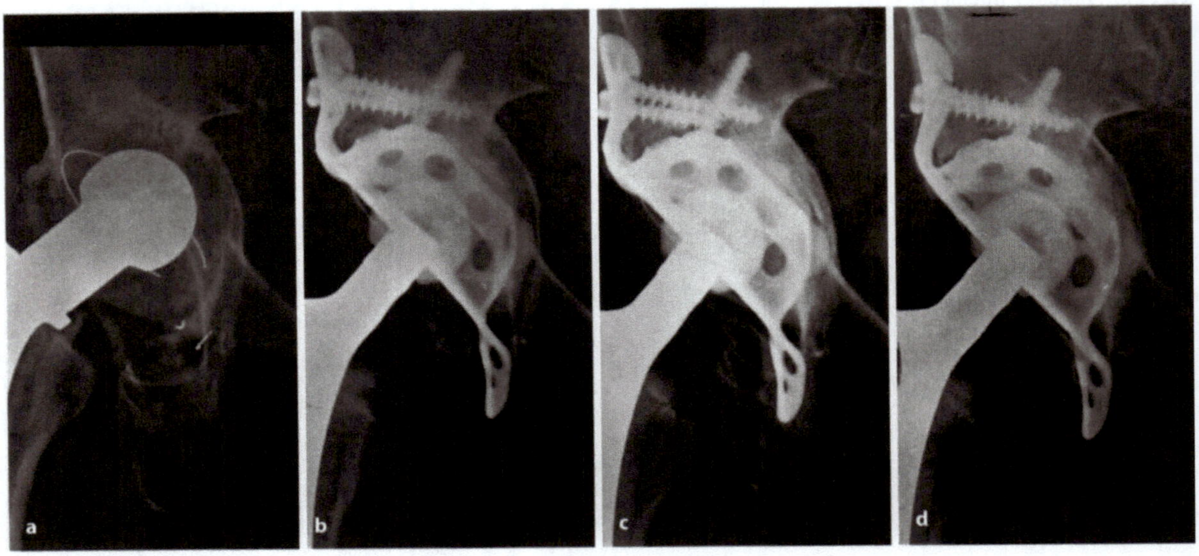

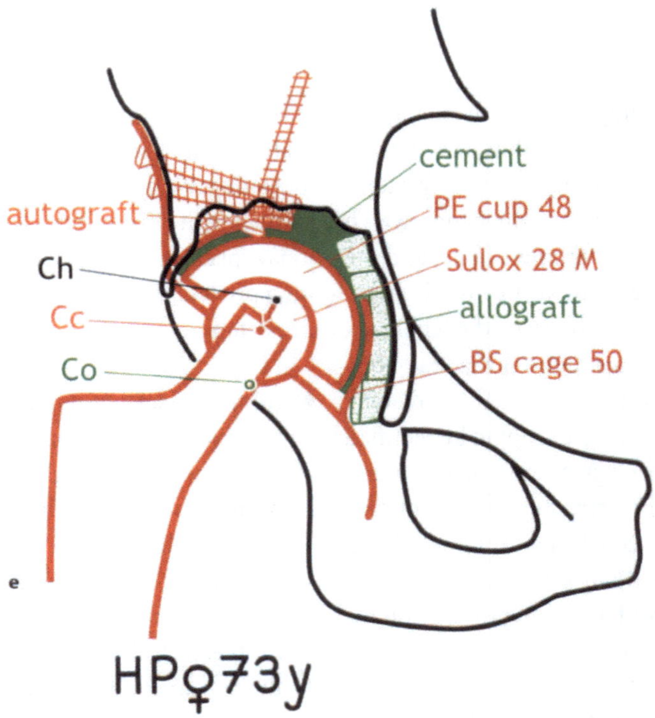

Fig. 3.11a–f. Acetabular management with a Burch-Schneider antiprotrusio cage. H.P., female, 73 years (0.5490)
a Substantial cup loosening and migration in the direction of the iliosacral joint
b Postoperative situation. Distinct, but not complete, distalisation of the cup centre. The antiprotrusio cage is shaped to match the local bone situation (see also Fig. 3.10). The remaining areas of subperiosteal bone are lined with bone grafts and do not come into direct contact with the bone cement. Mediocranially, a cement pillar supports the antiprotrusio cage and, together with the screw fixation, provides the primary stability
c Two years postoperatively, vigorous restructuring of the surrounding bone to produce secondary stability. Rather projecting bone formation around the medially placed bone grafts
d Five years postoperatively, largely balanced bone structure, no screw fracture
e Planning sketch: The preoperative head centre (*Ch*) has migrated distally (*Cc*), halfway toward the head centre copied from the opposite side (*Co*). The antiprotrusio cage is secured against migration to a subluxation position by the screws, which point in medial-distal-dorsal directions from the flange, and additionally against protrusion by the distal spur. The defects are filled cranially with autologous grafts and medially and distally with allogeneic grafts

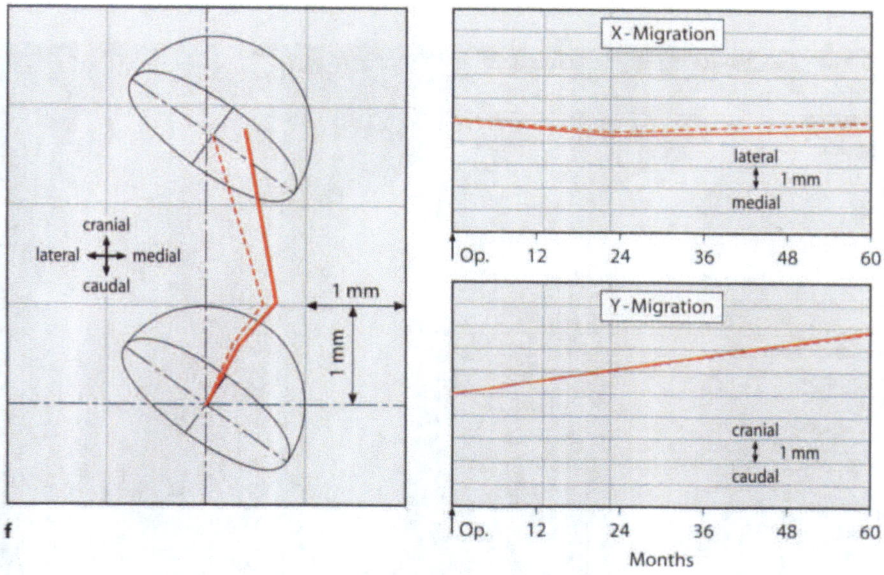

Fig. 3.11.
f EBRA migration analysis of the patient's cup over 4.8 years: The pseudo three-dimensional Simulgraph presentation shows a grid of squares, each side representing 1 mm in length. Overall, the cup centre (*red line*) migrates approx. 2.8 mm cranially and hardly at all medially. The degree of inclination and anteversion has remained almost constant. On four evaluable X-rays (*vertical lines* on the graphs on the *right*), significant, though hitherto very gradual and steady, migration in the cranial direction is apparent with no radiological evidence of loosening. This particular pattern very probably indicates reshaping of the acetabular bone stock under load. *Red dotted*: migration of the cup centre

sis, resulting in numerous point anchorages. Semi-tubular plates can also be inserted afterwards to effect deliberate positional corrections (Figs. 3.12g,h,i)

- Hazards: If cement manages to enter fracture clefts, bone remodelling will be incomplete in the long term since it has to bypass this cement (Fig. 7.1).

▪ **Femoral Side: Uncemented Revision.** The introduction in 1988 of the uncemented SL revision prosthesis according to Wagner opened up the possibility of bridging extensive defect zones [1]. This revision prosthesis is available in lengths ranging from 190 to 385 mm. Anchorage is based on a 2° taper which, if inserted with care, can also gain purchase distal to the femoral isthmus. The ideal anchorage length is approximately 8–10 cm. Given the antecurvation of the femur, longer anchorage lengths tend to be less protected against subsidence compared to shorter lengths (Fig. 3.13).

During the detailed planning (Fig. 3.14), the level of the femoral osteotomy is optimised so that, on the one hand, the cement and prosthesis can easily be removed and, on the other, the prosthesis can be anchored securely. If a prosthesis with a short neck is planned, lengthening up to an XL neck allows for possible compensation of up to 9 mm for offsetting any excessive subsidence of the prosthesis or any underestimated implant length.

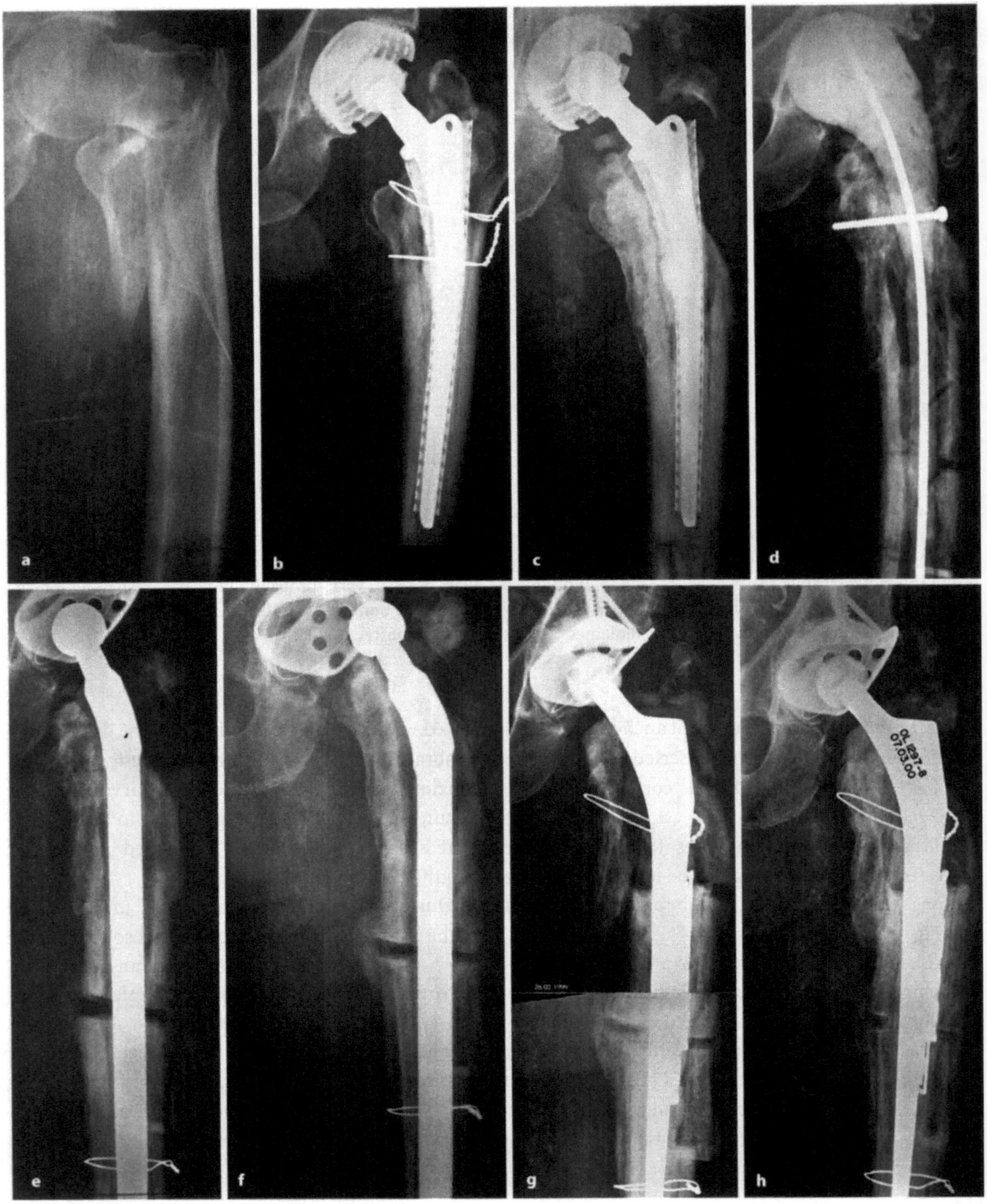

Fig. 3.12a–i. Plan for a partially cemented long-stem prosthesis to replace an uncemented prosthesis in a complex case of infection. E.H., male, 74 years (O.16710) blind, 190 cm, 107 kg

a Pertrochanteric fracture 3 years earlier

b Follow-up after 4 months. Dislocation shortly thereafter, hence the insertion of an XXL metal head. The patient underwent four revisions in a 2-year period because of infection. Although the prosthesis was not changed, the greater trochanter had to be sacrificed

c Situation prior to prosthesis removal. Two fistulas produced creamy pus (*Staph. aureus*)

d The cemented titanium funnel could only be removed by a very low-reaching lateral windowing procedure. Spacer (see also Chap. 5.5.2), irrigation-suction drainage, further drainage after 2 weeks following the accumulation of sterile fluid

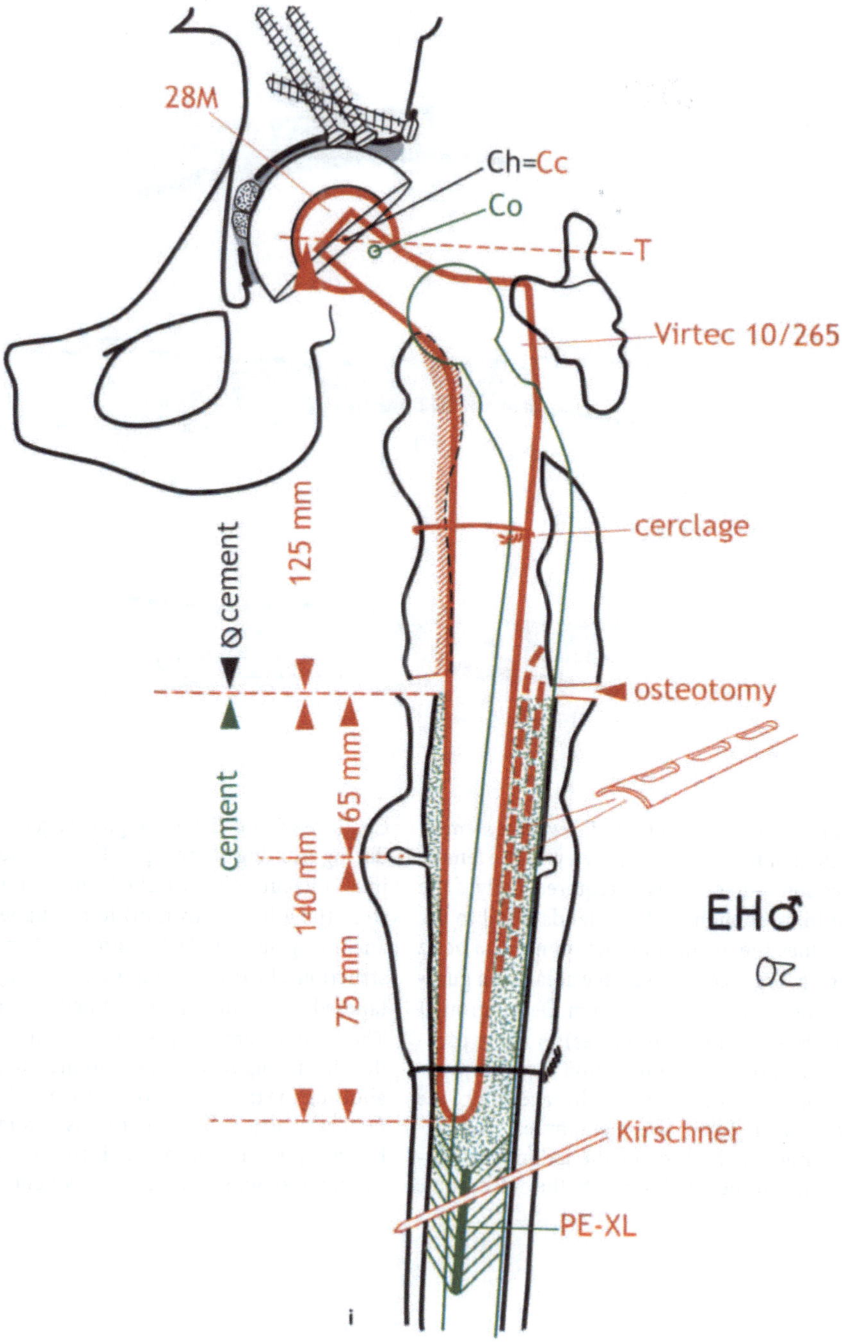

Fig. 3.12
e Reimplantation 4 weeks after prosthesis removal. Because a shorter implant was not thick enough, a longer one had to be selected (385/25), resulting in poor anchorage (Fig. 3.13)
f Prosthesis subsidence of 3.5 cm produced permanent internal dislocation. Revision necessary
g Cemented revision of the stem. The very rigid tissue prevented complete equalisation of leg lengths
h After 1 year, complete remodelling of the proximal femur is apparent all around the prosthesis. After 2 years, the patient was free of infection and able to walk with a stick, accompanied by his wife, for 2 h
i Plan for the cemented long-stem prosthesis: Osteotomy so as to create a 12- to 14-cm cemented anchoring section distally. The XL plug is secured against slippage distal to the femoral isthmus with a transcutaneous Kirschner wire. To ensure a slightly varus position, two semi-tubular plates are inserted laterally into the very wide medullary cavity

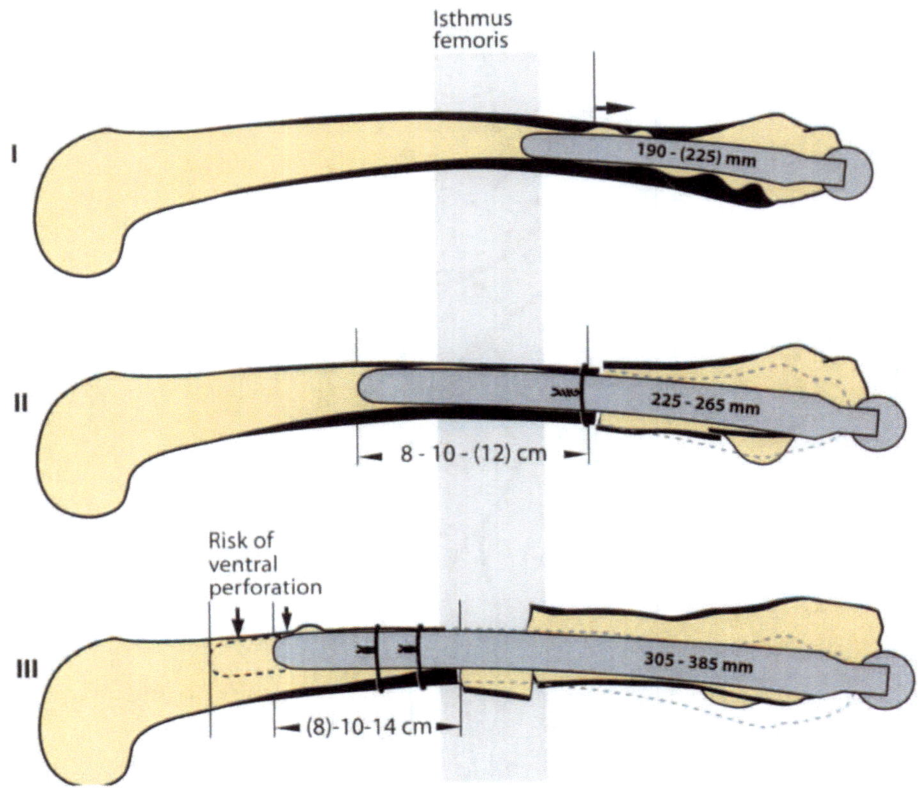

Fig. 3.13. Plan for the anchorage of an SL revision stem in relation to the extent of the defect, lateral view of the femur: An anchoring section 8–10 cm long is required. Only if the prosthesis is not thick enough or if it extends distal to the femoral isthmus does the anchoring section need to be 12 or 14 cm, although a larger contact surface area is not guaranteed in view of the femoral antecurvation. Defect group I (preserved bone sheath, thinned in places): A short prosthesis (190–225 mm) is selected for insertion from the proximal end without osteotomy and with anchorage before the isthmus. Defect group II (extensive metaphyseal destruction): With anchorage at the level of the isthmus, an osteotomy is performed immediately distal to the defect zone. Cerclage wiring distally to guard against fissures produced during reaming of the taper. This solution cancels the proximal antecurvation (dashed line), causing the prosthesis stem (length 225–265 mm) to be aligned parallel with the anchoring section. Defect group III (meta-diaphyseal destruction): Prosthesis lengths of 305–385 mm. In this case a tapered stem can only be reamed over a length of 3–4 cm. The double cerclage prevents any fissure from extending distally during reaming. Additional stability is provided by abutting the tip of the prosthesis distally against the ventral femoral cortical bone. If the osteotomy is too proximal, however, the tip will be inclined too steeply in relation to the cortical bone, with the consequent risk of perforation

Fig. 3.14a, b. Plan for an SL revision prosthesis (defect group II) B.J., female, 80 years (O.11131); see also Fig. 5.11
a Material removal: The proximal section of the femur has undergone substantial remodelling as a result of chronic infection. The osteotomy is planned distal to this section at the level of the medial fistula, the exact level being specified on the basis of measurements taken from the tip of the trochanter and the tip of the old prosthesis. The proximal section is split frontally for removal of the cement and prosthesis, see Sect. 3.7.1. The femur is secured distally with a double cerclage and the cement is then removed distally
b Prosthesis implantation: antiprotrusio cage plan as for Fig. 3.11. Stem planning: planning should be based on a short neck (28 S) since, if the stem subsides further than expected, the length underrun can subsequently be offset by up to 9 mm by selecting a longer neck. A 265-mm prosthesis is selected, since the cortical bone is also irregular distally. In the anchoring zone, the drawn prosthesis overlaps the cortical bone by about 1 mm on both sides. The estimated size is 18–21. With compensation of the preoperatively ascertained shortening, a taper is reamed distally over a length of 104 mm. During this reaming operation,

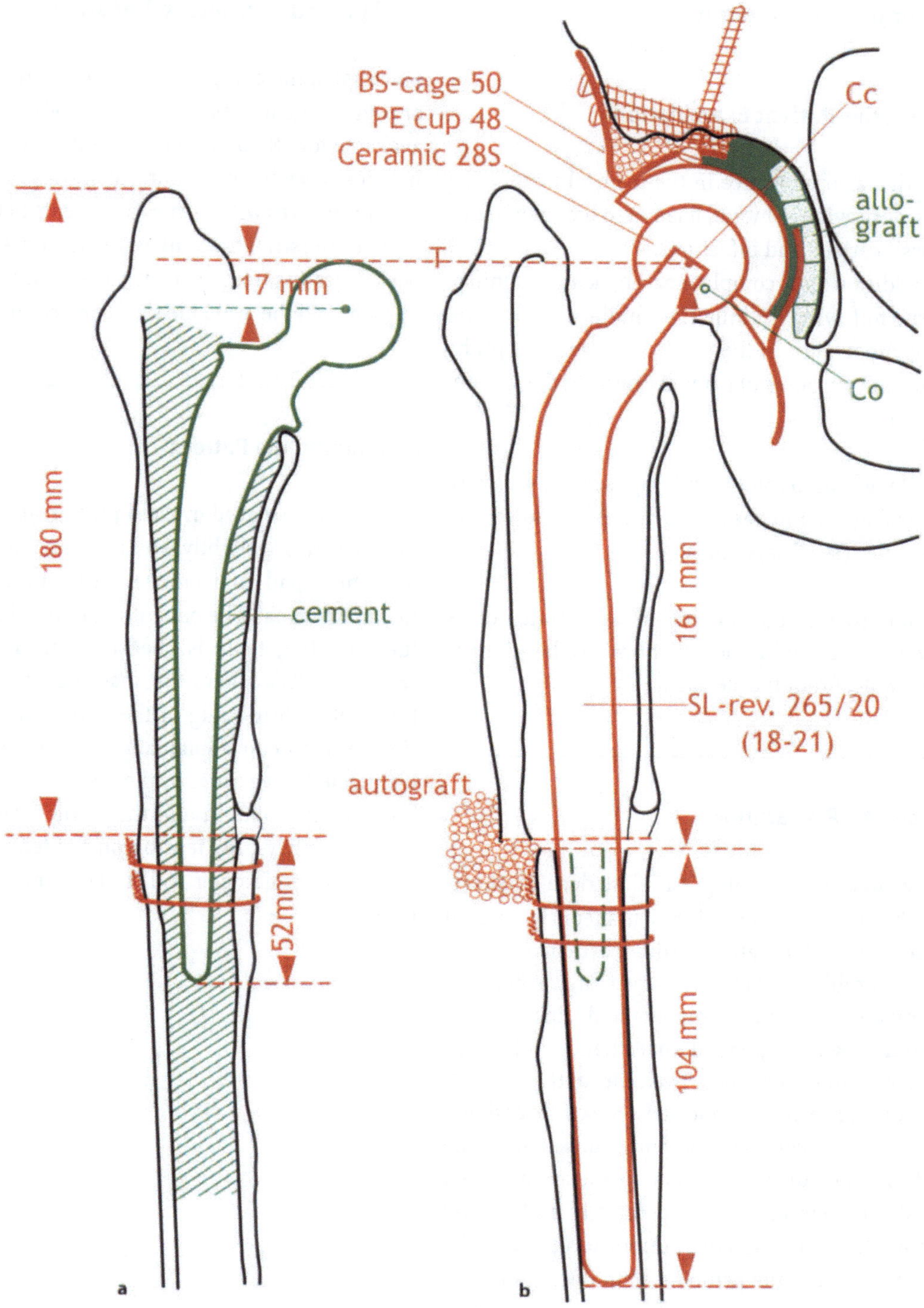

even the smaller reamers should only be advanced a few millimetres deeper, otherwise the taper will become distorted, thus reducing the contact surface area of the prosthesis. The gap produced in the lateral cortical bone at the level of the osteotomy should be filled with autologous bone material (e.g. using exostoses/ossifications comminuted in the bone mill, Fig. 3.20). Before the prosthesis is tapped into place, the impaction depth and points 5 and 10 mm cranial to this level are marked with a skin marker pen to prevent the prosthesis from being tapped in too deep. The antetorsion is adjusted to 10–15° or to a specific cup orientation

3.5 Preparing for the Operation

3.5.1 Preoperative Patient Examination

Of particular importance in the medical history are details of previous emboli, haemorrhages, periarticular ossifications and infections.

In addition to a complete orthopaedic examination, the following examination findings are of particular importance in the event of subsequent problems for the purposes of comparison with the 'before' situation:

- Leg length discrepancy, limping (see Chaps. 9, 10)
- Neurological and vascular status of the lower extremities (see Chaps. 11, 13)

To avoid any mix-ups, the hip to be operated on is marked, together with the patient, with a large cross, using a waterproof marker pen.

3.5.2 Anaesthetic Preparation

On the preceding evening, the first dose of short-chain heparins is injected subcutaneously. Special regimens exist for patients with particular blood-clotting problems. Generally-speaking, spinal or epidural anaesthesia is administered during primary procedures, while a general anaesthetic tends to be used in revision operations. Two units of the patient's own blood are usually collected on each occasion 3 and 2 weeks preoperatively. Since about 1990, the blood aspirated during revision operations has been washed and reinfused intraoperatively and during the immediate postoperative period. Additionally, the blood collected in the primary drain during the first four hours postoperatively is filtered and returned to the patient. During anaesthetic induction, 1 g Kefzol (cefazolin) is administered preoperatively as prophylaxis against infection. A second dose is administered 6 h later.

3.5.3 Implant and Instrument Preparation

Since 1984, the complete range of surgical implants and instruments designed by M.E. Müller has been available for all operations. We restrict the cups kept in stock (acetabular reinforcement ring, uncemented SL cup) to sizes with 4-mm increments between each size. For the straight stems we restrict ourselves to the basic sizes (7.5, 10, 12.5, 15, 17.5 and 20). For all other implants, all the available sizes are kept in stock.

3.5.4 Positioning the Patient

The patient is placed in the supine position. The buttocks are raised slightly with a 3- to 4-cm thick towel or a firm pad to facilitate access to the femoral medullary canal. The patient's horizontal position on the operating table is checked with a spirit level (Fig. 3.15). This allows the anaesthetist to check the horizontal positioning of the patient during operation prior to cup implantation. The surgical field is disinfected three times by the operator using an alcoholic iodine solution and the sterile drapes are applied. To relieve any tension on the femoral nerve a 10- to 15-cm diameter roll is placed under the knee (Fig. 3.16).

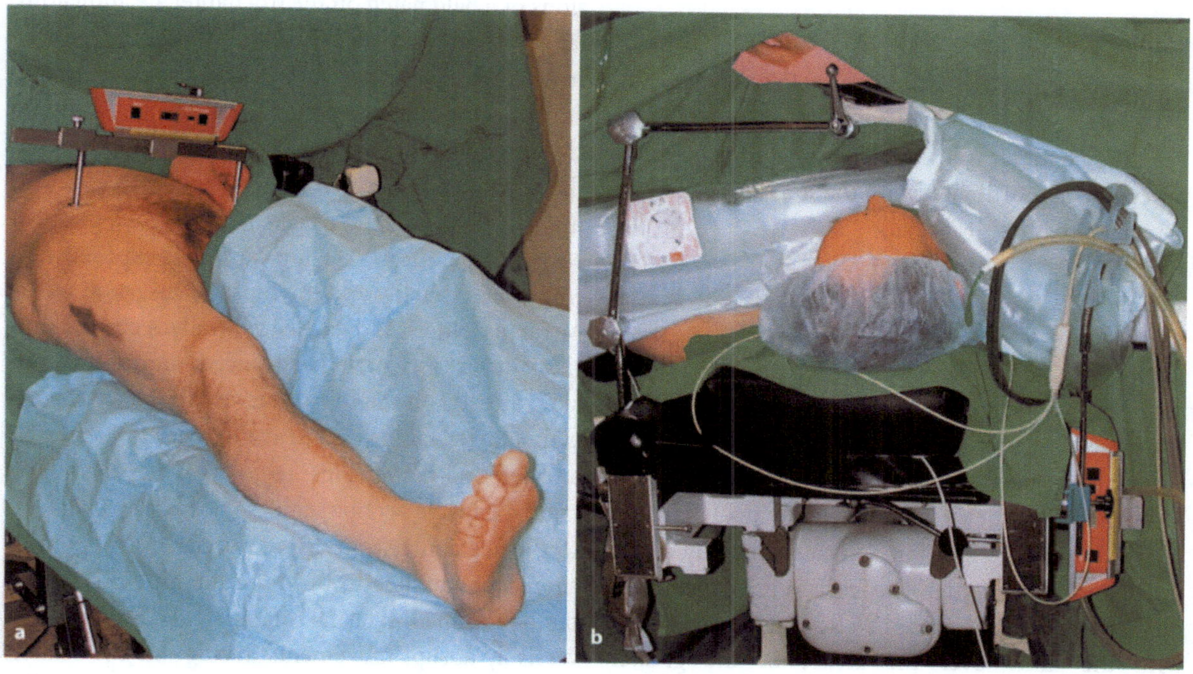

Fig. 3.15a, b. Positioning the patient with the spirit level. **a** The two ant. sup. iliac spines are linked by a metal bracket fitted with the spirit level and adjusted horizontally **b** After the patient is draped, the spirit level is mounted at right angles to the operating table next to the anaesthetist, so that the latter can adjust the table, and thus the patient, horizontally prior to cup implantation

Fig. 3.16. A roll placed under the knee should help relieve any tension on the femoral nerve, and thus reduce the risk of overstretching. For the same reason, the lever ventral to the acetabulum requires careful placement (Fig. 11.5)

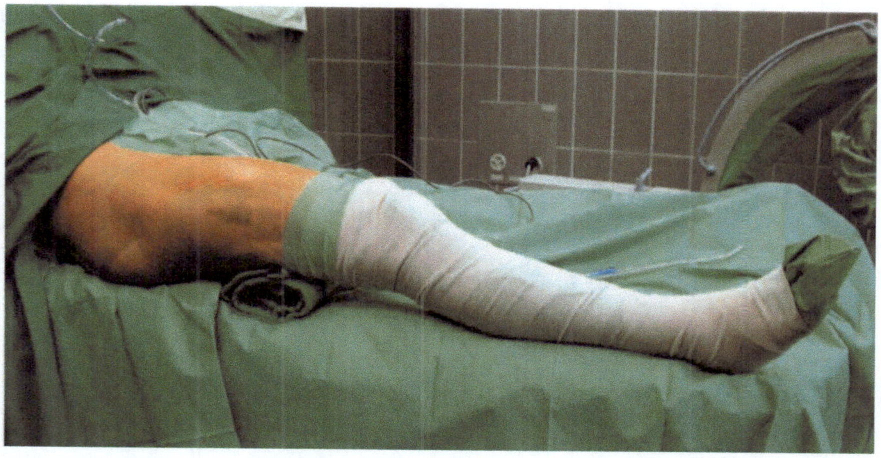

3.6 Operation Procedure for Primary Prostheses

For the sake of clearer understanding, the operation procedure is coordinated with the standard plan for a primary prosthesis (Fig. 3.6).

3.6.1 Approach

A straight skin incision is made over the centre of the greater trochanter. With an overall length of 15–25 cm – depending on the weight of the individual patient – the middle of the incision is located roughly above the tip of the trochanter. The fascia is divided and the greater trochanter exposed. Following a vertical cut with the knife over the centre of the greater trochanter, a sharply ground, curved chisel (Fig. 3.17a) is used to detach the ventral portions of M. gluteus medius and M. vastus lateralis and the whole of M. gluteus minimus ventrally from the trochanter. The aponeurosis that connects the muscles is preserved. The electric knife that we initially used for this detachment procedure is now no longer used following the observation during some revisions of a bald patch on the trochanter, i.e. indicating failed integration of the muscle with the greater trochanter. The small bone flakes raised by the curved chisel facilitate secure integration of the muscles. Any new osteophytes projecting ventrally from the trochanter (Fig. 7.2b) hardly have any effect on hip mobility, but can be used as autologous grafts in revision operations. The hip capsule is exposed ventrally and cranially and the capsular insertion of the M. rectus femoris is detached ventrally. A curved soft-tissue lever (Fig. 3.17f) is advanced, under direct vision, directly on the capsule across to the ventral acetabular rim, taking care to avoid injury to the vessels and femoral nerve (Figs. 11.5, 13.1). The ventral and cranial capsule sections and any osteophytes lateral to the acetabular roof are removed. At this point it should be possible to dislocate the hip with gentle, but determined, external rotation and adduction. Excessively abrupt movements during this dislocation can traumatise the knee. If excessive resistance to dislocation is met, the craniolateral osteophytes are removed more completely or else the femoral neck osteotomy is performed prior to dislocation. The soft-tissue fold linking the lesser trochanter to the femoral head dorsomedially is resected. While the lower leg is held horizontally by an assistant, we divide the femoral neck using an oscillating saw at the

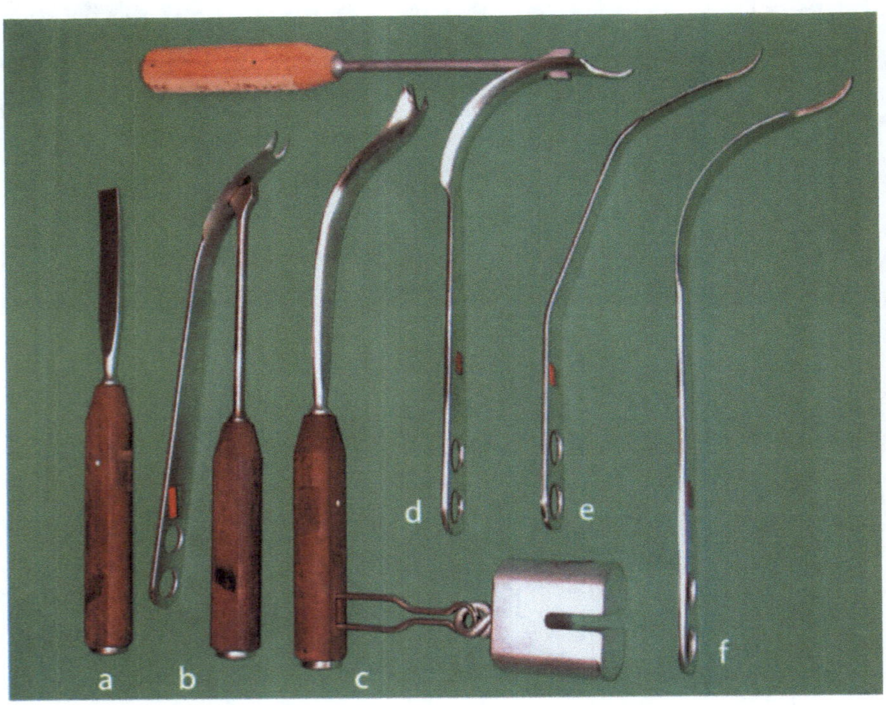

Fig. 3.17a–f. Selection of the most important instruments for exposing the acetabulum
a Sharply ground curved chisel. The length allows frequent regrinding
b Double-tipped soft tissue lever with driving hole and impactor
c Femoral lever with weight bracket and weight
d Lever with driving hole and impactor
e Double-angled bone lever
f Curved, long, soft tissue lever

planned level above the lesser trochanter (operation planning – Fig. 3.6f). To avoid division of the dorsolateral tip of the trochanter, particularly with varus hips, we start the osteotomy at the calcar on the medial side. The osteotomy is then carefully extended laterally until a fine movement in the gap indicates that the division of the femoral neck is complete. The head can now be grasped with forceps and any residual connections to soft tissues removed. The surgeon now has free access to the acetabulum and femoral shaft.

3.6.2 Cup Implantation

■ **Exposing the Acetabulum.** The curved bone lever (Fig. 3.17f) is again advanced over the ventral acetabular rim (Fig. 3.18a). Using scissors or a knife, the surgeon frees the hip capsule from the dorsal osteophytes until the base of the ischium is visible. The medial tip of the femoral lever (Fig. 3.17c) is tapped into the ischium using the hammer, the weight is attached and the lever is secured to the thigh with a small towel and clip (Fig. 3.18b). The limbus residues are separated cleanly from the acetabular rim. An elevator is used to push the soft tissues away from the acetabulum laterally and cranially. To produce self-retaining retraction, the lever with driving hole (Fig. 3.17d) is tapped into the exposed bone surface (Fig. 3.18c) using a broad-tipped impactor and secured to the drape with a towel clip.

■ **Preparation of the Acetabular Bed.** The curved chisel (Fig. 3.17a) is used to level the osteophytes along the acetabular rim and in the base of the acetabulum (Fig. 3.18, detail). A serrated, sharp curette is then used to remove the soft tissues from the acetabular fossa and scrape out any cartilage still remaining in the acetabulum. The acetabulum is widened spherically using increasingly larger acetabular reamers. During this operation, the head centre is generally shifted medially, dorsally and slightly distally in accordance with the surgical plan (Fig. 3.6b,c,e). Particularly if craniolateral defects of the acetabulum are present, the acetabular hollow is reamed so that the medial outline is directly over Köhler's radiographic teardrop (Fig. 3.6e). The operator should ensure that as much of the subchondral sclerosis zone as possible is preserved cranially (Fig. 3.1). Subchondral cysts are carefully curetted out and the resulting cavity is filled with autologous bone from the femoral head.

■ **Cup Placement.** A basic requirement for all cups is that the sliding component of the implant should maintain a precisely adjusted anteversion of 14–18°

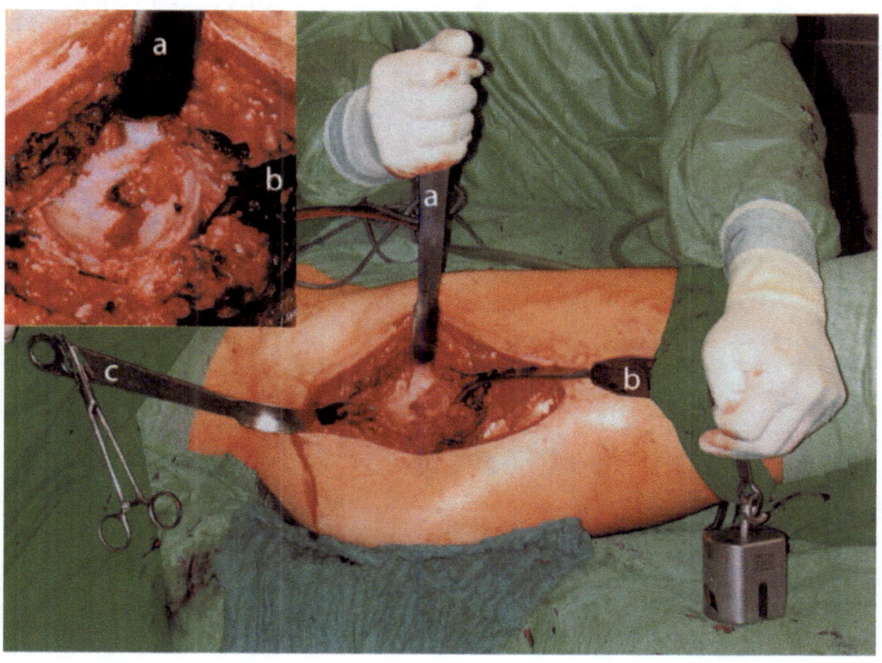

Fig. 3.18a–c. Standard exposure of the acetabulum with the
a curved soft tissue lever placed ventrally. The lever is advanced by finger over the ventral acetabular rim
b Weighted lever dorsomedially. Following removal of the dorsal osteophyte with the medial tip, this lever is tapped into the ischium. With the weight and securing towel, this acts as a self-retaining retractor
c Acetabular roof lever cranially. This lever is tapped into the iliac bone laterally with the impactor. Secured to the towel, this also acts as a self-retaining retractor

and an inclination of 35–40°. The other cup components, the surrounding bone stock and any cement projections must not restrict the range of motion permitted by the sliding component, otherwise impingement or even dislocation may be the result (Chap. 6). Before the trial prosthesis is implanted, and at the behest of the surgeon, the operating table is adjusted horizontally by the anaesthetist with the aid of the spirit level (Fig. 3.15b).

■ **Implantation of the Uncemented SL Cup** (see also Figs. 2.6, 3.1c). The trial cup is screwed onto the cup inserter with aiming device (Fig. 3.19) in line with the acetabular opening angle. The cup is first tapped in a medial direction by the assistant using the pointed impactor until it makes contact with the medial acetabular wall and then knocked into the definitive position in a cranial-medial direction by the operator. The alignment guide allows the cup orientation to be checked constantly during impaction (Fig. 3.19). If the SL cup is to be inserted, the centres of the future screw projections are marked with the drill so that, after the trial implant is removed, these points can be widened with a round burr. Bone from the femoral head that has been finely milled in the bone mill (Fig. 3.20) is inserted into the residual fossa, scraped out acetabular roof cysts and any remaining lateral acetabular defect. The definitive implant is then knocked firmly into place according to the procedure used for the trial cup (Fig. 3.19).

▸ *Screw fixation of the cup:* The holes used for screw fixation of the SL cup are positioned so as to avoid, insofar as possible, any likelihood of injury to vessels and nerves. A few basic principles can usefully be observed during screw fixation in order to prevent injuries (see also Sect. 13.4.2, Figs. 13.3, 13.7). In order to spare the adjacent structures it is advisable to drill the screw holes in the direction of the centre of the iliosacral joint (Fig. 3.1, 3.2). Drilling in stages has proved effective, since it allows the surgeon to identify any perforation of the bone surface before injury is caused to an adjacent structure (vessels, nerves) (Fig. 3.21). The central screw is tightened first in order to pull the implant centrally into the acetabular hollow.

▸ *Placement of the cup insert:* The implant rim is cleared of soft tissues around its full circumference using bone levers. The double-tipped bone lever is particularly suitable for the medial side (Fig. 3.17b). The cavity is irrigated and a special instrument is used to check that no screw head is projecting. The cup insert is loosely clicked into place in the SL shell using the inserter and then hammered home with a firm blow. The connection between the cup and insert should be visibly regular over its full circumference. As the polyethylene warms to body temperature, it expands to lock firmly in place.

■ **Acetabular Reinforcement Ring** (Fig. 3.1.d, Sect. 3.3.1). The number of the acetabular reinforcement ring to be selected is 2–4 mm smaller than the diam-

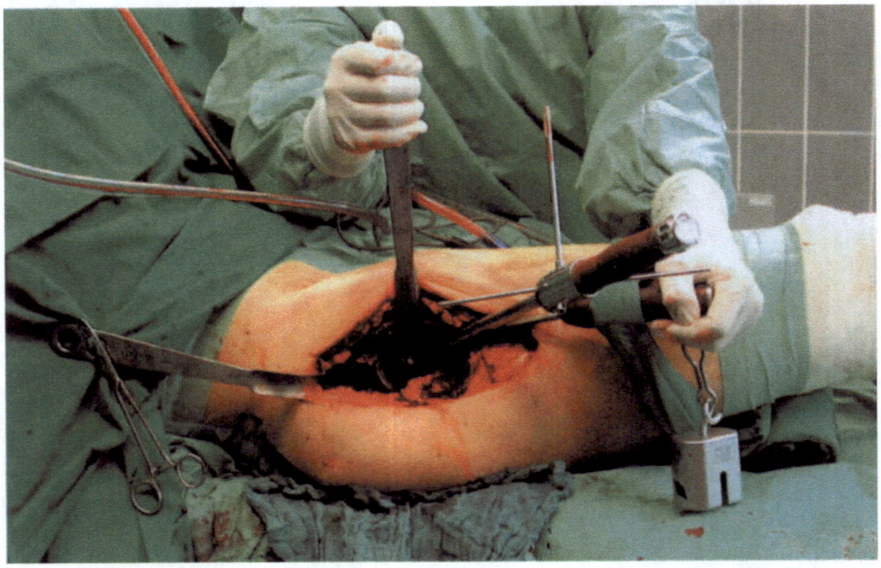

Fig. 3.19. The cup is inserted using the alignment instruments such that the horizontal arm of the alignment rod is parallel to the body's longitudinal axis while the vertical arm is perpendicular to the ground. The cup is normally implanted with an inclination of 35–40° and an anteversion of 14–18°

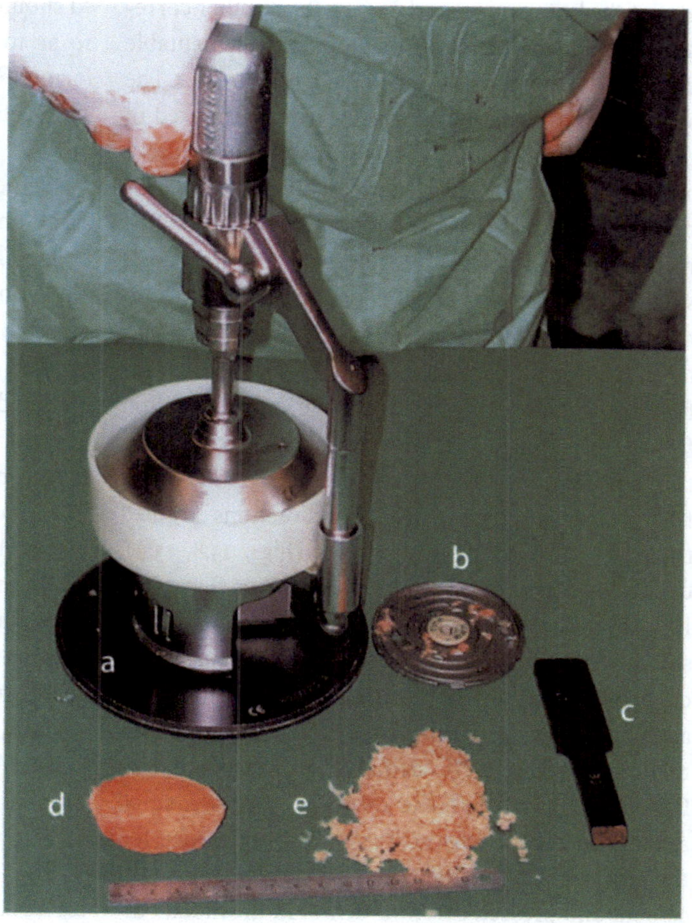

Fig. 3.20a–d. Bone mill for producing fine bone chips from autologous bone material. The drill available at the operating table is used to drive the mill
a The milled bone collects in a bone chip container
b Various cutting blades can be used to mill chips of differing coarseness, which are then picked up from the bone chip container using
c a spatula
d The section of femoral head produces
e the quantity of milled material shown here

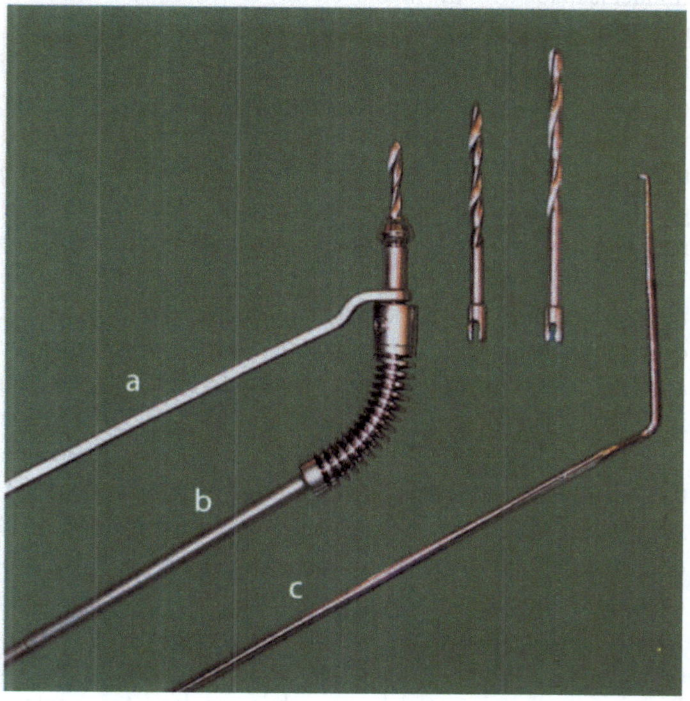

Fig. 3.21. Drill sleeve
a and drill shaft
b with three different sizes of short drill bits 40, 50 and 65 mm in length. If the drill is used first with, then without the drill sleeve, the maximum extension of the drilled hole for each step is 10–15 mm
c Angled screw measuring device

eter of the last reamer used. In fact, the number corresponds with the diameter of the largest cementable cup, while the external diameter is 4 mm greater. The selected acetabular reinforcement ring is knocked in the medial and proximal direction using a trial cup or a broad-tipped impactor/extractor until it is located directly over Köhler's radiographic teardrop on the medial side and against the bone stock on the cranial side. If a good wedge effect is present, the ring is removed, the remaining cavities are filled with bone material from the femoral head and the acetabular reinforcement ring is reinserted. The screw fixation follows the same procedure used for the SL cup. Here, too, it is vital that the first screw is placed in the central hole. Since screwing in certain directions can lead to injury of arteries and nerves (Figs. 13.8, 13.9), drilling in stages is particularly important (Fig. 3.21). If the bone stock is severely osteoporotic, it may occasionally be necessary to advance the screw tips to the cortical bone on the opposite side in order to obtain adequate screw purchase. After the horizontal alignment of the table is checked and the acetabular reinforcement ring dried, the operator inserts a small amount of high-viscosity cement. Using the inserter, the cup is placed in the correct position on the soft cement and pressed downward, first in the medial direction with the broad-tipped impactor until direct contact is made with the medial outline of the acetabular reinforcement ring. Only now is the cup pressed into the correct inclination and anteversion, where it engages with the projecting screw heads, which prevent any further positional correction. Cement protruding from the sides of the cup is pressed into the gap between the cup and acetabular reinforcement ring and any excess cement is completely removed. When the cement has hardened, any remaining cement projections are knocked off and the acetabular cavity is wiped out with a swab on a stick to wipe away any fine cement lamellae that may have entered. This is followed by irrigation.

■ **Cemented Polyethylene Cup** (Fig. 3.1b, Chap. 3.3.1). A short, self-limiting 6-mm drill is used to drill anchoring holes along the rim of the acetabulum. The cancellous bone in these holes is compressed using a tamp 5 mm in diameter. The operator must, at all costs, avoid drilling through to the lesser pelvis. Pressing cement into the lesser pelvis can lead to blood vessel injuries (Fig. 13.5). The cup to be selected should have approximately 2 mm of play all round so as to ensure that a certain cement thickness is formed. We use high-viscosity cement (e.g. Palacos). The acetabulum is irrigated with a strong, narrow jet of fluid, the cavity is dried with swabs on sticks and the cement is immediately inserted into the cavity as a ball and pressed down into the various anchoring holes. The table is aligned with the horizontal and any blood on the cement is swabbed away. The cup is placed on the cement using the alignment guide, and pressed down with the broad-tipped impactor in the medial direction until it abuts against the medial wall of the acetabulum, whereupon the cup is pressed, applying moderate pressure, in the cranial direction. The operator must ensure that the inclination (35–40°) and anteversion (14–18°) are adjusted correctly and that, craniolaterally, a sufficiently thick layer of cement of 2–4 mm remains in place. The protruding cement is wiped off and removed with a sharp curette. When the cement has hardened, any remaining cement projections are removed with the chisel. The acetabular cavity is wiped out with a swab on a stick to wipe away any flat-rolled fine cement layer. Irrigation.

3.6.3 Stem Implantation

■ **Ventilation Hole.** Studies suggest that fat emboli can form as a result of excessive pressure in the femoral canal during rasping, cement compaction and subsequent pressing down of the prosthesis [6]. In 1998, we initiated the practice of drilling a hole into the femoral canal percutaneously, using a 3.5-mm drill, approximately 4 cm distal to the planned location of the stem tip. This measure allows fat and air to escape into the soft tissues during rasping and cementing. To ascertain the level of this hole, the trial prosthesis of the planned size is held next to the proximal femur. A serrated drill sleeve with trocar is advanced through an incision 4 cm distal to the prosthesis tip until it abuts against the femoral shaft. The leg is protected against rotational movements by an assistant. Since the special drill is just 1 cm longer than the corresponding tissue protection sleeve, the hole cannot be drilled deeper than 1 cm. This prevents any tangential drilling along the edge of the canal and through the whole shaft.

■ **Shaft Adjustment.** The leg is turned outward and held horizontally from the other side by the assistant. Tension must be applied to the leg very carefully, particularly in patients with osteoporosis, obesity, coxa vara and powerfully developed muscles, in order to avoid trochanteric fractures (see also Sect. 8.4.2, Fig. 8.6). A double-tipped soft tissue lever (Fig. 3.17b) or femoral lever (Fig. 3.17c) is inserted between the muscle insertion of the abductors and the greater trochanter, while the abductors are held dorso-laterally away from the femoral entrance. The distance between the upper edge of the lesser trochanter and the neck osteotomy is checked with the ruler and any further resection performed. The dorsolateral base of the calcar cortex is removed with Lüer's bone forceps.

■ **Preparation of the Femoral Shaft.** Using an osteotome 1.5–2 cm in width, the operator prepares a slit, roughly 5 mm wide and with antetorsion of approximately 15°, proceeding in the dorsolateral to medioventral direction. This slit is extended downwards, towards the knee, using a sharp curette whose opening faces medially.

N.B.: If the operator fails to hold the curette exactly parallel to the femoral shaft at all times, there is a considerable risk of perforation of the shaft dorsolaterally, particularly in muscular patients with pronounced coxa vara. This can lead to a dangerously incorrect implantation of the femoral component in this direction. Whereas modular rasps were not available during the first phase of our review period, from 1991 onward, at first only occasionally but subsequently in every case, we used a motorised drive for the rasps. Starting with the smallest hammer rasp, the medullary cavity is gradually extended until the last rasp fits tightly. Fissure formation in the medial calcar area during rasping is a dangerous complication – particularly with cemented stems – and must be secured by cerclage wiring to guard against penetration of the cement in the fissure (Figs. 7.1, 7.2, 7.6). A sharply tapering or very narrow medullary cavity can lead to splitting of the shaft lower down, which only becomes apparent either on the postoperative radiograph (Fig. 7.10), or when a fracture occurs (Fig. 7.4). With cemented prostheses, any shaft fissures must be secured with cerclage wiring at operation before the stem is cemented in place (see also Sect. 7.5.1). The detachable rasp handle of the modular rasp is removed and the distance between the osteotomy and the edge of the cone is measured (Fig. 3.6f). If the measurement does not correspond with the drawing, the operator can either continue rasping deeper or select a smaller or larger prosthesis, as appropriate. When the desired depth is reached, the planned trial head is fitted and, after irrigation of the cup, a trial reduction is performed. To test for any dislocation tendency, the stability of the hip is checked by internal rotation of the hip in flexion (dislocation tendency dorsally?) and by adduction and external rotation of the hip in extension (dislocation tendency ventrolaterally?) (see also Chap. 6).

■ **Placement of the Intramedullary Plug.** Measuring rods are used to determine the diameter of the required intramedullary plug (Fig. 3.22c). The intramedullary plug should be placed approximately 0.5 cm distal to the tip of the femoral component (Fig. 3.6f). With primary prostheses, we fashion the plug from a piece of the femoral neck (Fig. 3.22). For easier insertion, the thicker side of the plug is given a slight oval shape using the bone forceps. With the thinner side facing forward, the plug is introduced into the femoral shaft and tapped down to the precisely desired depth using the graduated measuring rod and hammer. The trial prosthesis is loosely reinserted to check that no splintered fragments of the plug are blocking the medullary cavity. This plug costs nothing, is quickly prepared and placed and, after it has fulfilled its purpose, is almost completely resorbed because of the lack of mechanical loading (Fig. 3.4d,e). In contrast to polyethylene plugs – the bone plug will not become an obstacle in any subsequent revision procedure.

■ **Cementing the Femoral Component.** Throughout the period under review, we used a low-viscosity bone cement (Sulfix), which we pressed into the cavity from the proximal end, with ventilation via a plastic tube, using a manually operated syringe or gun. As a result of the experience acquired during Swedish studies [12], we changed over, in 1998, to the traditional Palacos bone cement with retrograde filling from a manually operated gun (Fig. 3.23).

Using copious quantities of Ringer's solution with Lavasept and a syringe with a long irrigation tube and a fine, angled metal nozzle, the operator washes out the fat from the medullary cavity and the cancellous trabeculae. The cement is now inserted in a ret-

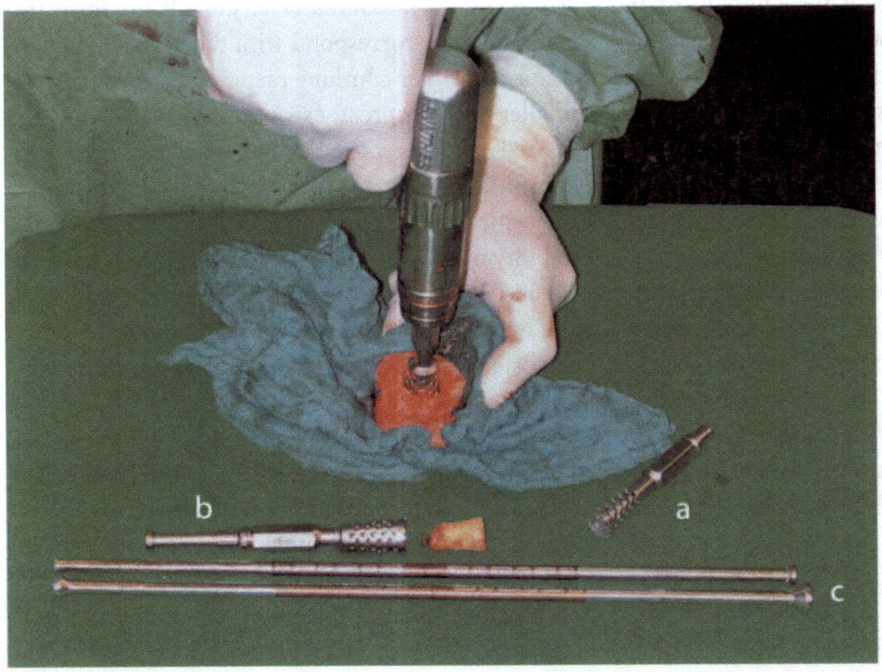

Fig. 3.22a–c. Preparation of intramedullary plugs from the removed femoral neck: An approximately 2-cm thick piece is sawn from the femoral neck fragment and placed on a tightly packed gauze pad with the end with the denser bone structure face down. The neck fragment is held securely with the hand, which is protected by the pad
a Depending on the measuring rods/tamps for intramedullary plugs (**c**), a choice of three sizes of conical reamer is available for reaming the tapered plug. The plug is ejected from the reamer with an ejector cylinder (**b**)

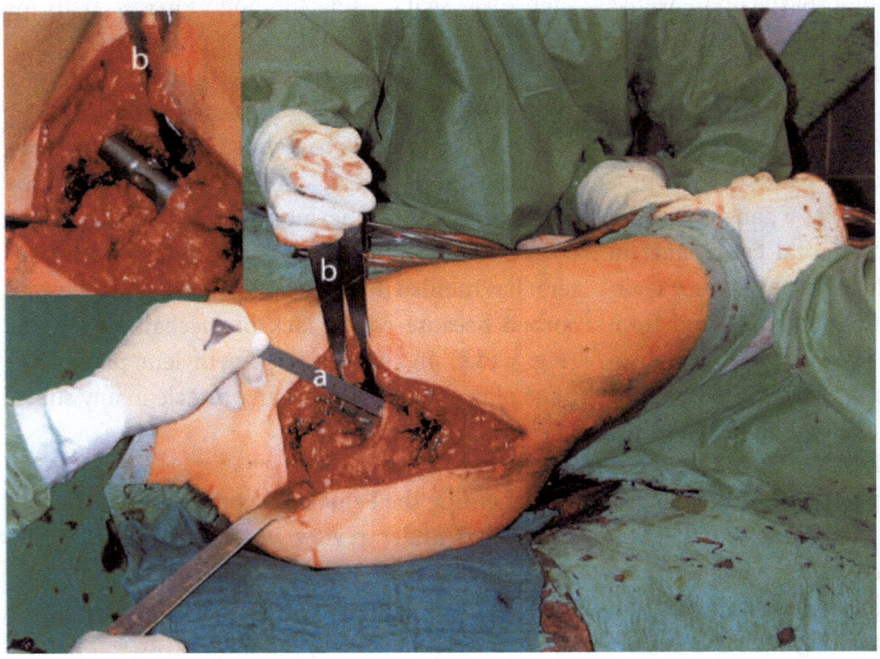

Fig. 3.23a, b. During cementing of the stem, the lower leg is held horizontally by the assistant and the stem entrance retracted laterally with a pointed lever (**b**). The ruler (**a**) is used to check the distance between the osteotomy and the edge of the cone. Looking from the dorsal side, the detailed view shows the retraction of the muscles away from the neck of the prosthesis by the pointed lever (**b**), which is designed to prevent twisting between the prosthesis and cement and consequent cracking

rograde manner with the gun. While maintaining an antetorsion of 10–15°, the selected prosthesis is advanced, first by hand and then with the impactor, and with simultaneous checking with a ruler (Fig. 3.23), until the distance between the edge of the cone and the femoral neck osteotomy matches that determined during planning (Fig. 3.6f). The excess cement is wiped off with a sharp curette, while the cement remaining in the shaft is pressed firmly against the prosthesis. The prosthesis is held in its correct position until the cement has hardened. The lower leg must be kept horizontal during this period (Fig. 3.23).

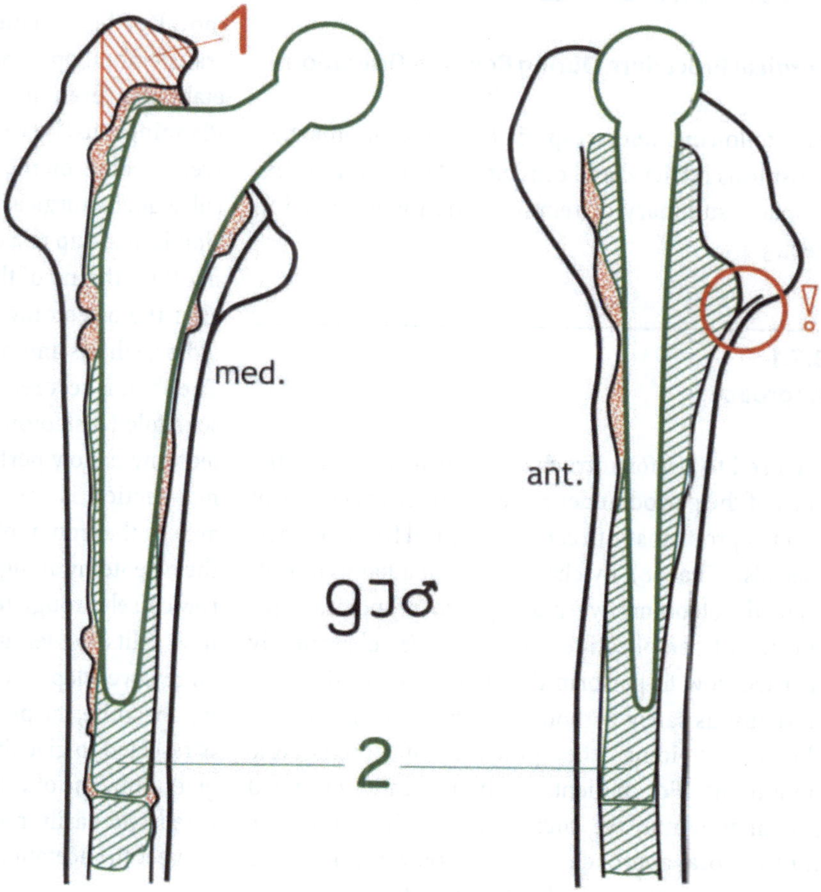

Fig. 3.24. Preparatory sketch for cement removal. The SL straight-stem prosthesis is loosened particularly at the proximal end, but has not undergone subsidence. Since the diaphyseal bone has hardly thinned at all, the transgluteal approach is to be used for the cemented revision. To enable the surgeon to remove the cement under direct vision, the canal in the greater trochanter is widened dorsolaterally using a gouge (1). The loose cement (2) is broken shortly above the firmly seated tip. During cement removal it is important to note that the cement is very thick proximally and dorsal to the prosthesis. There is a risk of perforation dorsally below the lesser trochanter (!). The ventral portion of cement becomes increasingly thicker distally near the tip of the prosthesis

A pointed lever inserted dorsal to the neck osteotomy should prevent the exertion of lateral pressure on the neck of the prosthesis (Fig. 3.23, detail). If the prosthesis is secure, the cup and cone are irrigated. A trial reduction is performed with the trial head of the desired length. The presence of any dislocation tendency is rechecked. Before the definitive head is fitted, the cone must be rinsed clean with meticulous care, particularly if ceramic heads are used. In extreme cases, substance residues can cause a ceramic head to fracture at a later date. If metal heads are used, particularly if these are paired with polyethylene, the operator must ensure that no scratches form on the articulating side, since these can result in increased wear in the long term.

■ **Marking the Greater Trochanter with Tantalum Balls.** Special measuring programs, such as Lund's RSA method or the PFA method developed by the Innsbruck group, can be used for more precise monitoring of stem subsidence. A very simple measuring method involves marking the greater trochanter at the level of, and in the same plane as, the prosthesis shoulder with one to three tantalum balls. Because the two parts to be compared are directly adjacent, this type of measurement is fairly position independent and provides a useful direct reading (Fig. 3.7).

3.6.4 Wound Closure

Following insertion of an intra-articular Redon drain, the ventral detached portion of M. gluteus medius and M. vastus lateralis are firmly sutured to the dorsal muscles connected with the greater trochanter using absorbable sutures. An additional suture is placed distal to the greater trochanter. The wound is closed in layers with subfascial and epifascial drains. A spica bandage, left in place for 2 days, should help minimise haematoma formation. Heel protection is provided for the first few days, particularly for elderly patients, to counter the excess loading.

3.7 Surgical Procedure During Revision Operations

The following refers especially to the approaches, prosthesis retrieval and cement removal, while an exemplary summary of reimplantation is provided in Sect. 3.4.5.

3.7.1 Approach

We used to perform trochanteric osteotomies at the start of the period under review, primarily because of fears of problems with cement removal from the shaft (see also Chap. 8). By changing from a flat to a roof-shaped osteotomy we managed to reduce the frequency of complications (Fig. 8.1). We subsequently learned how to perform the cement removal procedure just as safely without a trochanteric osteotomy, thereby avoiding the problem of trochanteric nonunions. For patients with a greatly modified proximal femur, we increasingly switched to the transfemoral approach from 1989 onward, since this results in better muscular control of the proximal femoral fragments (Fig. 8.2) and only rarely leads to nonunions (Fig. 6.2). The operator should plan carefully before the start of the operation to determine which type of prosthesis retrieval and cement removal is most appropriate (Figs. 3.14, 3.24).

■ **Transgluteal Approach.** The transgluteal approach is suitable primarily for cases involving a simple cup change or, if the bone stock of the proximal femur is good, planned provision with a standard prosthesis or a short SL revision prosthesis. Following transgluteal exposure of the greater trochanter, the pseudocapsule of the hip is removed, with gradually increasing adduction and external rotation of the leg, first ventrally, then laterally, medially and dorsally. The hip can now be dislocated and the stability of the shaft checked. Next, the acetabulum is adjusted as for primary prostheses (Fig. 3.18). If the acetabulum is strongly cranialised (Fig. 3.11a), a useful measure is to locate, early on, the lower edge of Köhler's radiographic teardrop and to adjust the acetabulum with the double-angled bone lever (Fig. 3.17e).

■ **Transfemoral Approach.** In addition to rapid removal of bone cement from the femoral shaft, the transfemoral approach offers a good view of the acetabulum, even in the presence of major defects. Planning must be very precise, otherwise reliable reference points on the femur will be lacking during the subsequent surgical procedure (Fig. 3.14d). An incision is made up to 4 cm distal to the planned osteotomy. With the aid of the image converter, the exact level of the osteotomy is measured from the tip of the old prosthesis and marked on the shaft with a chisel. The shaft is secured with cerclage wiring distal to the scheduled osteotomy. A transverse or oblique osteotomy is now performed on the femur. The proximal section is then osteotomied in the trochanter area in the frontal plane proceeding distally down to the osteotomy along the linea aspera. Inserting a narrow chisel through the M. vastus lateralis, the surgeon now splits the femur on the ventromedial aspect. A large cover flap can now be opened up ventrally. Using the knife, the pseudo-capsule of the artificial joint is resected to give the surgeon an overview of the acetabulum. The old stem component can now be dislocated and easily retrieved, allowing the operator to inspect the acetabulum and shaft.

3.7.2 Prosthesis Retrieval

■ **Acetabular Component.** After adjustment with the standard levers (Figs. 3.17, 3.18), all the granulation tissue covering the cup is carefully removed. If the bone ventral to the acetabulum is severely damaged, the use of a truncated, instead of the curved, soft tissue lever is recommended. If the cup is still firmly anchored in the bone, our most important instrument for cup retrieval is the "swan-neck chisel" (Fig. 3.25d). This asymmetrically ground, curved instrument is ideal for loosening an acetabular component just along its surface without bone loss, or with minimal bone loss. If the cup is firmly anchored in place it will need to be loosened very gradually all round its circumference. Bone loss can be reduced still further by starting the loosening processes on the mediodorsal side in the less crucial anchoring zones. Extensive cavities caused by the spreading granulation tissue are often present, and these can extend not only to the acetabular roof, but also far in the direction of the

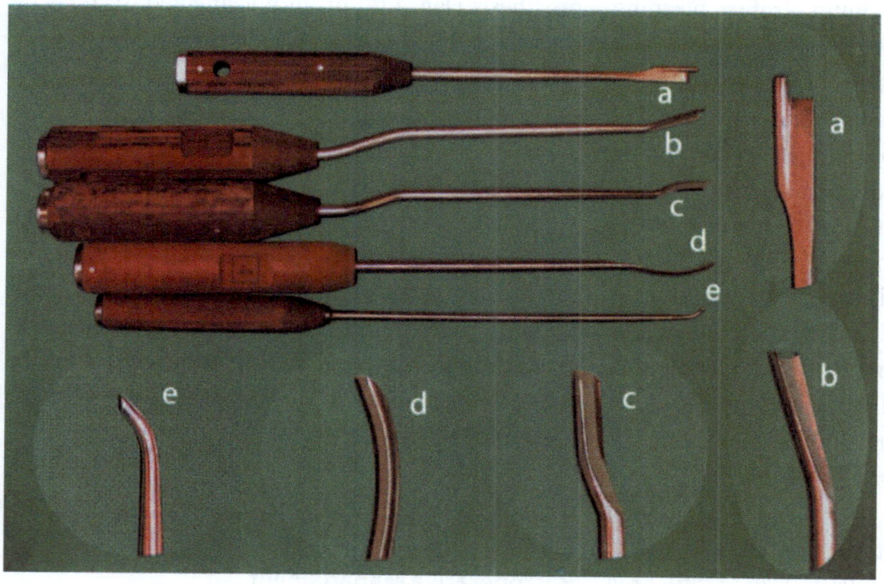

Fig. 3.25a–e. Chisels for prosthesis retrieval and cement removal
a cement splitting or pennant chisel. Used for splitting the cement in the femoral stem. When the chisel is in the central cavity, the "flagpole" makes it difficult to split the bony shaft at the same time
b, c Two cement removal chisels for loosening the cement from the bony femoral diaphysis
d Cup removal or swan-neck chisel. Used directly around the rim of the cup. Its specially shaped tip enables the chisel to follow the round outer contours of the cup and very rapidly loosen it from its anchorage
e Another cement removal chisel. Used for thin cement sections adhering firmly to the wall to create a new starting point for chisels b/c

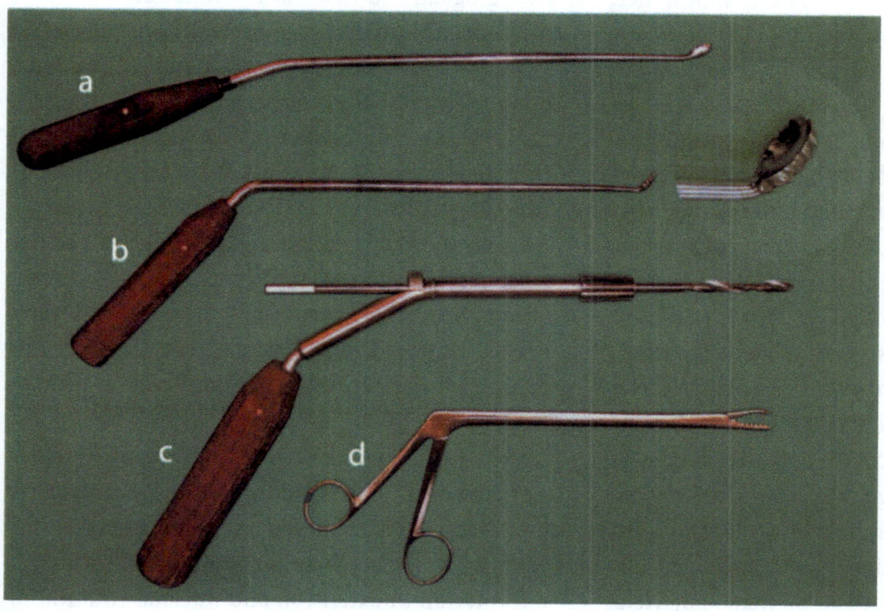

Fig. 3.26a–d. Instruments for cement removal
a, b Two specially shaped, sharp serrated curettes for removing cement and granulation tissue from the shaft (*a*) and acetabulum
c Drill guide with modular tapered attachment and front-cutting 6-mm drill bit. Following cement removal with the chisels down to the final cylindrical section, this instrument can be used under image intensifier control to drill through the centre of the cement
d Cement-holding forceps: used to pick out cement fragments from the medullary cavity

lesser pelvis and into the ischium. Profuse bleeding usually occurs during the removal of the granulation tissue and rapid curettage is useful, ideally with various sizes of sharp curettes. If the bone is destroyed in the direction of the lesser pelvis, the surgeon should at least attempt to preserve the periosteum. Large cement chunks should be left in place because of the risk of bleeding (see also Chap. 13). The angled sharp curette with serrated edges is particularly suitable for the curettage of granulation tissue from cavities (Fig. 3.26b). The surgeon can now decide whether the implant can be abutted directly against the bone stock using an acetabular reinforcement ring or whether an antiprotrusio cage is needed.

▪ **Femoral Component.** In the transgluteal approach, a double-tipped soft tissue lever (Fig. 3.17b) or a femoral lever (Fig. 3.17c) is used to adjust the greater trochanter so as to expose the whole width of the end of the femur. A gouge is used to open up a channel in the direction of the medullary cavity that will enable both the old prosthesis to be knocked straight out and the cement to be removed (Fig. 3.24). This gives the surgeon a clear view during cement removal, thereby substantially reducing the risk of shaft perforations. The chisels shown in Fig. 3.25 are used first to split the cement and then loosen it from the bony wall under direct vision. The operator maintains this clear view by regular irrigation and by having the operating luminaires directed through the shaft opening. The planning sketch (Fig. 3.24) will reveal the location of thick cement layers in particular. If the surgeon loses a clear view distally, it is worth extending the outwardly rotated leg and controlling the correct position of the chisel under the image converter. If the assistant alternately turns the leg through 90° in each case, an eccentric chisel can be used so as to avoid perforation. When the concluding cement cylinder is reached, the drill guide with tapered attachments (Fig. 3.26c) is inserted into the medullary cavity and the cement is drilled centrally under image intensifier control. The remaining cement can then simply be drilled out from the centre. The cement-holding forceps and sharp angled serrated curettes are used to meticulously clear the medullary cavity of cement fragments and granulation tissue, followed by liberal irrigation.

On the basis of a final assessment of the bone situation, the surgeon now decides whether to use a cemented normal prosthesis, a cemented long-stem prosthesis (Fig. 3.12) or an uncemented SL revision prosthesis (Fig. 3.14).

3.7.3 Reimplantation

The reimplantation procedure will depend greatly on the existing defects and the selected implants. Since the surgical technique is not particularly amenable to standardisation, there is little of relevance that can be stated at this point. In this connection we refer the reader to Sect. 3.4.5.

3.8 Postoperative Management

▪ **In the Operating Theatre.** A hip spica is placed over the patient's dressing. A filtering system is connected to the intra-articular drain to enable blood mixed with citrate to be retransfused during the first 4–5 h.

On the Ward. Several things must be done on the ward:

- Neurological and vascular examination
  As during the preoperative assessment, nerves and vessels are also carefully examined on the day of operation (see Sects. 11.3.1, 13.4.2, 13.5.2). If necessary, the vessels are additionally investigated by a Doppler scan or an appropriate specialist.
- Anticoagulation
  Each evening throughout the hospital stay, the patient is given short-chain heparins for anticoagulation purposes. If a particular risk of thrombosis exists, the patient is anticoagulated with dicumarols for the first 6 weeks of mobilisation.
- Hip movements
  Under normal circumstances, flexion and extension, internal rotation and abduction in extension and external rotation in flexion are permitted for exercise purposes. Caution is indicated for external rotation in extension and internal rotation in flexion. Difficulty with flexion is often a sign of excessive bleeding into the thigh muscles. In such cases, it is advisable to use the dynamic splint for continuous passive movements.

- Mobilisation
  On the first postoperative day, the patient is mobilized on the edge of the bed. Subsequently, depending on the individual patient's dexterity, mobilisation continues with a walking frame and then sticks, with gradually increasing weight-bearing. Stair-climbing is included in the programme as early as possible. A stay in a health spa or rehabilitation clinic on discharge from hospital is only envisaged if difficulties or additional problems are encountered.
- Special remarks
  - Transfemoral approach: Flexion is limited to 70° for 3–4 weeks to allow the proximal femoral fragments to knit together.
  - SL revision stem, extensive acetabular reconstruction with poor bone quality: in this exceptional case, partial weight-bearing is maintained for 6–10 weeks.

■ **After Discharge from Hospital.** The patient is advised to gradually increase his level of activity. Assistance with physiotherapy is only appropriate if the patient is otherwise unable to walk without limping. This is checked at the 6-week follow-up. Radiographic controls are implemented after 4 months and 1 year, with subsequent checks as described in Chap. 1.

References

1. Bircher HP, Riede U, Lüem M, Ochsner PE (2001) Der Wert der SL-Revisionsprothese nach Wagner zur Überbrückung großer Femurdefekte. Technik und Resultate. Orthopäde 30: 294–303
2. Brunazzi MG, Mcharo CN, Ochsner PE (1996) Hüfttotalprothesenwechsel – was erwartet den Patienten? Schweiz Med Wochenschr 126: 2013–2020
3. Draenert K, Draenert Y, Garde U, Ulrich CH (1999) Manual of cementing technique. Springer, Berlin
4. Dihlmann SW, Ochsner PE, Pfister A, Mayrhofer P (1994) Wanderungsanalyse verschraubter Hüftpfannen nach Revisionsarthroplastiken am Hüftgelenk. Z Orthop 132: 131–137
5. Hirakawa K, Mitsugo N, Koshino T, Saito T, Hirasawa Y, Toshikazu K (2001) Effect of acetabular cup position and orientation in cemented total hip arthroplasty. Clin Orthop 388: 135–142
6. Hirschnitz C, Ochsner PE (1996).Die klinische Relevanz von Fettembolien. Unfallchirurgie 22:57-73
7. Ilchmann T, Franzén H, Njöberg B, Wingstrand H (1992) Measurement accuracy in acetabular cup migration. J Arthroplasty 7: 121–127
8. Ilchmann T (1997) Radiographic assessment of cup migration and wear after hip replacement. Acta Orthop Scand Suppl 276
9. Krismer M, Bauer R, Tschupik J, Mayrhofer P (1995) EBRA: A method to measure migration of acetabular components. J Biomech 28: 1225–1236
10. Lequesne M (1967) Die Erkrankungen des Hüftgelenkes bei Erwachsenen 3. Teil. Folia rheumatologica 17a: 61
11. Lützner J, Ochsner PE (2000) Langzeitergebnisse mit der Orginal ME Müller-Geradschaftprothese aus CoNiCrMo-Schmiedelegierung (Protasul 10). Orthop Praxis 36: 416–421
12. Malchau H, Herberts P (2001) Prognosis of total hip replacement. The national hip arthroplasty registry (Sweden).
13. Müller ME (1966) Proceedings SICOT Congress Paris, pp 323–333
14. Müller ME, Jaberg H (1982) Total hip reconstruction. In: Evarts CM (ed) Surgery of the musculoskeletal system, 2nd edn. Churchill Livingstone, New York, pp 2979–3017
15. Sakalkale DK, Sharkey PF, Eng K, Hozack WJ, Rothman RH (2001) Effect of femoral component offset on polyethylene wear in total hip arthroplasty. Clin Orthop 388: 125–134
16. Schneider R (1989) Total prosthetic replacement of the hip. Huber, Bern

Chapter 4

Postoperative Haematomas

Mathias Klein, Damien Toia

In our own patient population, a haematoma requiring treatment occurred in 4% of cases after a primary total hip replacement and in 6% after a revision operation. If the patient complained of symptoms, the wound threatened to perforate, the haematoma liquefied or the wound remained moist, we managed these either by single or repeated aspiration or surgical revision. An early infection was involved in 5% of the revised haematomas. Haematoma prophylaxis consisted of intraoperative haemostasis, drain insertion in the various wound layers and a spica dressing for 2 days. A risk factor for haematoma is thromboprophylaxis, which we administered in the form of a low molecular weight heparin. We did not observe an increased risk of bleeding in orally anticoagulated patients.

We opted for aspiration in the case of closed haematomas and for surgical revision in the case of a moist wound, secondary decline in the haemoglobin level and a suspected infected haematoma. Embolisation of bleeding vessels by angiography is a modern option, especially in cases of acute blood loss.

After leg length discrepancies and limping, a postoperative haematoma requiring treatment is the commonest complication after primary and revision procedures. A haematoma prolongs the hospital stay and puts a strain on both the patient's mental state and the health insurance system. A haematoma revision should therefore be implemented as early as possible, between the 6th and 10th postoperative days.

4.1 Introduction

Postoperative haematomas are a familiar and common complication of hip replacement operations. We make a distinction between *immediate* and *delayed-onset* haematomas. The former are caused by factors arising directly at operation, whether in connection with inadequate haemostasis or poor blood clotting. Delayed-onset haematomas become apparent through subsequently occurring sensations of tautness as a result of delayed bleeding from a secondarily re-leaking blood vessel. The need for treating a haematoma is decided on the basis of clinical symptoms, e.g. weeping wounds, laboratory results indicative of inflammation, sensation of tautness and fluctuation.

In addition to intraoperative trauma, another risk factor is the standard thromboprophylaxis that is usually initiated at the preoperative stage. Closed drainage systems are used to prevent haematomas.

4.2 Frequency

4.2.1 Frequency in Our Own Patients

In this summary compilation we are particularly interested in the haematomas treated in the patient population defined in Chap. 2. We decided to proceed to a haematoma revision after 41 (4%) primary procedures and after 21 (6%) revisions (stem and/or cup change). In total, 27 women and 34 men were affected (Table 4.1). After leg length discrepancies and limping (Figs. 2.11, 2.12), haematomas are the commonest local complications (Fig. 4.1).

4.2.2 Frequency in the Literature

A figure of 1.1% of "massive" haematomas after primary operations is reported in the literature [7], i.e. the patients notice haematoma pain, the skin is very taut and the haematocrit level is reduced. Half of these patients underwent surgical revision which, according to our definition, gives a haematoma frequency of 0.6%. This percentage is not really comparable with our own, since we also performed a revision in cases where the findings were much less pronounced.

A literature review also reveals frequencies of 2.2% for haematomas after primary and revision total hip replacements [4] and 7.5% for treated haematomas after primary and revision total hip replacements [2]. In 3.0% of cases, the latter authors revised the haematomas openly in patients with a drainage system inserted after a total arthroplasty, but in no patients without a drainage system. Aspirations were performed in the remaining 4.5% of patients, 1.5% of whom had a postoperative drain, while the remaining 3.0% had none.

During postoperative ultrasound scans routinely performed on the 1st–3rd day after operation, other authors observed a frequency of 11.7% for haematomas in need of aspiration, i.e. containing >40 ml blood [5].

4.3 Preventive Measures

4.3.1 Haematoma Prevention

In our hip replacement procedures we normally employ a lateral approach with partial detachment of the middle gluteal muscle and incomplete joint capsule excision (Chap. 3). After each step in the operation, electrocoagulation is performed deep into the tissues to seal any leaking vessels. In our hospital, one "intra-articular" drain, i.e. close to the joint, one subfascial drain and one subcutaneous drain are inserted during wound closure. The intra-articular and subfascial drains are connected to the closed Handivac system (for drainage reinfusion) and the subcutaneous drain is attached to a Redon bottle. The drains are normally left in situ for 2 days to allow as much blood as possible to be aspirated from the wound area. We consider that the risk of infection as-

Table 4.1. Haematomas requiring treatment after primary total arthroplasty and prosthetic revision

	Primary total arthroplasty			Prosthesis revision		
	1 aspiration	>1 aspiration	Revision	1 aspiration	>1 aspiration	Revision
Number	18	5	18	15	3	3
Of which, orally anticoagulated	5	1	7	2	1	2
Time (days after operation)	16	–	14	15	–	11

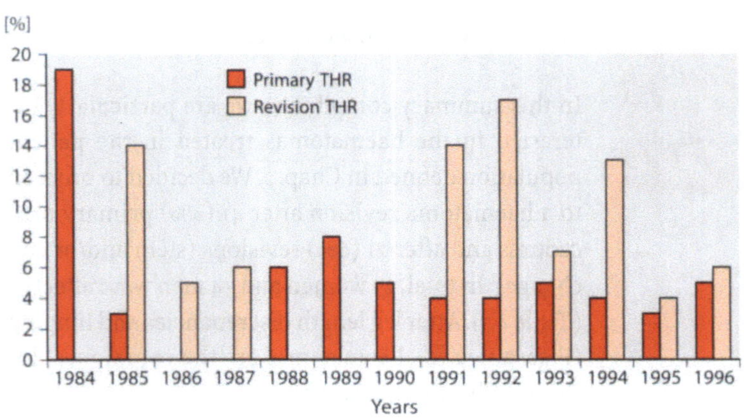

Fig. 4.1. Revised haematomas per year (%) after primary total hip replacements and revisions

sociated with a Redon drain left in situ for 48 h is less than the threat posed by a potential haematoma, even though bacterial colonisation of drain tips rises substantially, from 0% on the 1st to 20% on the 2nd postoperative day [3]. The latter authors consider a 24-h drainage period to be ideal.

We believe that the following measures are useful for avoiding a postoperative haematoma:

- Consistent haemostasis
- Drainage of the various wound compartments
- Compression dressing (hip spica) up to the 2nd postoperative day
- Conservative use of non-steroidal anti-inflammatory drugs (NSAID), since these prolong the bleeding time

4.3.2 Thromboprophylaxis

Up until the year 2000, patients received a single daily subcutaneous injection of low-molecular-weight heparin (Sandoparin) from the evening before the operation until discharge from hospital. Excluded were patients with an increased risk of thrombosis; in these cases a 6-week course of oral anticoagulation (Marcoumar) is initiated on the 3rd postoperative day. Until the Quick value [prothrombin time] falls below 30% (INR 2.2), the two drugs are overlapped. In our own patient population, oral anticoagulation did not affect the formation of haematomas.

Since 1984 we have experienced 5 phases of thromboprophylaxis:

1984–1986	subcutaneous low-dose Liquemin or heparin DHE three times daily,
1987–1990	Embolex or, if the vasoconstrictor component is contraindicated, heparin up to 1990
1990–1994	Embolex or Sandoparin
1994–2000	Sandoparin alone
from 2000	Fragmin

No relevant differences between the first four phases have been observed for haematoma frequency (Fig. 4.1). Insufficient data are currently available for Fragmin.

4.4 Treatment for Haematomas

The haematomas are treated by one or more aspirations or by open revision. Embolisation has recently been performed in some cases.

4.4.1 Aspiration

According to our regimen, aspiration is indicated if there is a distinctly palpable, liquefied haematoma surrounded by a blue-green ring, if the skin in the scar area has a glazed appearance as a result of haematoma pressure and there is a risk of penetration through the operation scar. Aspirations are usually carried out between the 8th and 15th days.

The aspiration is performed under aseptic conditions in the operating theatre anteroom with surgical gowns and masks. A local anaesthetic is first injected distally and dorsally at the lowest point of the haematoma. The aspiration needle is introduced through a stab incision, thereby avoiding the punching out of a skin cylinder, which might then be dragged deep into the tissues to form a potential source of contamination. The needle is inserted into the centre of the liquefied haematoma. After the procedure, a hip spica is applied for 24 h as a compression dressing. Only in rare cases does a haematoma fill up again after aspiration sufficiently to require a second aspiration. A third aspiration has been performed in only one instance (Table 4.1).

4.4.2 Revision

According to our regimen, open revision is indicated

- In the event of a rise, or absence of a reduction, in the C-reactive protein (CRP) level and leucocyte count, fever and pain with a suspected infected haematoma
- If a surgical wound is still moist after 6–8 days and risks becoming a portal of entry for germs
- In the event of a secondary drop in the haemoglobin level with assumed secondary bleeding with thigh tautness and pain

The surgical wound is retracted over its full length and opened down to the joint. The haematoma is aspirated. Any residues are removed with the Luer bone forceps and a sharp curette. Distinctly altered wound edges are excised. Two or three tissue samples are routinely collected from the wound area for bacteriological and histological investigation (see Chap. 5, Sects. 5.2.5, and 5.2.6). The whole wound area is irrigated extensively with an antiseptic solution (Lavasept; [6]). The wound is closed in layers with the insertion of two to four deep, wide drains and two superficial drains. These are successively removed over the next 3–5 days, depending on the amount of drainage in each case.

The revisions are performed, on average, after 11–14 days. In one case only was a revision required as early as the 2nd postoperative day because of a profusely bleeding vessel.

4.4.3 Embolisation of Bleeding Vessels

Modern angiographic techniques can now be used not only to produce a radiographic image of a bleeding vessel, but also to seal the vessel, or to reduce its blood flow sufficiently to induce thrombosis [1]. The method has been used in our hospital only in the past 3 years. The technique can even be used to stop bleeding from major vessels such as the superior gluteal artery (see also Chap. 13, Sect. 13.5.2).

Patient selection: Particularly suitable candidates for this treatment are patients with a suddenly deteriorating haematoma secondarily. A rapid response produces the best results.

Procedure: Selective aortography is performed to look for the sources of bleeding (Fig. 4.2). The extravasated fluid is particularly easy to see during the

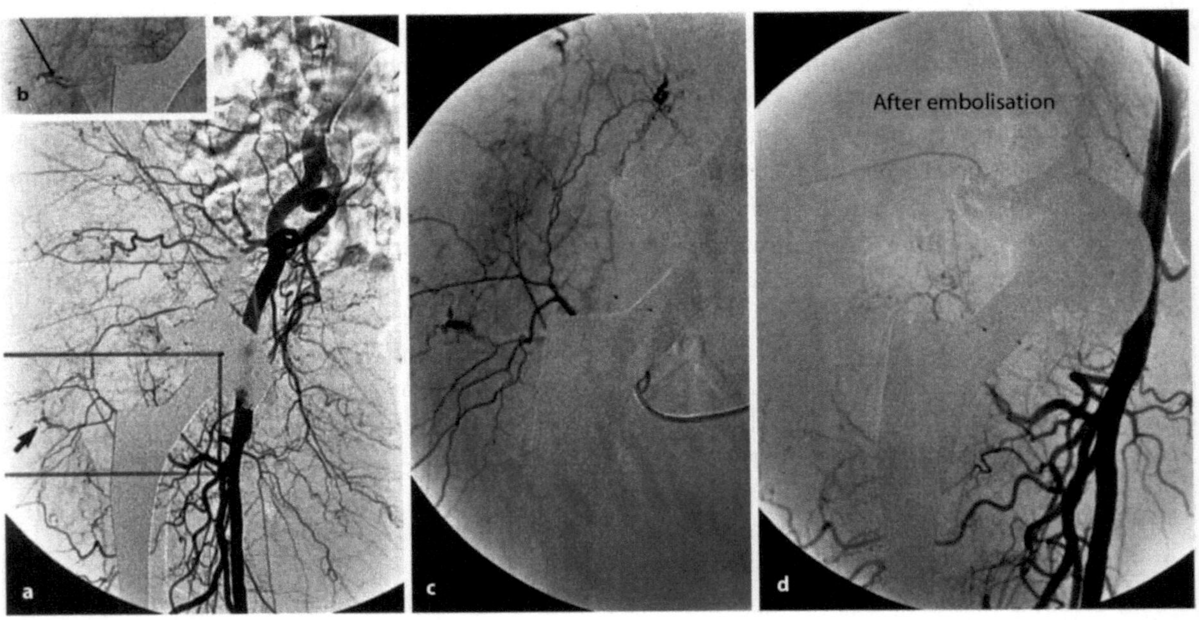

Fig. 4.2a–d. Selective embolisation of an acutely bleeding vessel. N.R., female, 76 years (O. 23519). Massively increased bleeding in the operation area 6 days after a total hip replacement (see also Fig. 13.1)
a The angiogram shows an amputated vessel (*arrow*) in the area of the ascending branch of the lateral circumflex femoral artery
b The extravasated fluid remains visible during the venous phase
c Catheterisation of the lateral circumflex femoral artery, injection of several particles measuring 300–1000 μm (Contour Emboli)
d The ascending branch is occluded. On the following day, the haematoma was evacuated during open revision. The wound subsequently healed without complications

venous phase (Fig. 4.2b), and the bleeding vessel is catheterised as peripherally as possible (Fig. 4.2c). Particles matching the diameter of the cannulated vessel are now introduced through the catheter to produce occlusion of the vessel (Fig. 4.2d). A wide variety of substances are used as particles, e.g. polyvinyl alcohol foam. If the vessel diameter is larger, the surgeon must resort to embolisation coils.

Haematoma revision: An open haematoma revision may follow after 1 or 2 days (see also Sect. 4.4.2).

4.4.4 Infected Haematomas

Two of the 41 haematomas (5%) revised after a primary total hip replacement and one of the 21 (5%) haematomas treated after a revision operation became infected. All three haematomas were openly revised. In one case, the revision was only carried out after an aspiration had confirmed the presence of bacteria. Subsequent management was in accordance with the guidelines for early infections (see Chap. 5). An aggressive approach to haematomas can be useful for identifying and successfully treating early infections in good time without the need for a change of prosthesis.

The frequency of infection in patients suffering a haematoma after primary and revision operations, 5% in each case, contrasts with frequencies of 0.45% and 0.35%, respectively, in an unselected patient population during the first 2 years, and is a non-statistically confirmed indication of increased infections in the presence of a haematoma.

In routine, sonographically controlled haematoma aspirations of >40 ml blood on the 1st–3rd postoperative days, bacteria were found in 16.6% of cases (1.9% of all patients) [5]. In the control group of patients not sonographically controlled, an infected haematoma was present in 5.2% of cases.

4.4.5 Duration of Hospitalisation

Patients attending the Liestal Cantonal Hospital have traditionally been kept in hospital for relatively long periods (Fig. 2.3). After a primary implantation, the hospital stay used to be 22.4 days, compared with 25.9 days after revisions. Only during the past few years has this period been appreciably shortened. In general, however, patients are rehabilitated until they are able to climb stairs and are often then discharged home directly. An aspiration after a primary operation prolonged hospitalisation by an average of 6.7 days, whereas an aspiration after a revision procedure did not affect the length of hospital stay. Repeated aspiration extended the hospitalisation to 28.8 and 46.5 days, respectively (small number of patients). Surgical revision after primary and revision operations prolonged hospitalisation by 16.4 and 13.9 days, respectively.

These data show that a haematoma usually results in conspicuous lengthening of the period of hospitalisation, i.e. a haematoma has a negative impact not only on the well-being and mental state of the patient, but also on the health insurance system. Accordingly, early, i.e. aggressive, intervention in the presence of a haematoma is justified.

4.5 Conclusion

Our current practice is to endeavour to aspirate or revise a haematoma after a total hip arthroplasty between the 6th and 10th postoperative days. However, our figures have shown (Table 4.1) that any delay can significantly prolong the hospital stay.

References

1. Coldwell DM, Stokes KR, Yakes WF (1994) Embolotherapy: Agents, clinical applications and techniques. Radiographics 14: 623–643
2. Crevoisier XM, Reber P, Noesberger B (1998) Is suction drainage necessary after total joint arthroplasty? Arch Orthop Trauma Surg 117: 121–124
3. Drinkwater CJ, Neil MJ (1995) Optimal timing of wound drain removal following total joint arthroplasty. J Arthroplasty 10: 185–189
4. Lieberman JR, Wollaeger J, Dorey F, Thomas BJ, Kilgus DJ, Grecula MJ, Finerman GA, Amstutz HC (1997) The efficacy of prophylaxis with low-dose warfarin for prevention of pulmonary embolism following total hip arthroplasty. J Bone Joint Surg Am 79: 319–325
5. Möllenhoff G, Walz M, Muhr G (1995) Kontrolle von Wundheilungsstörungen mittels Sonographie anhand postoperativer Kontrollen nach TEP-Implantation. Chirurg 66: 188–191

6. Roth B, Müller J, Willenegger H (1985) Intraoperative Wundspülung mit einem neuartigen Antiseptikum. Helv Chir Acta 52: 61–65
7. Suomalainen O, Mäkelä AE, Harju A, Jaroma H (1996) Prevention of fatal pulmonary embolism with warfarin after total hip replacement. Int Orthop (SICOT) 20: 75–79

CHAPTER 5

Infections

MATHIAS SCHAFROTH, WERNER ZIMMERLI,
MARCO BRUNAZZI, PETER E. OCHSNER

Infections after total hip replacements are serious complications. They can be triggered either exogenously (intra- or perioperatively) or endogenously (haematogenously). In our own patient population, the infection rate was 0.82% in 1098 primary prostheses and 1.16% in 330 revisions. Considering just the predominantly exogenous infections, which almost always manifested themselves during the first 2 years, the respective infection rates were 0.4% and 0.35%. We distinguish between three types depending on the interval between operation and the manifestation of the infection:

- Early infection: manifestation up to the end of the 3rd month
- Delayed infection (mostly low-grade infection): from the 4th month up to 2 years after operation
- Late infection: from the 3rd year after operation

A distinction is also made between a monoinfection and a mixed infection. The commonest pathogen in both groups is *Staphylococcus aureus*. While the diagnosis is initially made on the basis of clinical and radiological findings, the microbiological and histological tissue investigations are decisive. Treatment consists, on the one hand, of systemic, resistance-matched antimicrobial therapy and, on the other, of surgical treatment, which will largely depend on the time of manifestation of the infection.

Three surgical procedures are possible:
- Hip revision, leaving the prosthesis in situ
- One-stage exchange of the total hip prosthesis
- Removal of the total hip prosthesis without replacement (Girdlestone hip) or with a two-stage reimplantation of a new prosthesis

In our hospital, 94.5% of all hip prosthesis infections were successfully treated, 71% of them during a single in-patient stay.

5.1 Classification, Definitions

Infections can be classified according to five criteria:
- Infection route: exogenous or haematogenous/endogenous infections
- Interval: period between the operation and first manifestation of the infection
- Pathogens: type, pathogenicity and virulence of the pathogens
- Tissues: soft tissue situation when the infection is diagnosed
- Diagnosis: probability of the presence of an infection

5.1.1 Exogenous vs. Haematogenous Infection

▪ **Exogenous infections** are triggered by pathogens that penetrate the prosthesis area from the outside. Portals of entry are local open wounds, local decubital ulcers and surgical wounds. Following implantation of a hip prosthesis, germs can be introduced, either during or immediately after operation, through a wound infection as a result of a wound healing problem. An exogenous infection can manifest itself after just a few days or – particularly in the case of a low-grade infection – may only be recognised after periods ranging from a few months to 2 years.

▪ **Haematogenous infections** of a prosthesis are caused by a focus of infection that primarily affects another part of the body. These bacteria then reach the prosthesis via the bloodstream. Although haematogenous infections can occur at any time, they tend to be overshadowed numerically by exogenous infections during the first 2 years.

Sepsis is rarely detected clinically in these patients prior to the infection of the prosthesis. The main foci for dissemination of a haematogenous infection can be found in the skin (erysipelas, infected decubital ulcer), the genitourinary system and the respiratory tract [31]. Typical pathogens include streptococci, *S. aureus* (skin), *Escherichia coli* (genitourinary tract) and pneumococci (respiratory tract), although other bacteria such as salmonellae (enterocolitis) and anaerobes (periodontitis) can also lead to prosthesis infections via the haematogenous route. Since they weaken the body's defences, long-term steroid therapy, HIV infection, diabetes mellitus, immunosuppression after transplantation, old age and terminal renal failure are associated with an increased risk of infection.

5.1.2 Implant-Associated Infection

In terms of pathogenesis, infections occurring in the presence of implants, e.g. prostheses, internal fixation materials, pacemakers, etc., behave differently from infections in which no foreign body is present. This is best illustrated in infections with *S. aureus* [33]. While staphylococci, when not associated with an implant, are completely destroyed by flucloxacillin, for example, even the highest dose of this antibiotic is not sufficient for eliminating bacteria adhering to a foreign body. They can be eliminated, however, with rifampicin, though this drug can rapidly lead to the development of resistance when used as monotherapy. In a clinical study we showed that implant-associated staphylococcal infections can be cured using a combination of the two drugs, followed by the oral administration of ciprofloxacin plus rifampicin [34].

5.1.3 Time of Manifestation of the Infection

We define the time of manifestation of an infection as the point at which an infection is unambiguously diagnosed for the first time by microbiological and histological investigation. The interval after the prosthesis operation will determine the corresponding group classification. The time of microbial inoculation can precede the manifestation of the infection by periods ranging from a few days up to 2 years [27].

Three groups are distinguished:

- Early manifestation: manifestation within the first 3 months after operation
- Delayed manifestation: manifestation of an exogenous infection in the period between 3 months and 2 years after operation (low-grade infection)
- Late infection: start of the (haematogenous) infection more than 2 years after operation

An *early manifestation* of an infection generally involves an exogenous bacterial colonisation associated with an infected haematoma or wound healing problem that occurs directly at operation or during the immediate postoperative period. Clinically, and often as early as the wound healing stage, the wound appears red and swollen. Although early haematogenous infections are rare, they have been described, for example, during acute urinary tract infections [31]. The cemented prosthesis remains securely seated in early infections. If it is not cemented then bony integration will not yet be concluded.

In a *delayed manifestation* the infection, usually exogenous, will have been simmering for several months, frequently resulting in loosening of the prosthesis and consequent weight-bearing-related pain. While cemented prostheses may remain integrated with the bone to a certain extent, this does not prevent the prosthesis from being surrounded in many cases by large sections of infected tissue. The onset of individual acute or subacute haematogenous infections is also possible during this period.

In *late infections* haematogenous colonisation is assumed to be present. A late infection can first manifest itself acutely in the form of sepsis, leading to an acute onset in the affected joint, or else can start gradually and lead to a deep-seated abscess. If sepsis is initially present (as occurs particularly with *S. aureus*), the disease can even prove fatal.

Chronological distribution of infections: Infections are observed more frequently during the first 2 years postoperatively than in later periods (Fig. 5.1). Since the exogenous infections acquired perioperatively manifest themselves during this period, a conclusive view on the operation-associated infection rate can be expressed 2 years after operation (Fig. 5.2; see also Sect. 5.2.1). Haematogenous infections in later years,

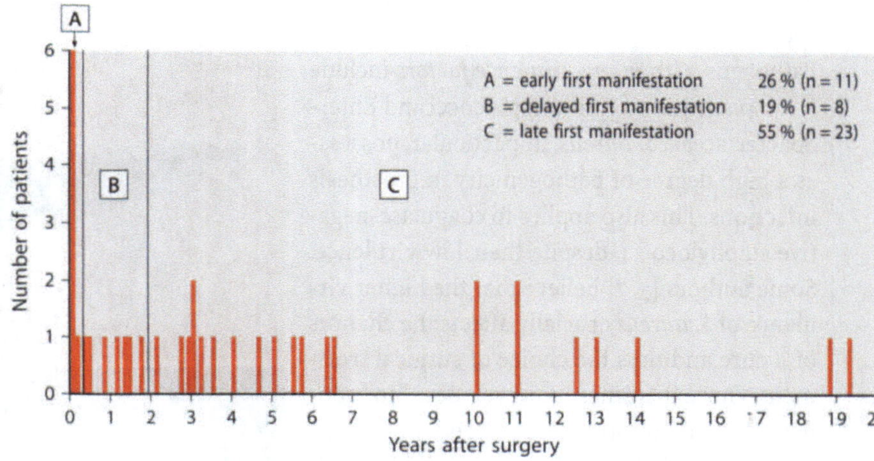

Fig. 5.1. Time of manifestation of the infections after total hip replacements treated in the period 1984–1996 in Liestal, in some cases jointly with the Medical Unit (n=44). More than half of the cases concern late infections occurring more than 2 years after the operation

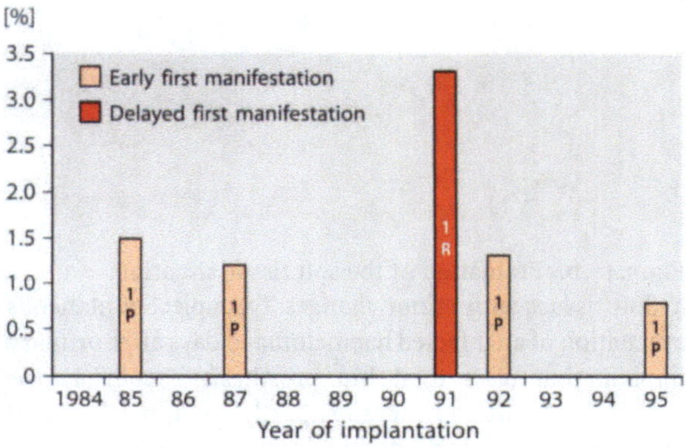

Fig. 5.2. Early and delayed infection manifestation. The percentages relate to the year of implantation and are shown separately for primary (*P*) and revision operations (*R*). The figures presented here on the operation-related infection rate are definitive, since all the patients undergoing surgery during the period under review (1984–1995) either died free of infection or were followed up almost without exception during a postoperative observation period of at least 2 years

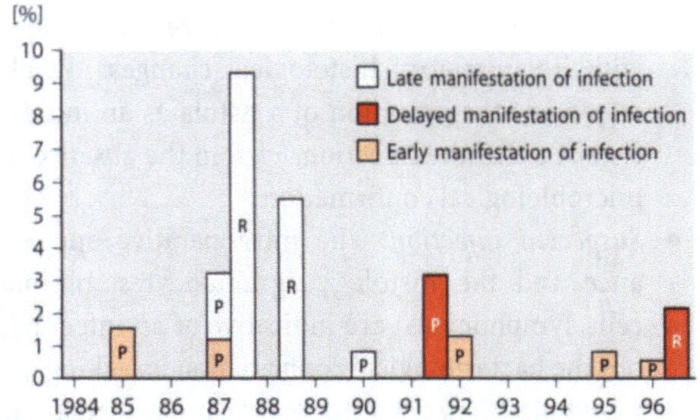

Fig. 5.3. Total infection rates after hip implantation. Presentation analogous to Fig. 5.2. The percentages will continue to grow in future, since additional late infections can occur up until the patient's death

in terms of the percentage distribution over the individual years, are less frequent. However, if the patient survives for a long time after operation, the risk of a haematogenous infection is greater than the risk of a complicating exogenous infection (Figs. 5.1–5.3).

Willenegger and Roth [27] showed that infections tend to occur earlier after internal fixation procedures than after prosthesis implantations. Consequently, the chronological classification as an early or delayed manifestation of an infection differs from that after the implantation of a total hip prosthesis.

5.1.4 Pathogenicity and Virulence of the Pathogens

Two definitions are important in evaluating the pathogens:

- *Pathogenicity*: The pathogenicity is the basic ability of a pathogen to produce clinical disease after inoculation in the body. This ability is also dependent on the conditions prevailing in the host. Thus, for example, coagulase-negative staphylococci are, for practical purposes, only pathogenic in the presence of a foreign body.
- *Virulence*: The virulence is the degree of pathogenicity of a population of microorganisms. A pathogenic species can include virulent and less virulent strains. Pathogens connected with implant infections can be subdivided into two groups:
  - Pathogens with *few virulence factors* are, principally, coagulase-negative staphylococci, *Pro-*

pionibacterium acnes and *Corynebacterium* spp.
- Pathogens with *many virulence factors* include *S. aureus*, β-haemolytic streptococci and Enterobacteriaceae. *S. aureus*, in particular, possesses a high degree of pathogenicity in prosthesis infections. This also applies to coagulase-negative staphylococci, despite their low virulence. Some authors [3, 7] believe that the higher virulence of *S. aureus* crucially affects the chances of a cure and thus the choice of surgical treatment. Our experience, however, does not confirm this assumption (see Sects. 5.1.5, 5.6.2, 5.6.3;) [19, 20]. A much more crucial factor is probably the availability of suitable antibiotics which are effective against bacteria adhering to the implants and which possess good bioavailability [33, 35].

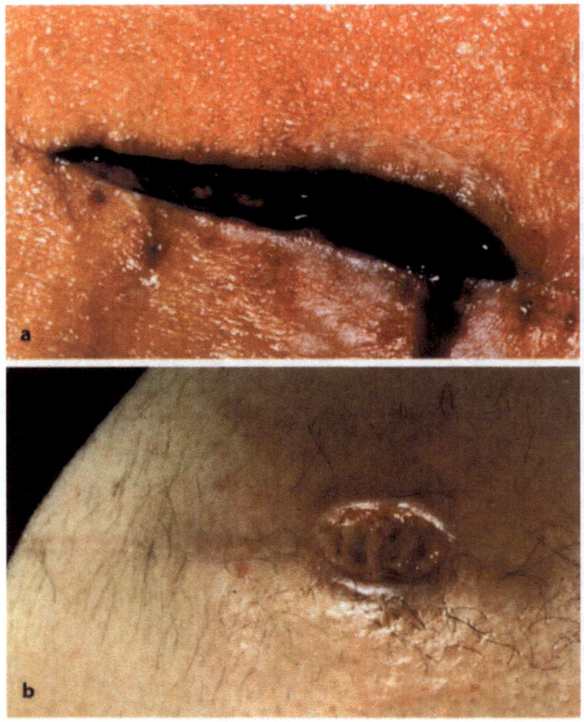

Fig. 5.4a, b. Evaluation of the soft tissue situation:
a Soft tissues with minor changes: Example: Spontaneous evacuation of an infected haematoma 10 days after primary implantation of a total hip prosthesis. *Staphylococcus aureus*. Clean wound margins, partly solid, partly liquid haematoma. Revision without implant replacement (see also Fig. 5.9)
b Soft tissues with major changes: Several weeks after a fall with massive haematoma, rapidly increasing swelling and eruption of a productive fistula 14 months after implantation of a total prosthesis. β-haemolytic streptococci as evidence of haematogenous dissemination. Two-stage replacement of the prosthesis

5.1.5 Soft Tissue Conditions

In relation to the soft tissue situation we distinguish between two groups of patients:
- Soft tissues with minor changes: The soft tissues are normal and the wound margins/scar are not greatly affected by the infection (Fig. 5.4a).
- Soft tissues with major changes: swollen, glazed-oedematous soft tissues, abscess cavity systems (arthrography)/fistulae, pronounced pus production (Figs. 5.4b, 5.12b,c).

If the soft tissues are substantially changed as a result of the infection, we proceed to a two-stage prosthesis exchange procedure.

5.1.6 Probability of Infection

An infection is not always microbiologically documented. Since bacteria occasionally remain unidentified, even in extensive tissue samples, we define three groups:

- *Definite infection (acute or chronic)*: signs and symptoms of clinical infection such as redness, swelling and excessive warmth, coupled with specific infection-related findings, e.g. positive cultures or positive eubacterial PCR result together with inflammatory histological changes. We always view the detection of a fistula as an indication of a definite infection, even in the absence of microbiological confirmation.
- *Suspected infection*: The intraoperative appearance and the histology (granulocytes, plasma cells, lymphocytes) are indicative of an infection, but the bacteriological confirmation is lacking.
- *Contamination:* Bacterial growth is detected in the culture, but the clinical and histological signs of infection are lacking.

5.2 Diagnosis

During the detection and evaluation of an infected hip prosthesis, we investigate six criteria: history and clinical findings, laboratory investigations, imaging procedures, intraoperative findings, microbiological findings and histological investigations [8].

5.2.1 History and Clinical Findings

In the patient's history, the social integration and degree of independence, or need for care, particularly influence the subsequent therapeutic management. Equally important are the presence of any other illnesses and the expectations of the patient.

Clinically, the following signs are decisive:

- *Pain*: typically including pain at rest, sensation of tautness, dull pain and sensation of warmth. If implant loosening is present, weight-bearing-related pain, or pain during rotational movements, e.g. in bed, predominate.
- *Redness*: Of particular interest are the extent, localisation (scar area, groin, thigh and buttocks) and the change in redness over time.
- *Swelling*: glazed, oedematous skin, palpable accumulations of fluid (haematoma, abscess).
- *Fistulae*: Time of onset, extent (fistulography), retention, type and quantity of secretion (serous, purulent, blood-tinged) (Fig. 5.4b).
- *Soft tissue conditions*: These are particularly important for the decision concerning therapeutic management (see also Sect. 5.1.5).

■ **Diagnostic value:** The above-mentioned clinical signs are rated differently. A fistula definitely confirms the diagnosis of infection. All other signs, e.g. pain at rest, redness, swelling, are indicators possessing only moderate sensitivity and specificity.

5.2.2 Laboratory Investigations

The erythrocyte sedimentation rate (ESR), C-reactive protein (CRP) and leucocyte count may be raised. While the absolute figures are of interest, a more important consideration is their change over time. The CRP is primarily an appropriate parameter for checking the efficacy of antibiotic treatment. No controlled studies have yet provided any evidence about the validity of procalcitonin in orthopaedic infections.

■ **Diagnostic value:** The laboratory values possess only moderate sensitivity and specificity.

5.2.3 Imaging Procedures

We expect these procedures to give as clear an indication as possible concerning the presence of an infection and implant loosening. Loosening is easier to detect for cemented than for uncemented prostheses.

▸ *Standard radiographs* (see also Fig. 3.1): New subperiosteal bone growth in the diaphyseal area on standard radiographs can provide direct evidence of an infection. Any migration detected on conventional x-rays is direct confirmation of prosthetic loosening. Double outlines at the border with the bone is an indication of loosening of cemented prostheses only. Uncemented prostheses can be loose without any visible radiological signs. In a corresponding investigation, evaluable radiological signs were lacking in half the cases of prosthesis infection, while a quarter of the patients in each case showed non-specific and specific signs [23].

▸ *Arthrography and fistulography* (Fig. 5.7): These two methods are also used in the diagnosis of infection and loosening. Typical signs of infection are joint capsule outpouchings and abscesses, which together can form large cavity systems. If substantial wear is apparent on radiographs, the possibility of cavities filled with detritus should be considered in the differential diagnosis.

▸ *Magnetic resonance imaging and computer tomography*: Since both techniques produce massive artefacts as a result of the implants and the actual operation, they are not usually able to provide any diagnostically relevant information in the immediate surroundings of the prosthesis, although they can detect abscess formation in the pelvic area cranial to the prosthesis.

▸ *Scintigraphy*: A technetium scan can be used to detect increased bone remodelling around the prosthesis. Since this increases in any case during the first year after implantation of the prosthesis, the validity of this method is irrelevant during this period. Antigranulocyte scintigraphy is not suitable for hip prostheses because of the accumulation of these antibodies in the area of the blood-forming bone marrow. Though expensive, leukocyte scintigraphy can detect the infection in its acute and subacute phases [4]. The informative value of scintigraphy is generally overestimated.

■ **Diagnostic Value:** A typical arthrogram (Fig. 5.7) is very valuable in diagnostic respects. Important indicators are new subperiosteal bone formation and signs of loosening during the first 2 years.

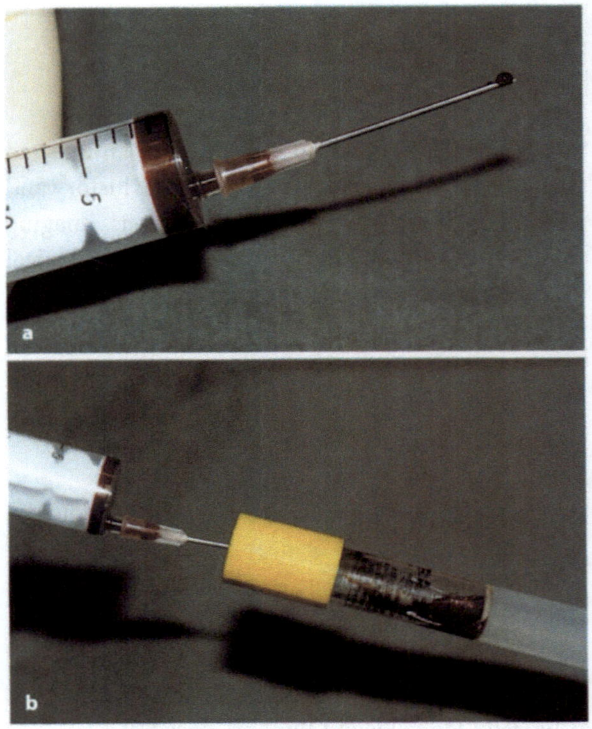

Fig. 5.5a,b. Management of aspirated fluids, pus
a After the fluid is withdrawn through a wide-bore needle, the additionally aspirated air is removed
b The fluid, without air, is transferred to an oxygen-free tube with a colour indicator for detecting any introduced oxygen

5.2.4 Intraoperative Findings

Important factors noted at operation are the description of the extent and localisation of cavity and fistula systems, the presence of pus, granulation tissue, sequestra, loose foreign bodies, the observed blood supply and the mechanical resistance of the bone.

■ **Diagnostic Value:** Evaluating the intraoperative findings is simple in the case of acute infections. In low-grade infections, however, the clinical impression often fails.

5.2.5 Microbiological Investigations

A positive microbiological culture or PCR performed on a correctly taken sample is necessary for the reliable confirmation of infection. The following methods are relevant in this context:

▸ *Aspiration of the hip joint*: Local anaesthetisation of the planned puncture channel is advisable. The sharply ground aspiration needle is introduced through a stab incision, thereby avoiding the punching out of a skin cylinder and its subsequent transport into the joint along with any included bacteria. To check the intraarticular location of the aspiration needle it is advisable to inject some contrast medium into the joint space under image intensifier control (see also Sect. 5.2.3). So that anaerobes can also be detected, the aspirated fluid is injected into an anaerobic transport medium (Fig. 5.5). A colour indicator shows whether oxygen enters the container (e.g. Portagerm) during inoculation. While hip aspirations repeatedly produce false-negative results, only occasionally will a false-positive culture result from a correctly implemented aspiration. If previous bacteriological results are already available, the validity of this investigation is greatly enhanced if the same germs and resistances are found. False-positive results can occur with coagulase-negative staphylococci or propionibacteria since these germs are regularly found in the area around the puncture site. In two different papers on preoperative hip aspiration, Cheung et al. [3] and Taylor and Beggs [22] attested to the very high degree of accuracy of this procedure in detecting infected hip prostheses.

▸ *Intraoperatively collected tissue samples*: These provide the most reliable means for detecting pathogens, and also form the basis for deciding on the appropriate antimicrobial therapy. Tissue samples should be collected from three to six sites. The surgeon should select areas at various points around the surgical wound that look infected. At least one sample in each case should originate from the capsule, the floor of the acetabulum and the femoral medullary cavity. We collect a double sample in each case for bacteriological and histological investigation. If the presence of an organism that is difficult to culture is suspected, collection of a third sample in each case is recommended for investigation by eubacterial PCR [24]. The collected tissue portions should measure approximately 0.5 cm on each side and should be transported to the laboratory in sterile plastic containers as quickly as possible (Fig. 5.6). The microorganisms are then enriched in broth for 24 h, and the result is then subcultured with aerobic and anaerobic incubation. If no growth occurs, the broth is incubated again for 9 days prior to the preparation of new subcultures.

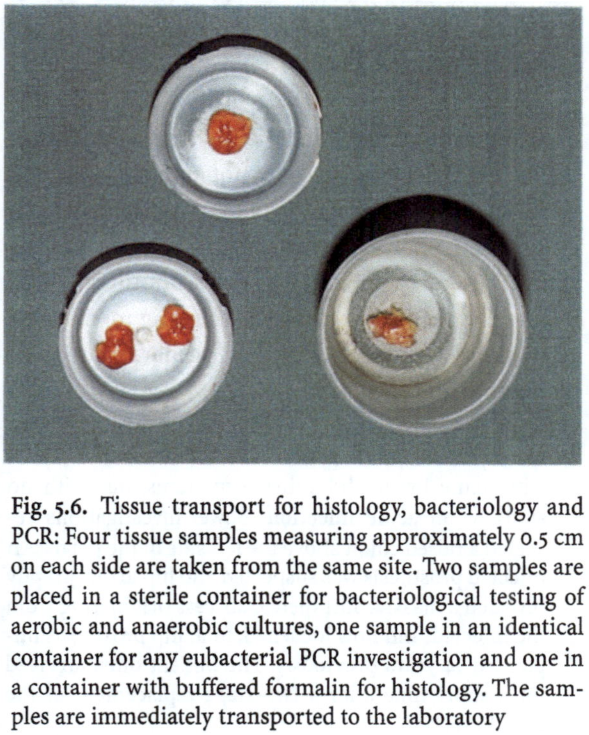

Fig. 5.6. Tissue transport for histology, bacteriology and PCR: Four tissue samples measuring approximately 0.5 cm on each side are taken from the same site. Two samples are placed in a sterile container for bacteriological testing of aerobic and anaerobic cultures, one sample in an identical container for any eubacterial PCR investigation and one in a container with buffered formalin for histology. The samples are immediately transported to the laboratory

▸ *Removed implants/cement fragments*: It is also a good idea to culture individual screws, a cup or cement fragments, so that the growing bacteria exclusively adhering to these items can also be identified [25].

▸ *Wound and fistula swabs*: Particularly if several germs or typical skin bacteria are detected, swab investigations should not be used as a basis for antibiotic therapy since contamination cannot be ruled out.

The following conditions should be observed to prevent distortion of the microbiological analysis by previous antibiotic treatments:

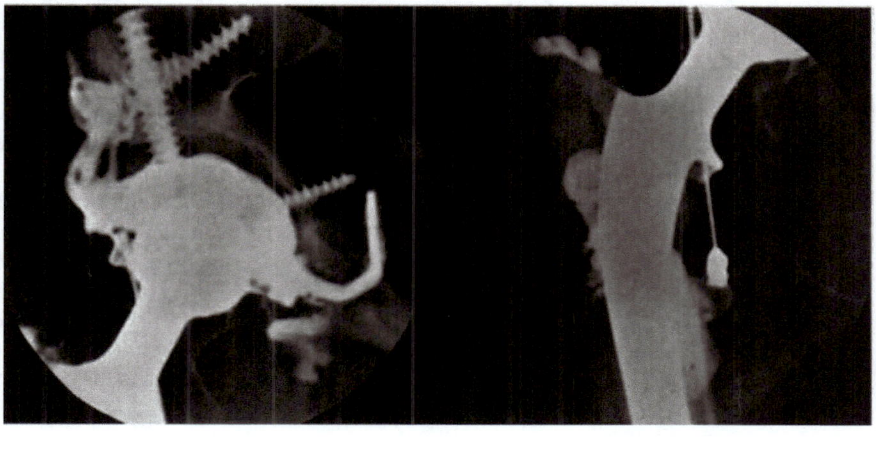

Fig. 5.7. Arthrogram of an infected hip during bacteriological sample collection (B.J., female, see also Fig. 6.11). The cup implant and the proximal section of the femoral component are irrigated with contrast medium. The local cystic outpouchings and the outlier near the greater trochanter are indications of infection

1. *Preoperatively known germ*: A specific antibiotic treatment can be initiated even before operation if there is no doubt about the preoperative bacterial diagnosis.
2. *Preoperatively unknown germ*: Preoperative empirical treatment without collection of a tissue sample for culture is not appropriate in this case. If antibiotics have been given, however, these should be discontinued at least 4 days before operation so that the samples taken at operation do not contain any antibiotic.

■ **Diagnostic Value.** Bacteriological samples collected in the above-mentioned manner are the most important way of confirming the diagnosis. Tissue samples taken at operation are much more reliable than a preoperative hip aspiration. The outcome is also much more reliable if several samples and the cultured implant components produce the same results and the histological investigation confirms the infection findings. The specificity of the result is very high, although false-negative reports still occur. In individual cases, the eubacterial PCR test can be used for bacterial detection purposes.

5.2.6 Histological Investigation

■ **Sample Collection.** Standard practice during each revision is to collect several tissue samples for histology, if possible from the same collection sites used for the microbiological samples (see also Sect. 5.2.5).

■ **Preparation.** The samples are decalcified if necessary, routinely prepared (HE staining) and evaluated immediately by a pathologist.

■ **Evaluation.** Everyday clinical experience has revealed five main groups of findings:

- Acutely inflammatory, infection-specific infiltrates (granulocytic) in all samples
- Partly acute (granulocytic), partly chronic (lympho-plasmacytic) infection-specific infiltrates
- Only chronically inflammatory (lymphoplasmacytic) infiltrates
- Only individual samples show chronically inflammatory infiltrates
- None of the samples shows inflammatory infiltrates

These findings allow certain conclusions to be drawn about the duration of the infection and thus, possibly, about the infection route. If no germs are detected, the diagnosis of infection is occasionally based solely on the histological findings.

■ **Diagnostic Value.** A very high degree of specificity is achieved if the bacteriological and histological tests produce the same result. If the bacteriology is negative, then only histology can provide adequate confirmation of the diagnosis.

5.2.7 (Missed) Infection in Old Age

In the case of very elderly patients admitted to hospital for acute illnesses, one does not immediately think of an infection complicating a total hip replacement undertaken many years in the past. There are increasing reports of, in some cases life-threatening, haematogenous hip infections occurring 10–20 years after implantation (Fig. 5.1). This scenario can be illustrated with three cases:

- A 69-year-old male patient was admitted to hospital with acute lower abdominal symptoms, but with no signs of an acute infection. Bowel investigations revealed a raised colon above the left side of the pelvis. An infected prosthesis was suspected and hip arthrography revealed a massive intrapelvic abscess originating from the infected, and now loosened, total hip prosthesis implanted 14 years previously. The patient only survived for a short time after a two-stage replacement of the prosthesis [17].

- An 83-year-old female patient (V.M., O. 7609) with syncope was investigated for a possible pulmonary embolism or cerebrovascular accident. Recurrent fever and disseminated skin defects did not respond either to parenteral antibiotics or local measures. Also present were melaena, reductions in the haemoglobin level and thrombocytopenia. The C-reactive protein level rose to 186 mg/l and the white cell count to >20,000/µl, but no focus of infection could be located. The patient's general condition steadily deteriorated and she became increasingly confused. She died after 6 weeks with no diagnosis having been made. The autopsy (Professor W. Wegmann, Liestal) revealed an infected, but not loosened, total hip prosthesis (Fig. 5.8c), from which a huge abscess extended down to the knee. The prosthesis had been implanted

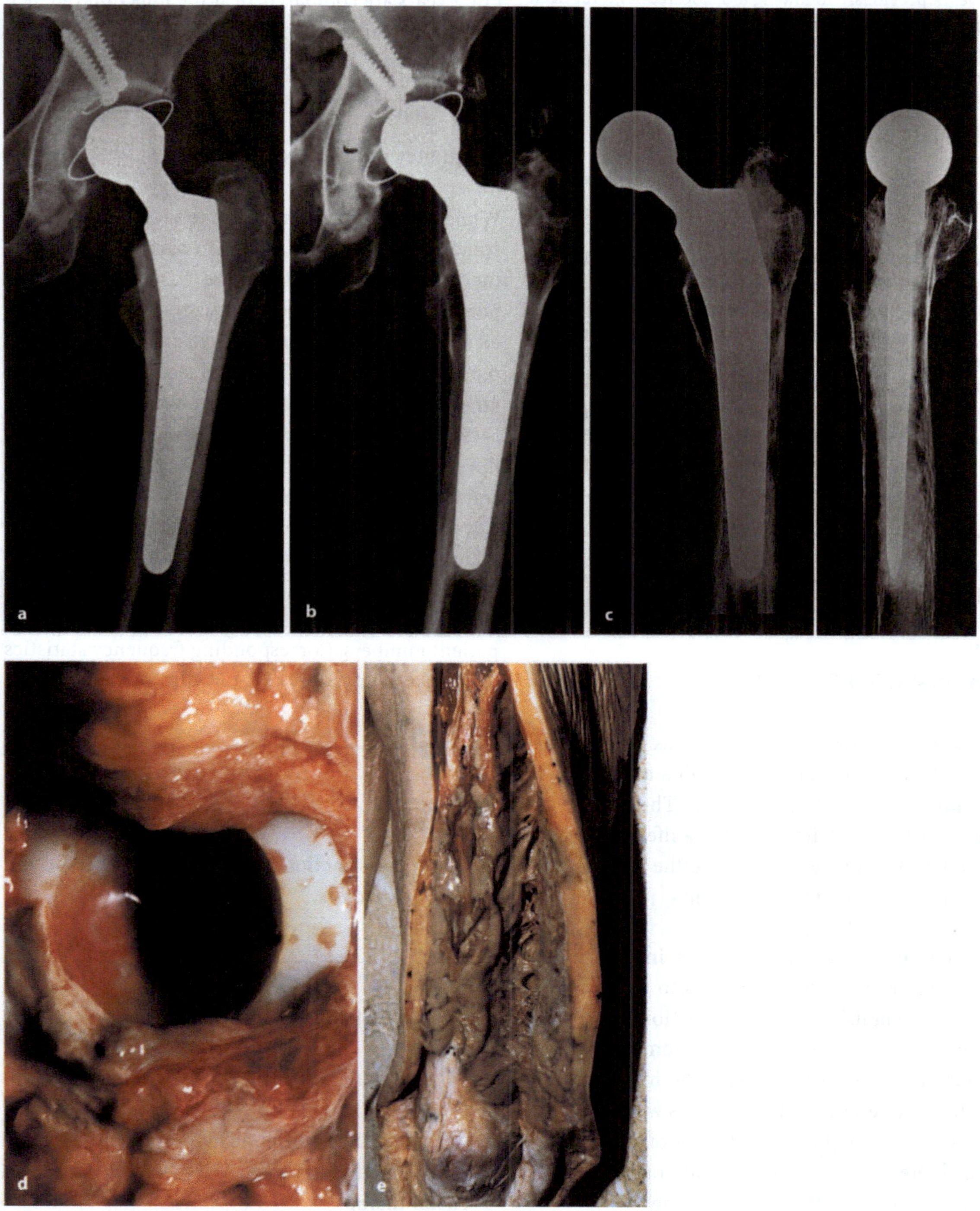

Fig. 5.8a–e. Overlooked late infection in old age with fatal outcome

a Postoperatively, after insertion of a slightly over-medialised polyethylene cup with armament screws and a well-placed straight-stem femoral prosthesis with a fixed 32-mm head

b After 10 years, cup wear of a good 1 mm, with consequent craniolateral seam between cement and acetabulum. No migration detected using the EBRA method (see p. 20). Loosening of the cortical bone around the prosthesis as evidence of stress protection

c At autopsy after 11 years, seamlessly integrated straight stem with no osteolysis

d The polyethylene cup is filled with pus and surrounded by thick granulation tissue

e From the ventrally exposed thigh: Extensively necrotising and abscess-forming myositis with disintegration cavity near the gluteal muscles and subsidence abscess distally along the muscle compartments down to the knee

11 years previously following a dislocated femoral neck fracture (Fig. 5.8a). At the 10-year follow-up, the patient had been free of pain, could walk without limping for 1 h and climb stairs without difficulty (Fig. 5.8b). No migration of the cup was detected by the EBRA method 5 years after revision (see also Sect. 3.3.1)

- In a male diabetic with bilateral total hip replacements (W.O., O. 2738), an aseptic stem had to be replaced on one side and the total hip prosthesis on the other after 4 and 3 years, respectively, because of infection with coagulase-negative staphylococci. Nine months later, the patient was admitted to hospital with sepsis, infection of a necrotic toe and arthritis in the shoulder. *S. aureus*, *Proteus*, *E. coli* and enterococci were found. Despite a toe amputation, shoulder aspiration and open shoulder revision on two occasions, and drainage of a recently revised hip that was also affected, the patient died. The autopsy also revealed involvement of the other hip.

5.3 Frequency

5.3.1 Frequency in Our Own Patients

Among our own patients, 13 infections occurred between 1984 and the end of 1996, nine after primary procedures and four after revisions. The average age of the patients at the time of first manifestation of the infection was 74 (46–84) years, and the average period until the infection manifested itself was 34 (1/2–68) months (Fig. 5.1).

To determine the infection rate in our patient population, we restricted ourselves to the predominantly exogenously induced infections occurring during the first 2 years after operation, i.e. early infections and delayed infections. The infection rates for primary operations and revisions were 0.4% and 0.35%, respectively (Fig. 5.2). Analysis of all infections revealed infection rates after primary operations and revisions of 0.8% and 1.2%, respectively.

Because of the lifelong risk of haematogenous infections, the latter figures continue to increase right up to the deaths of the relevant patients (Fig. 5.3). Consequently, they are not particularly meaningful for evaluating the quality of the operation and must be calculated in relation to prosthesis years (see also Sect. 5.1.3). Figures enabling comparisons to be made between studies can therefore be produced only if those infections occurring exclusively during the first 1 or 2 years are compared, or if the infection rate per prosthesis year is stated [1].

5.3.2 Frequency in the Literature

While infection rates as high as 10% were observed in some cases before 1970, infection rates of less than 1% for primary implantations are currently being reported in the literature [6, 9, 14, 29]. A study conducted at the Mayo Clinic [1] reported an infection rate of 0.6% for the first year. From the second year onward, an average of <0.2% infections occur each year. Observations covering a period of many years have produced an annual infection rate of 0.13%. As also illustrated in Fig. 5.1, there is an initially rapid, followed by a gradually ever decreasing, rate of increase in the total infection rates. This trend can be explained partly by the relative rarity of haematogenous infections and partly by the mortality-related gradual decline in patient numbers. Corresponding frequency statistics for revision procedures are not currently available.

5.4 Risk Factors

We make a distinction between patient-specific and general risk factors.

5.4.1 Patient-Specific Risk Factors

- Patient's nutritional and general condition (obesity, cachexia, old age)
- Immune status (immunosuppression after organ transplantation, rarely: HIV, steroid therapy, chemotherapy)
- Systemic illnesses and their sequelae, e.g. diabetes mellitus, renal insufficiency [18], inflammatory rheumatic arthritis (rheumatoid arthritis, psoriatic arthritis etc.)
- Number and type of previous operations
- Soft tissue conditions
- Blood supply (peripheral arterial occlusive disease)
- Any pre-existing or previous infections in the operation area

5.4.2 General Risk Factors

- Sterility, preoperative preparations, draping
- Surgical technique
- Design of the operating theatre (e.g. type of air flow, see also Sect. 5.5.1)
- Absent or inadequate antibiotic prophylaxis

▪ **Clinical Significance.** Whereas many studies have shown that a specific operating theatre design and antibiotic prophylaxis can make a significant and important difference, other investigations have shown only a slight, albeit significant, influence for the other factors.

5.5 Preventive Measures

As a general rule, preventive measures are primarily suitable for avoiding exogenous infections. Haematogenous infections are much more difficult to prevent. While it is possible to clean up chronic infection foci preoperatively, and thus exclude sources of haematogenous dissemination, it is highly unlikely that such measures would reduce the number of haematogenous infections to any significant extent. Inadequate data are available on the benefits of antibiotic prophylaxis during dental procedures [5].

5.5.1 Proven Effective Measures

▪ **Clean Room technique.** If the surgeon operates on the supine patient from the side, the air falling from above in a vertical laminar air flow does not directly enter the wound. With this technique, the operator stands to one side and does not lean across the operation wound, thereby keeping the non-sterile covered part of his head outside the air flow.

▪ **Antibiotic Prophylaxis.** The best results have been recorded for prophylaxis with a first- or second-generation cephalosporin [36]. We administer a dose (1 g i.v.) of cefazolin (Kefzol) immediately before operating and again 6 h later. This provides effective protection primarily against the spectrum of staphylococci and streptococci, but also against certain gram-negative microorganisms (e.g. *E. coli*). These are the pathogens responsible for most prosthesis infections. Many hospitals prefer a single antibiotic dose. Possible alternatives include cefamandole (Mandokef) or cefuroxime (Zinacef). The administration of a glycopeptide (vancomycin, teicoplanin) is only acceptable in hospitals with a prevalence of methicillin-resistant *S. aureus* (MRSA). The development of resistance to glycopeptides as well has already been observed in the USA and Japan [21] and is a consequence of the inappropriate use of these substances.

▪ **Disinfectant.**Alcohol plus iodine (combined in Betaseptic) is suitable for disinfecting the operation area because of its rapid onset of action, lack of resistance and reasonable cost. For the hands we use alcohol with moisturising additives. These combine rapid action with good skin tolerance, are economical and are likewise not associated with resistance.

▪ **Double Gloves.** Even a very small hole can easily be detected by the ring of fluid that forms between the two gloves.

▪ **Drains.** Deep and superficial drains are left in situ for only 2 days. The superficial drains also promote rapid, leak-proof wound closure.

▪ **Dressings.** Unless the wound is dry, it should be sprayed with a disinfectant (in our case Lavasept) whenever the dressing is changed (antiseptic coverage). Important: If the wound secretions penetrate the outermost layer of the dressing, the dressing must be changed immediately in order to prevent germs, including nosocomial pathogens, migrating from the outside into the wound via the resulting wet track.

5.5.2 Presumed Effective Measures

The following two measures are not employed in our hospital:

- Draping with a sterile surgical film: Films protect the skin from mechanical influences and prevent the deeper, non-disinfected horny layers of the epidermis from being exposed by the instruments. Unfortunately, however, skin films tend to come off during the course of the operation, often directly at the skin incision. As a result, the uppermost disinfected skin layers are torn off, placing the germs in the lower layers directly adjacent to the operation wound at the surface.

- Special suits and hoods: The wearing of surgical hoods and suits incorporating an air exhaust system can reduce the number of microorganisms in the operating theatre air.

5.6 Treatment of Infected Total Hip Prostheses

5.6.1 Surgical Management

Our therapeutic regimen is based on the following elements (see also Fig. 5.9):

- Loose prostheses associated with infections must always be replaced.
- During the first 3 months after the start of an infection, the prosthesis can generally be assumed to remain firmly seated. If, when the infection first manifests itself, the infection is thought to have been present for longer than this, then a complete change of prosthesis is indicated (Fig. 3.12a–c).
- We assume that the virulence of the bacteria is of secondary importance for the healing chances of an implant infection, though this applies only if the antibiotic treatment takes account of the specific situation of an implant-associated infection [34]. We have obtained clinical data to support this assumption [19, 20].
- Poor soft tissue conditions are important.
- Exogenous infections predominate during the period of early and delayed manifestation (up to 2 years). Haematogenous infections can occur at any time. Even as a late infection, they can occur acutely with a stable prosthesis and can therefore be treated in the same way as an early infection.
- Even if the soft tissue conditions are poor and the bone is badly affected, the local infection situation can be sufficiently cleared up within 2–4 weeks after implant removal as to allow reimplantation.

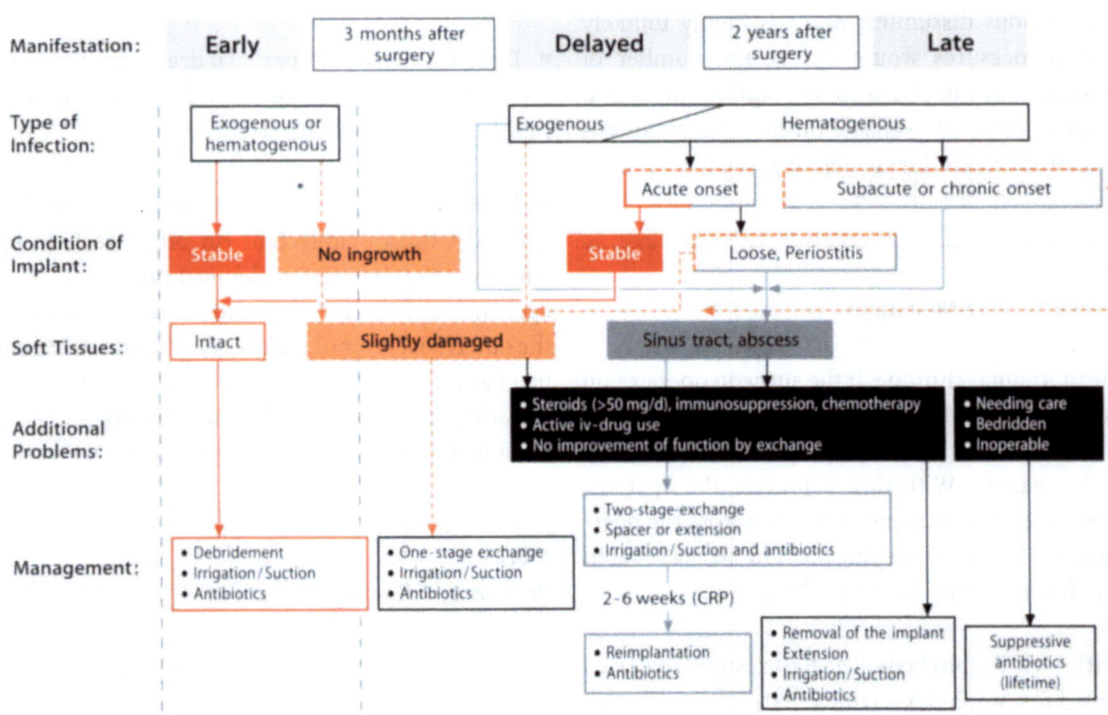

* in case of early infection after partial revision of a cup or a stem, the retained part should be replaced at the time of debridement

Fig. 5.9. Algorithm for the treatment of infections after total hip replacements. This plan cannot be applied without reservation in patients with MRSA or recurrences occurring after adequate previous treatments (see Table 5.1).

Our algorithm (Fig. 5.9) is derived from these guidelines.

In cases of early manifestation of infection (Fig. 5.9), the prosthesis may be considered to be firmly seated. We opt for débridement without exchanging the prosthesis, supplemented by irrigation-suction drainage [15] (Fig. 5.10).

- Case study 1: Débridement and irrigation-suction drainage in early infection. F.E., male, 65 years (O. 9652). Because he suffered from severe pain, this overweight patient underwent total hip replacement on the left side (Fig. 5.10a,b). An extensive haematoma was observed postoperatively. After 13 days the wound started secreting again, though the patient remained afebrile. The leucocyte count was 11,200/µl and the C-reactive protein 9 mg/l. The revision performed on the same day revealed a large haematoma with no definite pus (Fig. 5.4a). All six samples contained *S. aureus*. The patient was given a 2-week antibiotic treatment with flucloxacillin (4 2 g/day i.v.), followed by a 10-week course of oral ciprofloxacin (2 750 mg/day) and rifampicin (2 450 mg/day). Five years later the patient remained free of pain. Flexion/extension was 90°–0°–0°. The patient was able to continue wind-surfing, even during the last 2 years with 2 prostheses (Fig. 5.10c).

A haematogenous prosthesis infection occurring suddenly in connection with sepsis, or at any time after implantation in the presence of a stable prosthetic system with no signs of loosening, may be treated surgically like an early manifesting infection without a change of prosthesis.

In the event of a delayed infection manifestation, or if a late infection occurs in the presence of an already loosened prosthesis, a revision procedure without a change of prosthesis should not be undertaken (Fig. 3.12). In these cases a gradual onset of the infection must be assumed. Even if uncemented prostheses appear stable, some prosthetic components will almost always be in direct contact with infected areas in this situation. The most important decision is whether to replace the prosthesis in a one- or two-stage procedure (Table 5.1). Special risks to be mentioned in this scenario apply to two unfavourable groups, i.e. patients with a recurrence after apparently adequate previous treatment and patients with methicillin-resistant *S. aureus* (MRSA). A two-stage replacement, and possibly a Girdlestone hip procedure depending on the respective microbial status or local

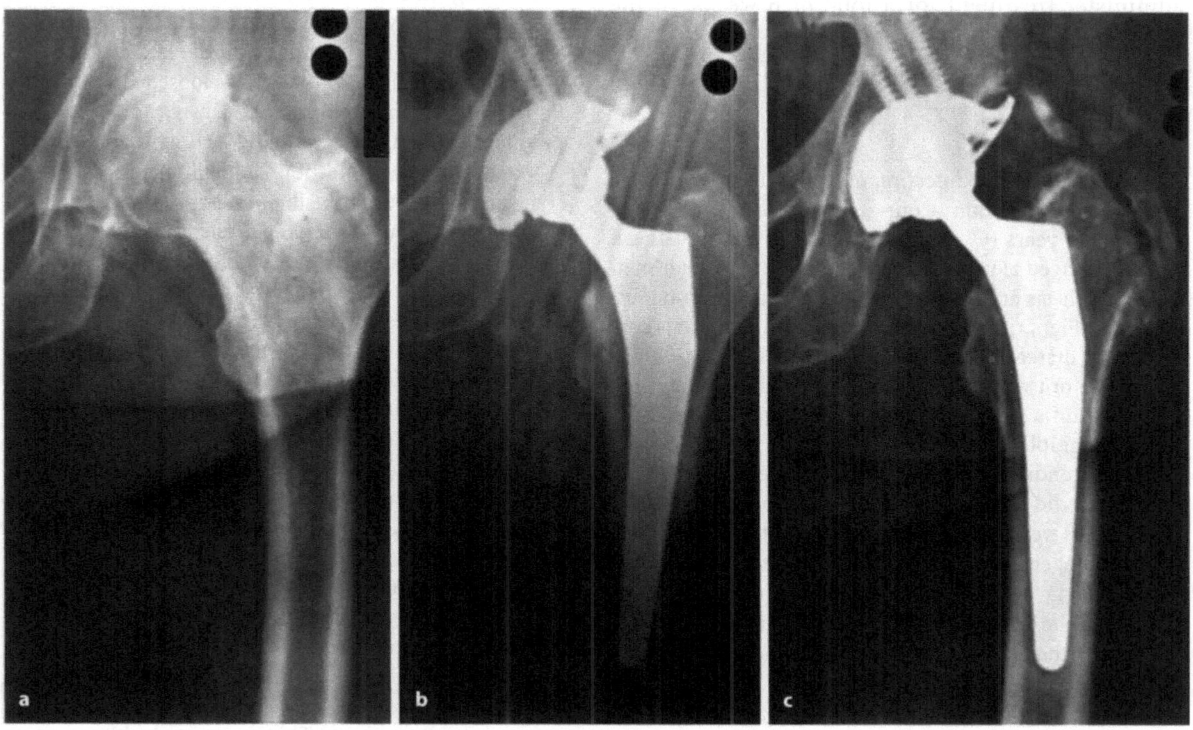

Fig. 5.10a–c. Débridement and irrigation-suction drainage for an early infection (case study 1)
a Mild dysplastic coxarthrosis
b Postoperative view after implantation of a hybrid prosthesis (SL cup, Metasul joint, SL straight stem made from chromium-cobalt)
c 5-year follow-up: No signs of loosening, a few periarticular ossifications

Table 5.1. Indications for one-stage/two-stage prosthesis replacement

One-stage replacement	Two-stage replacement
Soft tissues with minor changes (Fig. 5.4a)	Soft tissues with major changes (Fig. 5.4b)
Recurrent infection after inadequate therapy	Recurrent infection after adequate therapy
	MRSA and other pathogens for which no adequate oral treatment is available (e.g. enterococci).

situation, should be performed for these patients. In order to leave the options open after implant removal, we do not use a spacer in these specific cases during the often protracted intervening period of antibiotic treatment, thereby avoiding the need to take into account the presence of a foreign body.

A one-stage revision is the preferred option for patients with favourable soft tissue conditions. In these cases it is desirable to administer a 2- to 6-week course of targeted antibiotic treatment, based on aspiration findings, prior to the surgical revision. The antibiotic therapy should be discontinued 4 days before the procedure in order to enable a reliable microbiological diagnosis to be made when the prosthesis is changed. If the cultures prove negative, we administer treatment for a total of 6 weeks. In the event of positive cultures, on the other hand, we prescribe an additional 3-month course of treatment postoperatively.

- Case study 2: Late infection or protracted and delayed low-grade infection – one-stage replacement. B.J., female, 80 years (O. 11131; Fig. 5.11). The total prosthesis was changed 21 years after implantation of a metal-metal prosthesis according to M.E. Müller due to cup loosening (Fig. 5.11a,b). The patient suffered symptoms constantly thereafter, experiencing increasing pain despite the use of two sticks. Suspected septic loosening is apparent on a radiograph taken after 3 years (Fig. 5.11c). Arthrography revealed a joint capsule with outpouchings extending to the greater trochanter (Fig. 5.7). The aspirate did not show any bacterial growth. The existing implants were replaced with an antiprotrusio cage lined with allogeneic bone blocks and an SL revision stem inserted via a transfemoral approach (Fig. 5.11d). Although the samples collected at revision also showed no growth, the histological examination did reveal a partly chronic, partly purulent-fibrinous non-specific inflammation. The patient was treated with a 2-week course of intravenous cefazolin (3 × 1 g/day) followed by a 10-week course of oral ciprofloxacin (2 × 750 mg/day) and rifampicin (2 × 450 mg/day). Five years later the 85-year old patient was living independently in her own home and walking without sticks (Fig. 5.11e).

If a two-stage revision is planned for a patient with poor soft tissue conditions, the period before reimplantation of a prosthesis should be made tolerable for the patient. Traditionally, an extension was inserted (Fig. 5.11), but today we generally implant a spacer (see below). In our hospital, the average interval in the two-stage revision between prosthesis removal and reimplantation is 2.5 weeks. Intervals of between 1 and 6 months are cited in the literature [18, 26, 30]. In our experience, such prolonged waiting times are unnecessary, pose a considerable burden on the patient and are associated with substantial additional costs.

- Case study 3: Late infection – two-stage revision with intervening extension. F.E., female, 67 years (O. 5782; Fig. 5.12). At 57 years of age this patient received an uncemented total hip prosthesis on the left side (Endler-Zweymüller). Eight years later, the loosened cup was replaced by a cemented implant. During this procedure cement entered the acetabulum. Three years later, the patient's general condition suddenly deteriorated and she showed distinct swelling and abnormal adduction of the left hip, suggesting the presence of a septic status (Fig. 5.12a,b). During removal of the prosthesis, approximately 1 l of pus (*S. aureus*) was evacuated from the implant bed and lesser pelvis (Fig. 5.12c,d). After 5 days of irrigation-suction drainage and with insertion of an extension, conditions returned to normal within 2 weeks, at which point a new prosthesis was implanted (Fig. 5.12e). Antibiotics were administered according to Table 5.2. The patient has been free of infection for 5 years and is hampered by general muscle weakness of the left leg (Fig. 5.12f).

- Case study 4: Late infection – two-stage revision with intervening spacer. S.S., female, 71 years (O. 19229; Fig. 5.13). Shaft perforation occurred during the replacement of a prosthesis that had been inserted 12 years previously. Somewhat later, a fatigue fracture occurred under the inserted short prosthesis. This was treated with a cemented long-stem prosthesis and a concurrently inserted plate. Residual pain became worse during the following 6 years and ended with the outbreak of a fistula six months before hospitalisation. In view of the very sub-

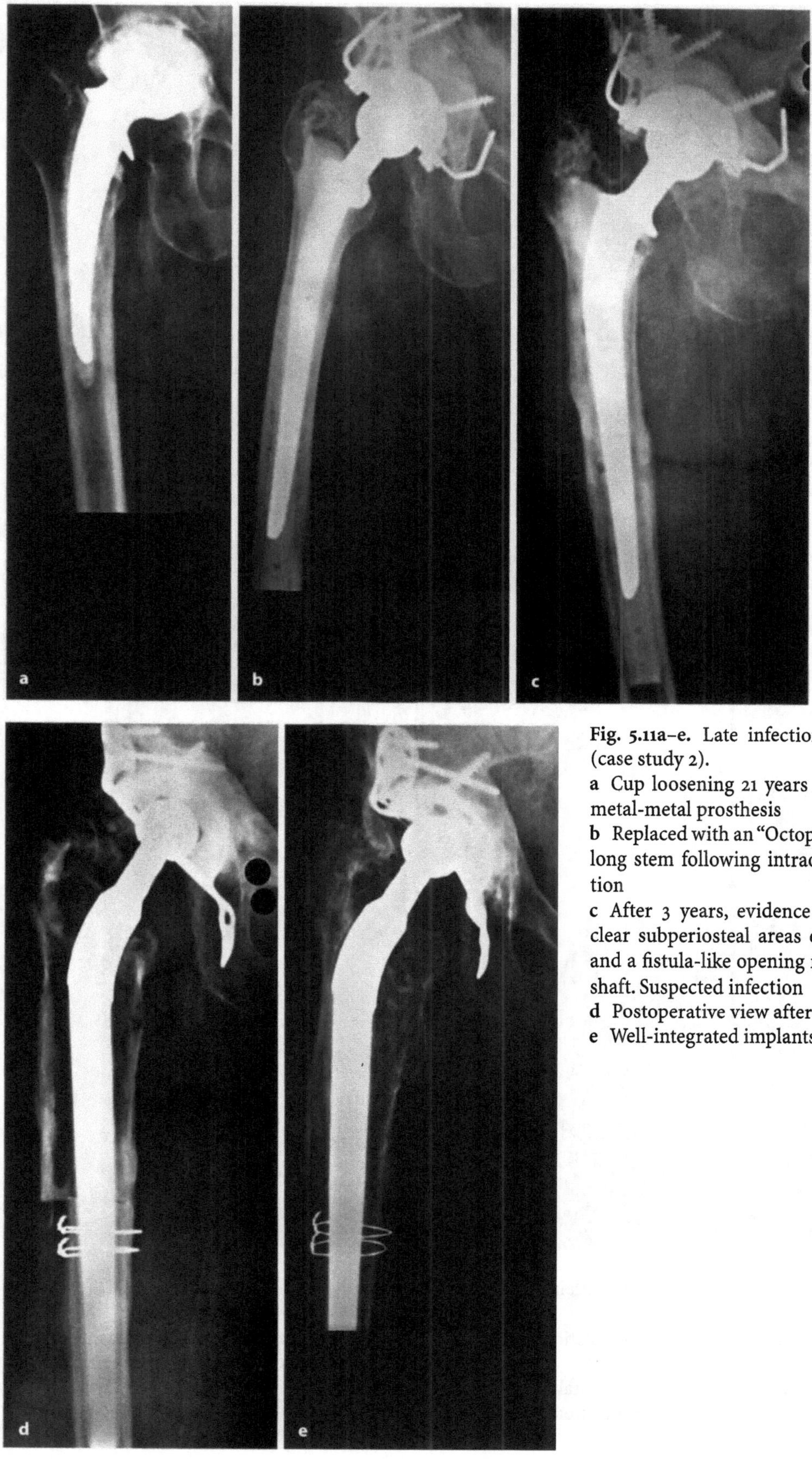

Fig. 5.11a–e. Late infection – one-stage revision (case study 2).

a Cup loosening 21 years after implantation of a metal-metal prosthesis

b Replaced with an "Octopus" cup and a cemented long stem following intraoperative shaft perforation

c After 3 years, evidence of cup loosening and clear subperiosteal areas of new bone formation and a fistula-like opening medially-distally on the shaft. Suspected infection

d Postoperative view after transfemoral revision

e Well-integrated implants 5 years later

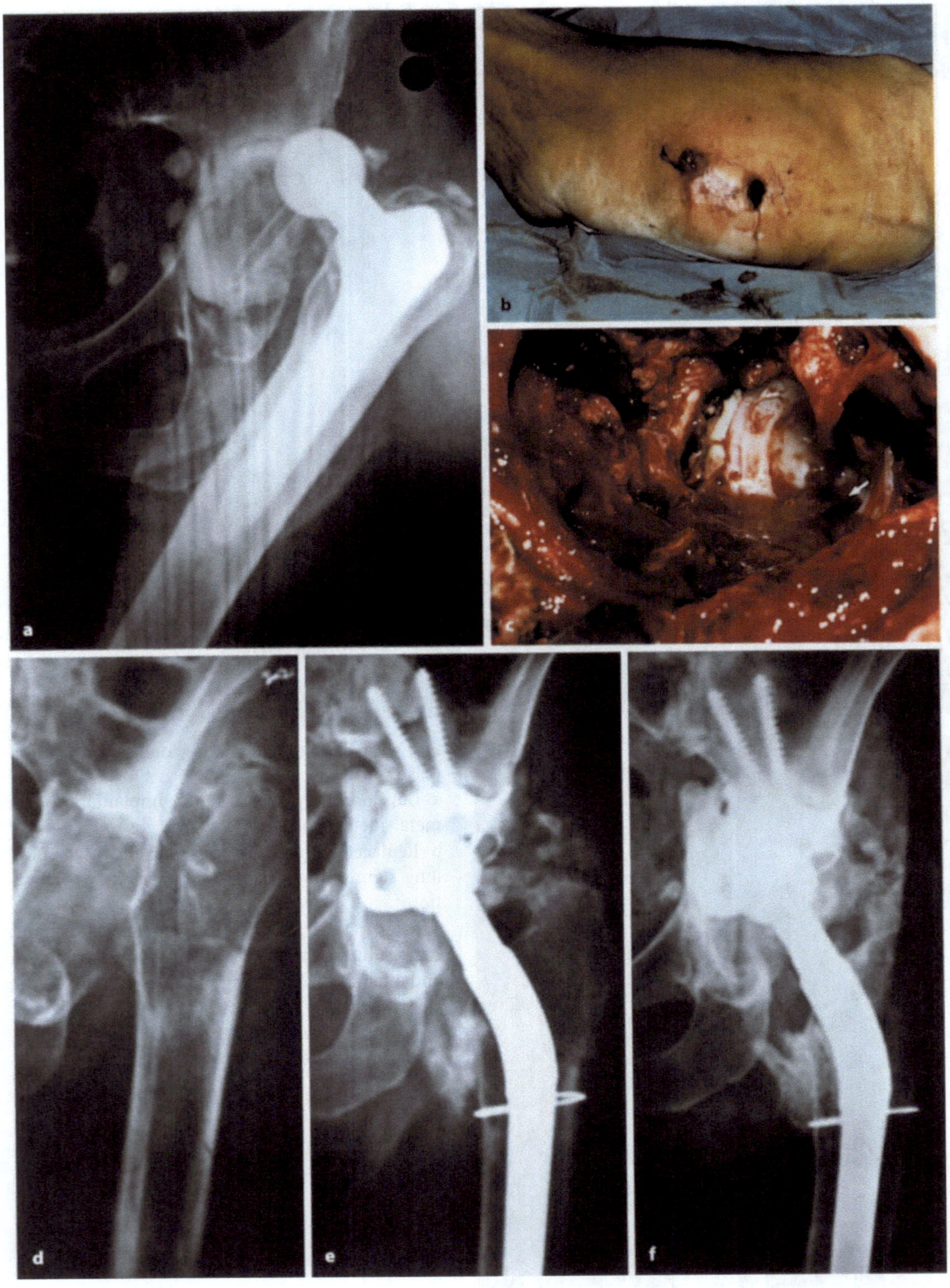

Fig. 5.12a–f. Late infection – two-stage revision with interim extension (case study 3)

a Septic dislocation in connection with accumulation of pus in the greatly dilated joint

b Penetrating double fistula on admission to hospital

c Acetabular component surrounded by granulation tissue. Pus originating from an intrapelvic abscess flows out of a drilled hole in the acetabular floor (*arrow*)

d Temporary Girdlestone situation with extension

e Reimplantation of an acetabular reinforcement ring with shortening and an SL revision stem

f Check radiograph after 3 years with good integration

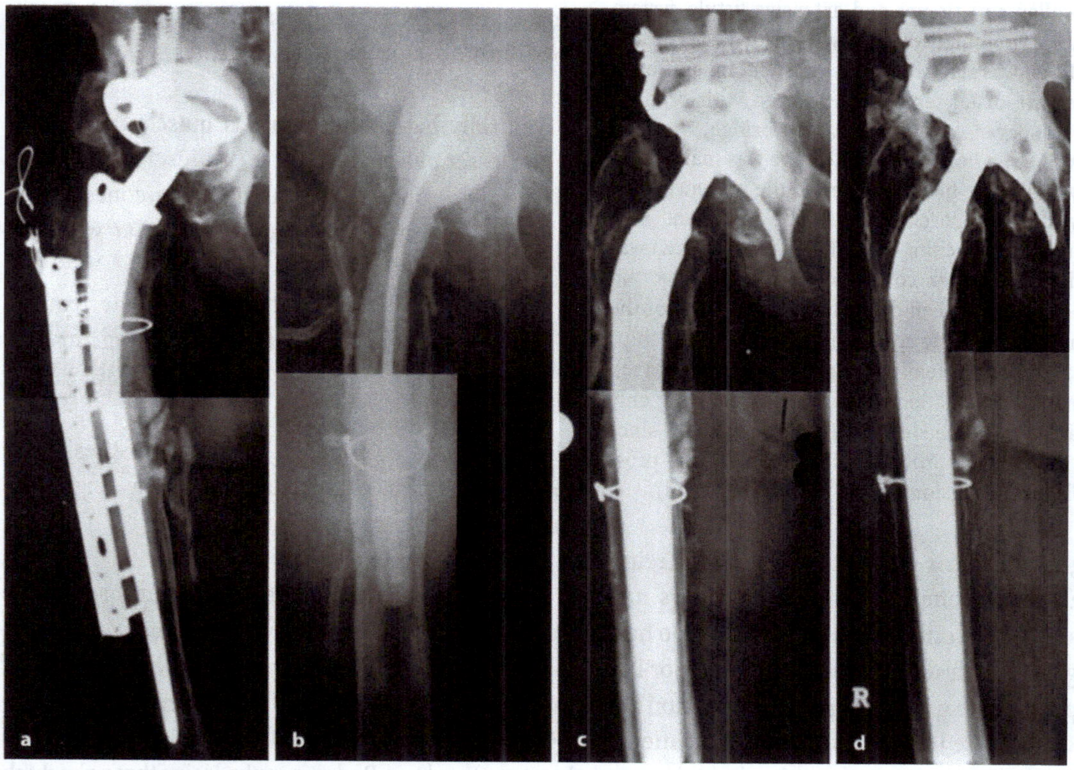

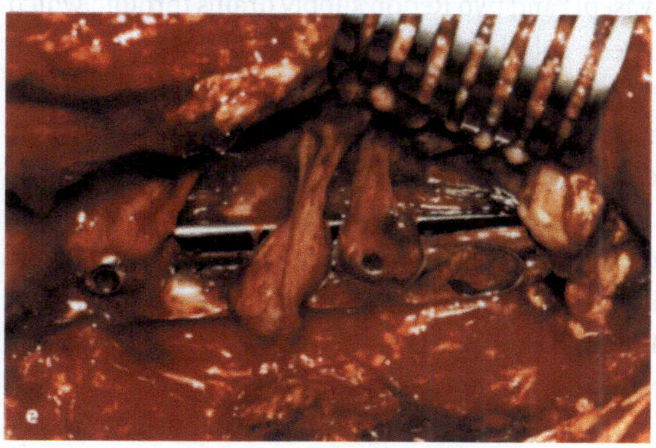

Fig. 5.13a–f. Late infection – two-stage revision with spacer. (case study 4)

a Preoperative situation with trochanteric nonunion, loose acetabular reinforcement ring and cement that has leaked from the shaft medially

b The spacer inserted between the two stages is provided with a ball-shaped tip (see also Fig. 5.15) and inserted into the reamed acetabulum. It is inserted loosely into the distal end of the medullary cavity, and its upper edge is supported by a collar

c Antiprotrusio cage and SL revision stem immediately after reimplantation

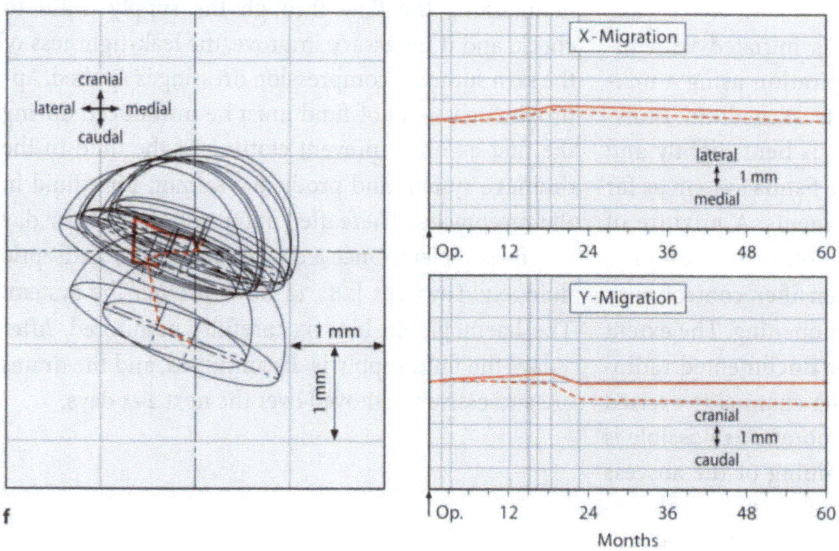

d 5-year follow-up. Seamless remodelling of the bone around the antiprotrusio cage. The osteoporosis of the diaphysis has increased around the shaft

e Intraoperative findings during implant removal: Prosthesis bed with a large quantity of purulent granulation tissue

f Analysis of cup migration by the EBRA method (see also Sect. 3.3.1). No significant migration of the head or cup centre detected over a period of 4.8 years. The nine measurements of the cup centre oscillate around a zero position stantial implants, widely disseminated cement (Fig. 5.13a), swollen soft tissues and extensive fistula system (Fig. 5.13e), a two-stage revision was performed. The foreign material was removed via a transfemoral approach and, after the distal femur was secured with cerclage wiring, a spacer was inserted to bridge the gap (Fig. 5.13b). Irrigation-suction drainage was maintained for 3 days. All three biopsies revealed the presence of β-haemolytic streptococci. As antibiotic treatment, a 4-week course of penicillin (20 million units/day i.v.) was followed by a 10-week course of amoxicillin (3 × 750 mg/day orally). Eighteen days after implantation of the spacer, an antiprotrusio cage lined with allogeneic chips and an SL revision stem were reimplanted (Fig. 5.12c). Five years later the patient was satisfied, reporting only slight pain, but still needed to walk with two sticks since she was also having problems with the other hip prosthesis. Flexion/extension was 90°–0°–0° (Fig. 5.13d).

Removing a prosthesis without a subsequent reimplantation (Girdlestone hip) is rare nowadays and represents a solution only if reimplantation is too hazardous, e.g. with high-dose steroid therapy, major immunosuppression (e.g. following transplantation) or active i.v. drug abuse [11]. In other cases, the patient's general situation may suggest that reimplantation can no longer be expected to offer any benefit and a Girdlestone hip is therefore the appropriate solution.

Abstaining from surgical correction, possibly combined with suppressant antibiotic cover and a long-term fistula, may be appropriate for patients in a poor general condition requiring nursing care [16].

5.6.2 Therapeutic Elements

■ **Débridement.** Débridement is initiated with renewed fistula filling or joint aspiration using a mixture of methylene blue and contrast medium. In fistulography, an olive tip cannula is bent slightly and advanced carefully deep into the fistula system as far as possible with rotating movements. A mixture of 50% methylene blue and 50% contrast medium is then injected under image intensifier control with concurrent sealing of the fistula opening. The extent of the cavity system can now be documented radiologically. The blue-stained fistula channel is excised and as much of the abscess membrane as possible is carefully removed. The blue staining of the abscess membrane serves as a guide. In extensive fistula/abscess systems however, the fistula- or joint-filling procedure is often not sufficient for reaching all the corners. The surgeon should also search carefully for possible outliers at the following sites:

- Ventrally below the iliopsoas muscle through to the lesser pelvis
- The area around the acetabular fossa, concealed by the cup, through the medial acetabular wall into the lesser pelvis
- Distal to the lesser trochanter from the femoral medullary cavity out into the surrounding muscles, with or without a connection with the main cavity

The prosthesis is removed and the prosthesis bed carefully cleared of granulation tissue, e.g. with sharp, serrated curettes (Fig. 3. 26a,b).

■ **Irrigation-Suction Drainage.** The purpose of irrigation-suction drainage is to prevent haematoma formation in the large wound cavity following removal of the diffusely bleeding abscess membrane [15] (Fig. 5.14). The wound is liberally irrigated (e.g. with Lavasept) and two Redon supply drains through which Ringer's solution flows into the wound are inserted. Next, two to four thick drains are inserted, distributed across the wound cavity – but not in the immediate vicinity of the supply drains, and all are fixed to the skin. The skin is now closed, with constant irrigation, by apposing both the fascia and skin in a single layer with thick, deep-reaching, monofilament sutures. An additional skin suture is added, the irrigation-suction drainage is switched on and checked for correct functioning. All draining drains are clamped off while maintaining the flow through the supply drain to check, and if necessary improve, the leak-tightness of the skin suture. A compression dressing is applied. Approximately 4–6 l of fluid must be introduced during the first 4–6 h to prevent clotting of the fluid in the drainage system and produce a salmon-pink fluid in the receptacles. Thereafter, about 6 l of fluid per day will be sufficient. Once a day we allow 1 l of antiseptic fluid, e.g. Lavasept [28], to flow through the system. The haemoglobin level is carefully monitored. After 3 days the fluid supply is discontinued, and the drains are successively removed over the next 2–4 days.

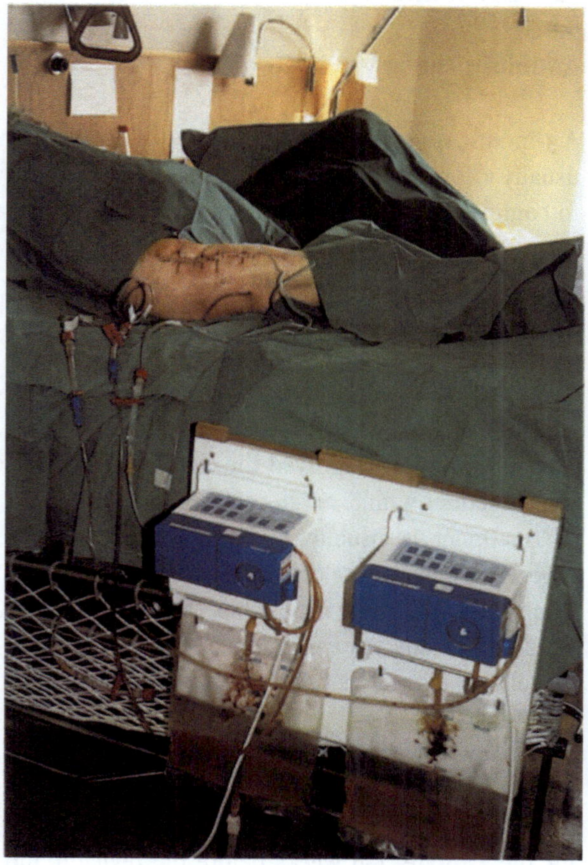

Fig. 5.14. Irrigation-suction drainage. Following débridement and, if applicable, prosthesis removal, irrigation fluid is supplied via two drains and mixes with the haematoma. This fluid is then sucked out by two roller pumps operating with constant suction. This prevents the formation of haematoma-filled cavities

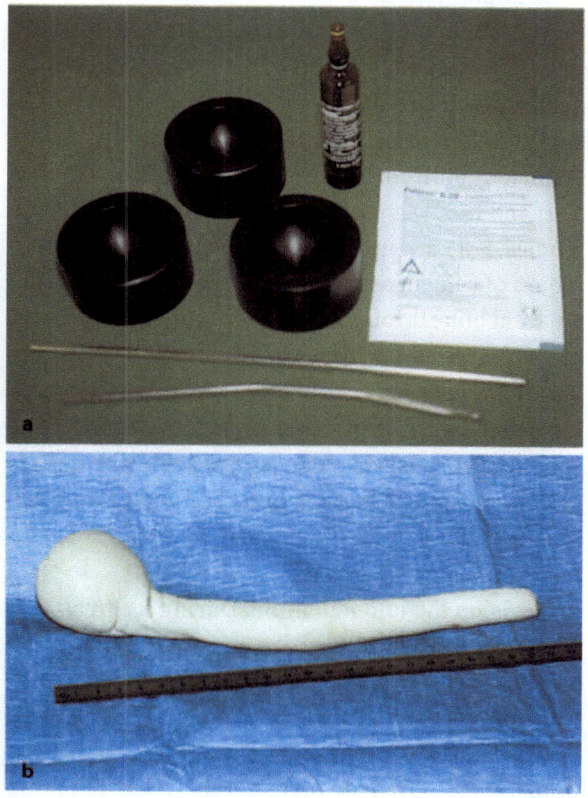

Fig. 5.15a, b. Spacer preparation.
a As a basis we use about three portions of Palacos mixed with gentamicin, fragments of old Ender nails for reinforcement and spherical shells in 2-mm increments for preparing a head of the desired diameter
b The finished spacer is checked for length

■ **Spacer Preparation.** In the two-stage revision, a substantial gap is often left after removal of the prosthesis between the acetabulum and the femoral stump, hence the regular practice, in the past, of inserting an extension. Nowadays, an internal spacer is generally used (Fig. 5.15). The spacer releases gentamicin locally, but has the disadvantage of constituting a foreign body to resistant microorganisms which can hamper the infection control with antibiotics. If an appropriate technique is employed, the patient can, to a certain extent, move freely in bed and be mobilised with little pain. Heel-toe walking is possible in many cases [30]. Neither the acetabulum nor the femoral medullary cavity should be sealed off by the spacer sufficient to block fluid outflow. We ream the cleaned acetabulum conservatively with a not too large reamer (Fig. 3.12c,d). The reamer diameter determines the diameter of the spacer head (Fig. 5.15a). On the femoral side, we measure the lumen with standard trial prostheses. The largest fitting trial prosthesis serves as the model for the diameter of the spacer stem. With the leg extended, the gap between the femoral stump and acetabulum is measured. The selected head shaper (a plastic shell with the appropriate internal diameter for preparing a round spacer head, Fig. 5.15a) is rubbed with Vaseline. The spacer is fashioned from three or so portions of Palacos with gentamicin and reinforced with a piece of Ender nail. A slight shoulder prevents the spacer from sinking too deeply into the shaft. The spacer (Fig. 5.15b) is inserted into the shaft and reduced (Fig. 3.12, Fig. 5.13b).

■ **Reimplantation.** During reimplantation we believe in the importance of striving for both primary and long-term stability. Since the bone stock is often severely damaged by the infective process and the associated loosening, implants such as the Burch-Schneider antiprotrusio cage (Fig. 2.9a, case studies 2, 4) and the Wagner SL revision stem (Fig.2.9a, case studies 2–4) are used particularly frequently. Large blocks of cement are avoided so as not to damage the adjacent bone through the resulting liberation of heat of polymerisation. In younger patients, we fill any large gaps in the weight-bearing area of bone with an autologous graft if possible. Frozen allogeneic bone samples are used in older patients, and for defects away from weight-bearing bone sections (case studies 2, 4).

■ **Revision in Fluid Retention.** During the treatment of infection, the débridement and antibiotic therapy lead to a marked reduction in local oedema. Not infrequently, however, further accumulations of fluid deep inside the tissues can occur, particularly if the drains are removed too prematurely. If fluid retention is suspected an ultrasound scan can be helpful. To avoid breakthrough to the outside and thus a threatened superinfection, the hip must be surgically drained again and a compression dressing applied. The drains may be removed completely 4 days, at the earliest, after insertion.

■ **Reimplantation Long After a Girdlestone Hip.** After living with a Girdlestone situation [7] for many years, some patients occasionally request reimplantation of an implant. Provided any infection has cleared up and hip function remains poor, this is possible in principle if the pelvitrochanteric muscles are adequately preserved [7, 16]. However, compared with a reimplantation as part of a two-stage prosthesis replacement with an interval of just 2–4 weeks, this is a much more radical operation in which complete leg length matching cannot be guaranteed, and the patient is usually left with a limp.

We have abided by the above therapeutic regimen in nearly all cases bar one (disarticulation with a pre-existing femoral stump, Table 5.4). As the results show, this regimen (Fig. 5.5) is an appropriate solution for the successful management of infections.

5.6.3 Antibiotic Therapy

A 3-month, resistance-matched course of antibiotics, usually a combination therapy, should be prescribed to complement the surgical management of hip implant infections. Certain antibiotics are viewed as standards in combating various important pathogens (Table 5.2). The antibiotic selection should take particular account of those microorganisms that adhere to the implants [implant-associated infections 33, 34, 35] (see also Sect. 5.1.2). These findings in themselves have considerably improved the chances of controlling infections with *S. aureus*.

Treatment is usually initiated parenterally for 2 weeks. If appropriate drugs are available, continuation via the oral route is possible. Otherwise, the use of a "Port-a-cath" system should be considered, since this allows antibiotics to be administered on an outpatient basis [10].

In a one-stage, and occasionally in a two-stage, revision, parenteral antibiotics should generally be started, in the event of a positive bacteriology result for the aspirate, 2–6 weeks before the revision and then discontinued 4 days before the procedure. A 6-week course is indicated if the bacteriology result is negative, and a 3-month course in the event of a positive result.

■ **Definition of Cure.** We consider a patient to be cured if the CRP and leucocyte count have returned to normal and the patient is apyrexial and free of symptoms. There should be no more local signs of inflammation (excessive warmth, swelling, fistula). Recurrences can occur at any time, but are particularly frequent during the first 2 years. We therefore require a follow-up period of at least 2 years before confirming that the patient is cured [34].

Table 5.2. Systemic antimicrobial treatment of the most common pathogens causing orthopaedic/trauma-related implant infections*

Pathogen	Drug	Dosage[b]/administration route	
Staphylococcus aureus or coagulase-negative staphylococci			
Methicillin-sensitive	Nafcillin or flucloxacillin	4×2 g/day	i.v.
	+ Rifampicin	2×450 mg/day	Oral
	× 2 weeks, followed by		
	Ciprofloxacin	2×750 mg/day	Oral[a]
	+ Rifampicin	2×450 mg/day	Oral[a]
Methicillin-resistant	Vancomycin	2×1 g/day	i.v.
	+ Rifampicin	2×450 mg/day	Oral
	× 2 weeks, followed by		
	Ciprofloxacin	2×750 mg/day	Oral[a]
	Or fusidic acid	3×500 mg/day	Oral[a]
	Or teicoplanin	400 mg/day	i.v.
	Or co-trimoxazole	3–4 tabs. forte/day	Oral[a]
	+ Rifampicin	2×450 mg/day	Oral[a]
Streptococcus spp.	Penicillin G	4×5 mill. IU/day	i.v.
	× 4 weeks, followed by		
	Amoxicillin	3×750 mg/day	Oral[a]
Anaerobes	Clindamycin	4×600 mg/day	i.v.
	× 2–4 weeks, followed by		
	Clindamycin	4×300 mg/day	Oral[a]
Quinolone-sensitive gram-negative bacilli (excluding Pseudomonas aeruginosa)	Ciprofloxacin	2 750 mg/day	Oral[a]
Pseudomonas aeruginosa	Ceftazidim or cefepime	3×2g/day	i.v.
	+ Tobramycin 2–4 weeks, followed by	based on clearance	i.v.
	Ciprofloxacin	2×750 mg/day	Oral[a]
Mixed flora	Imipenem	2×750 mg/day	i.v.
	× 2–4 weeks, followed by various treatments, depending on the results of resistance testing		

* The sensitivity of the microorganisms must be confirmed by resistance testing.

[a] Duration: At least 3 months or longer, up to 1 month after normalisation of the clinical signs of infection and laboratory results.

[b] Dosage stated for patients with normal kidney and liver function. Quinolones should not be used for infections with methicillin-resistant S. aureus because of the risk of resistance development, which occurs frequently.

5.6.4 Our Own Results

■ **Patients.** During the period from 1984 to 1996, we treated a total of 38 patients with infected hip prostheses (Fig. 5.16). Thirteen cases originated from our own patient population (nine primary operations, four revisions; six women and seven men). 25 hips (12 primary operations, 13 revisions; ten women and 15 men) were referrals. The average age at the time of infection was 70 (44–84) years, and there were 11 early, six delayed and 21 late infections. The infection occurred, on average, 4.5 years (1 week to 16 years) after the hip operation. Given the differing origins of the patients, a variety of prosthesis types were involved.

■ **Pathogen Spectrum.** We found 27 monoinfections and nine mixed infections (Table 5.3). *S. aureus* was detected in 21 cases. No pathogen was detected in two cases (suspected infections according to Sect. 5.1.6). We did not encounter any cases of methicillin-resist-

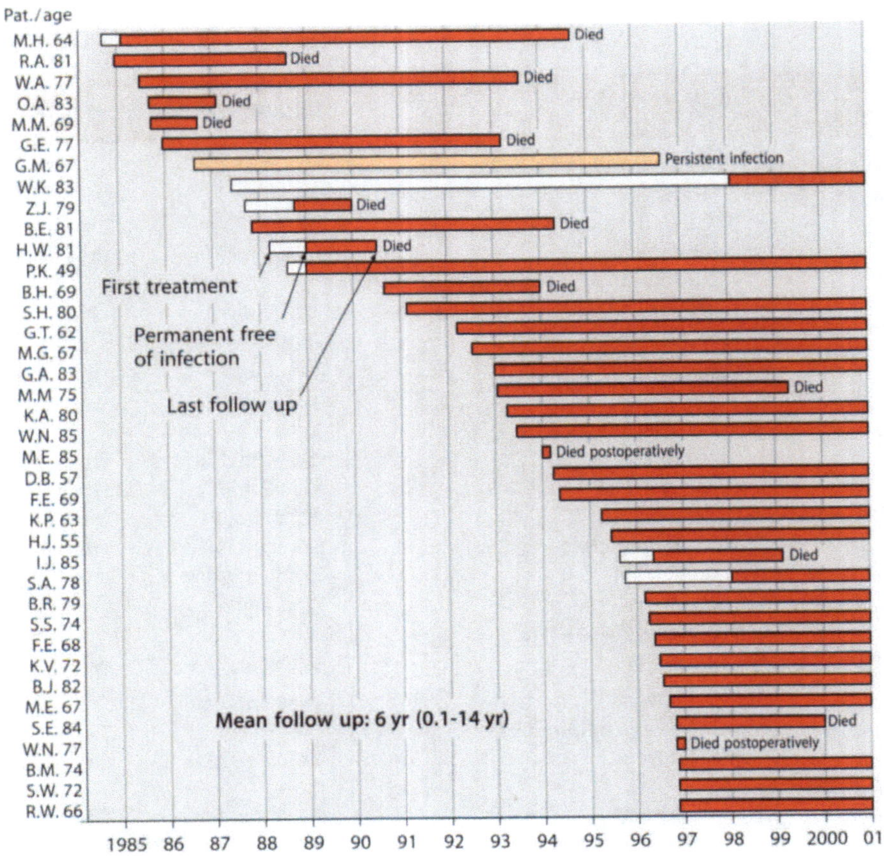

Fig. 5.16. Therapeutic success in total hip prosthesis infections. All cases treated in our hospital during the period 1984–1996 are included (n=38), listed chronologically and up-dated to the end of 2000. A *solid red bar* signifies an infection-free interval from the start of treatment to the final checkpoint (follow-up appointment, written or telephone query or death). A *white bar* signifies a period of one or more recurrences during the interval between the start of treatment and the start of the red bar. A *pink bar* signifies a persistent infection. Deaths connected with treatment are identified as such (died postoperatively)

Table 5.3. Pathogen spectrum, subdivided according to in-house (n=13) and external cases (n=25)

	In-house	Referred
Monoinfections		
S. aureus	7	7
β-haemolytic streptococci	2	2
Coagulase-negative staphylococci	–	3
Enterobacter faecalis	1	–
Enterococci	2	1
Salmonella heidelbergii	–	1
Staphylococcus xylosus	–	1
Other streptococci	–	1
Mixed infections		
S. aureus + β-haem. streptococci	–	2
+ Pseudomonas aeruginos	–	2
+ Proteus + enterococci	–	1
+ Enterobacter sakazakii	–	1
+ Micrococcus luteus	–	1
Enterococci + Morganella morganii	1	–
No microorganism detected	–	2
Total	13	25

ant staphylococci (MRSA) at the start of our treatment. One instance of *Salmonella heidelbergii* was observed in a late infection after sepsis.

In our own infection cases we analysed the pathogens after their appearance. In early infections (n=4) we detected three cases of *S. aureus* and one case of *Enterobacter faecalis*. *S. aureus* and β-haemolytic streptococci, respectively, were detected in the two patients with delayed first manifestation. The latter patient was almost certainly suffering from a haematogenous infection. In the patients with a late first manifestation (n=7), we detected three cases of *S. aureus*, two of enterococci, one of enterococci with *Morganella morganii* and one case of β-haemolytic streptococci. The antibiotics were definitively selected on the basis of the results of resistance testing (Table 5.2), which were generally available 3 days after operation.

▪ **Duration of Hospitalisation, Number of Operations.** On average, 1.3 hospital stays and two operations were needed to resolve the prosthesis infections. The average total duration of hospitalisation was 2.2 (0.5–4) months. While the comparison of patients who had *S. aureus* infections with patients who had other germs did not reveal any significant differences for the aforementioned parameters, 77% in the former category were cured after the first hospitalisation, compared with just 63% in the latter group.

▪ **Follow-up.** Of the 38 patients, we followed up 28 regularly and three on a partial basis. Seven patients died without any signs of infection during the follow-up period.

▪ **Infection Resolution.** Of the 38 infections treated, 34 resolved completely during the review period (Fig. 5.16). Two patients with considerable co-morbidity died during the postoperative phase, one 4 days after prosthesis removal (W.N.), the other a few days after reimplantation (M.E.). In one patient, the infection was only cured after three treatments (S.A.). A persistent infection, which was still present at the end of the study period (β-haemolytic streptococci and *S. aureus*), occurred in just one patient (G.M.), who declined further treatments. This resulted in a success rate of 89.5% for all patients, if the postoperative deaths are considered as failures. On the basis of infection resolution alone, we achieved a success rate of 94.5%. After the first stay in hospital, 27 patients (71%) were free of infection, while nine patients (26%) had to be admitted to hospital a second time. The surgical measures were in line with the therapeutic strategy presented above and are summarised in Table 5.4. A two-stage revision had to be performed secondarily following a recurrence in two cases, in one case after 2 years (S.A.) and in one case secondarily following recurrent loosening after 8 years and a fistula after 10 years (W.K.). Only one patient required three hospital admissions in order to achieve definitive resolution of the infection. All patients subsequently remained free of any signs of infection for an average follow-up period of 6 (0.1–14) years.

▪ **Clinical Results.** We checked the results in respect of pain and walking ability. An improvement in walking ability is often hampered by the very protracted nature of the event and the numerous preceding operations. The following findings were recorded at the

Table 5.4. Therapeutic measures, 1984–1996. The different treatments used in the external cases is reflected in the wide variety of preoperative scenarios [4]

Infected total hip prostheses	In-house	Referred	Total
Revision without replacement	6	–	6
One-stage replacement of prosthesis	1	6	7
Two-stage replacement of prosthesis	6	11	17
Prosthesis removal		1	1
Infection revision for Girdlestone hip		4	4
Disarticulation		1	1
Reimplantation nach Girdlestone-Hüfte		2	2
Total	13	25	38

final follow-up of the 34 patients with a resolved infection:

- Pain relief was achieved in most patients, 59% experiencing no pain at all and 26% slight pain. 12% were suffering from moderate pain and 3% from severe pain.
- Walking ability was considerably restricted in a good quarter of cases. 32% of patients were able to walk well. Walking ability was slightly restricted in 26%, moderately restricted in 15% and severely restricted in 21% of patients. Two patients were unable to walk.

  Specific technical problems:
- During the reimplantation of a cementless SL revision prosthesis, a supracondylar femoral fracture occurred below the prosthesis tip during reaming of the taper. This required the insertion of a condylar plate (Fig. 7.10). We have since introduced the practice of grasping the femoral diaphysis where the taper is reamed with two reduction forceps with prongs applied transmuscularly. This prevents any torsional force from acting on the metaphysis.
- One SL revision stem had to be replaced with a cemented long-stem prosthesis in a patient weighing over 100 kg (Fig. 3.12).
- One incompletely cemented long-stem prosthesis subsided and was successfully replaced by an SL revision implant. However, problems with fragment healing after a transfemoral approach resulted in a dorsal hip dislocation, which required revision (Fig. 6.2).
- In one patient with nonunion after a flip osteotomy of the greater trochanter and a previous Girdlestone hip procedure for MRSA infection, considerable difficulties were encountered during reimplantation in the attempt to put back the ventrally displaced greater trochanter. Consequently, an autologous bone graft and a second fixation were additionally required (Fig. 8.11).

5.6.5 Comparison with Published Data

Infection Classification. Certain deviations from our own concept can be found in the literature. Some authors attach great importance to the type of pathogen. Thus, a two-stage procedure is recommended for infections with *S. aureus* [6, 12, 13]. Since the introduction of rifampicin for the treatment of *S. aureus*, this germ no longer poses an increased risk for our patients and we therefore consider that a two-stage operation is no longer necessary provided the soft tissues are not greatly changed. Occasionally, antibiotic therapy without surgery is mentioned as a possible treatment option [6], although we cannot support this suggestion, because an operative inspection is required in order to be able to assess the local conditions. Otherwise the infection cannot be properly evaluated. We therefore consider antibiotic treatment without débridement to be inadequate.

The literature confirms the significantly increased risk of an implant infection in HIV-infected patients and intravenous drug users [11].

■ **Cure Rates.** The success rates cited in the literature for the resolution of total hip prosthesis infections range from 33% to 100% for a one-stage revision [6]. Figures between 13% and 100% are given for the two-stage revision [6]. However, direct comparison is not possible because the evaluation criteria for the success rates differ very widely. It is very important, therefore, to check the results of one's own revisions with care.

■ **Clinical Results.** The results achieved for pain and walking ability are inferior to those reported after revisions for aseptic loosening [2].

5.7 Concluding Remarks

Infection after a total hip replacement continues to pose a serious problem. Whereas, in the early days of prosthetics, infections frequently ended with a Girdlestone hip, most of today's infections can be cured, enabling the patient to retain a properly functioning hip implant. The following significant advances have been made over the years:

- Subdivision into exogenous and haematogenous infections
- Systematic bacteriological and histological tissue investigation
- Clear definition of the various possible infection states

- Definition and antibiotic treatment of implant-associated infections
- Synergistic use of surgical and medical treatment
- Systematic débridement
- Introduction of the spacer in surgical treatment

The therapeutic algorithm presented in Fig. 5.9 should help surgeons find the optimal treatment. But it also illustrates the importance of providing such highly complex treatment exclusively in centres with experience in this field.

References

1. Berbari EF, Hanssen AD, Duffy MC, Steckelberg JM, Ilstrup DM, Harmsen WS, Osmon DR (1998) Risk factors for prosthetic joint infection: case control study. Clin Infect Dis 27: 1247–1254
2. Brunazzi M, Mcharo C, Ochsner PE (1996) Hüfttotalprothesenwechsel – was erwartet den Patienten? Schweiz Med Wochenschr 126: 2013–2020
3. Cheung A, Lachiewicz P, Renner J (1997) The role of aspiration and contrast-enhanced arthrography in evaluating the uncemented hip arthroplasty. AJR 168: 1305–1309
4. Corstens FHM, Meer JWM van der (1999) Nuclear medicine's role in infection and inflammation. Lancet 354: 765–770
5. Deacon JM, Pagliaro AJ, Zelicof SB, Horowitz HW (1998) Prophylactic use of antibiotics for procedures after total joint replacement. J Bone Joint Surg 78 (A): 1755–1770
6. Elke R, Zimmerli W, Morscher E (1997) Das infizierte Implantat und die septische Lockerung. In: Die Hüfte. Enke, Stuttgart, S 274–283
7. Engelbrecht E, Siegel A, Kappus M (1995) Totale Hüftendoprothese nach Resektions-arthroplastik. Orthopäde 24: 344–352
8. Fitzgerald R (1995) Diagnosis and management of the infected hip prostheses. Orthopedics 18: 833–835
9. Hauser R, Berchtold W, Schreiber A (1996) Incidence of deep sepsis in uncemented total hip arthroplasty using clean air facility as a function of antibiotic prophylaxis. Bull Hosp Jt Dis 54: 175–179
10. Hunger T, Gösele A, Ochsner PE (1993) Implantierbares Venenkathetersystem zur ambulanten Langzeit-Antibiotikatherapie bei chronischer Osteomyelitis. Hefte Unfallchir 230: 1032–1035
11. Lehman CR, Ries MD, Paiement GD, Davidson AB (2001) Infection after total joint arthroplasty in patients with human immunodeficiency virus or intraveneous drug use. J Arthroplasty 16: 330–335
12. Liebermann J, Callaway G, Salvati E, Pellicci P, Brause B (1994) Treatment of the infected total hip arthroplasty with a two-stage reimplantation protocol. Clin Orthop 301: 205–212
13. Morscher E, Herzog R, Babst R, Zimmerli W (1995) Management of infected hip arthroplasty. Orthop Int 3: 343–351
14. Morscher E, Babst R, Jenny H (1990) Treatment of infected joint arthroplasty. Int Orthop 14: 161–165, 18: 833–835
15. Pfister A, Ochsner PE (1993) Erfahrungen mit geschlossenen Spül-Saug-Drainagen und gleichzeitiger Anwendung eines Antiseptikums. Unfallchirurg 96: 332–340
16. Ochsner PE, Brunazzi M, Picard C (1995) Rettungseingriffe bei chronischem Infekt nach Hüfttotalprothesen. Orthopäde 24: 353–359
17. Ochsner PE, Hauser R, Lotz M (1987) Diagnostik und Therapie der Skelettinfektionen aus orthopädischer Sicht. Praxis 76:532–542
18. Salvati E (1994) Diagnosis and management of the infected hip. Orthopedics 17: 811–814
19. Schafroth MU, Ochsner PE (1999) Does Staphylococcus aureus infection worsen the prognosis for treatment of infected total hip replacement? Eur J Orthop Surg Traumatol 9: 241–244
20. Schafroth MU, Zimmerli W, Ochsner PE (1999) Das infizierte künstliche Hüftgelenk: Möglichkeiten, Verlauf und Resultate der Behandlung. Praxis 88: 2101–2105
21. Smith TL, Pearson ML, Wilcox KR, Cruz C, Lancaster MV et al. (1999) Emergence of vancomycin resistance in *Staphylococcus aureus*. N Engl J Med 340: 493–501
22. Taylor T, Beggs I (1995) Fine needle aspiration in infected hip replacements. Clin Radiol 50: 149–152
23. Tigges S, Stiles R, Roberson J (1994) Appearance of septic hip prostheses on plain radiographs. AJR 163: 377–380
24. Tunney MM, Patrick S, Curran MD, Ramage G, Hanna D, Nixon JR, Gorman SP, Davis RI, Anderson N (1999) Detection of prosthetic hip infection at revision arthroplasty by immunofluorescence microscopy and PCR amplification of the bacterial 16S rRNA gene. J Clin Microbiol 37: 3281–3290
25. Widmer AF, Colombo VE, Gächter A, Thiel G, Zimmerli W (1990) Salmonella infection in total hip replacement: tests to predict the outcome of antimicrobial therapy. Scand J Infect Dis 22: 611–618
26. Wilde A (1994) Management of infected knee and hip prosthesis. Rheumatology 6: 172–176
27. Willenegger H, Roth B (1986) Behandlungstaktik und Spätergebnisse bei Frühinfekt nach Osteosynthese. Unfallchirurgie 12: 241–246
28. Willenegger H, Roth B, Ochsner PE (1995) The return of local antiseptics in surgery. Injury 26: Suppl 1
29. Wroblewski B, Siney P (1993) Charnley low-friction arthroplasty of the hip. Long-term results. Clin Orthop 292: 191–201
30. Younger A, Duncan C, Masri B, McGraw R (1997) The outcome of two-stage arthroplasty using a custom-made interval spacer to treat the infected hip. J Arthroplasty 12: 615–623
31. Zimmerli W (1984) Hämatogener Protheseninfekt beim Menschen und im Tiermodell. Schweiz Med Wochenschr 114: 1756–1757

32. Zimmerli W, Zak O, Vosbeck K (1985) Experimental hematogenous infection of subcutaneously implanted foreign bodies. Scand J Infect Dis 17: 303–310
33. Zimmerli W, Frei R, Widmer AF, Rajacic Z (1994) Microbiological tests to predict treatment outcome in experimental device-related infections due to Staphylococcus aureus. J Antimicrob Chemother 33: 959–967
34. Zimmerli W, Widmer A, Blatter M, Frei R, Ochsner PE (1998) Role of rifampicin for treatment of orthopedic implant-related staphylococcal infections. JAMA 279: 1537–1541
35. Zimmerli W (1999) Prosthetic device infection. In: Root RK et al. (eds) Clinical infectious diseases: a practical approach. Oxford Univ Press, London, pp 801–808
36. Zimmerli W (2000) Antibiotic prophylaxis. In: Rüedi TP et al. (eds) AO principles of fracture management. Thieme, Stuttgart, pp 699–707

Chapter 6

Dislocations After Total Hip Replacement

Gregor Kohler

The minimum information required for describing a dislocation after total hip replacement are the dislocation mechanism, the dislocation position and the time of dislocation after operation. Dislocation is frequently accompanied by impingement, i.e. encroachment of the rim of the acetabular cup against the neck of the femoral implant, which is particularly important in the case of hard bearing couples (metal-metal or ceramic-ceramic). 1.8% of our patients receiving a total hip replacement experienced a dislocation of their implant. The dislocations can be divided into early dislocations (up to the 6th week postoperatively) and late dislocations (after the 6th week). This chronological classification correlates with the formation of the new joint capsule, which is generally completed after 6 weeks.

Over 90% of our patients suffering a dislocation experienced this event as an early dislocation during their stay in hospital. In such cases, this was successfully treated by simple reduction under short-term anaesthesia. Although this prolonged the period of hospitalisation, it did not adversely affect prosthesis life. If dislocation occurs repeatedly, or if a late dislocation is involved, the causes must be sought and rectified. The most common causes are faulty placement of the cup or malrotation of the stem.

To avoid the risk of faulty placement, a standardised, controlled positioning technique is needed during surgery in order to facilitate the control of implant orientation. Alignment rods on insertion instruments facilitate the accurate positioning of the cup. Polyethylene cups with an antidislocation rim are one possible option, but in this case particular care should be taken to avoid impingement.

To minimise the frequency of early dislocation, patients, nursing staff and physiotherapists, not forgetting the doctors responsible for follow-up, must be given precise instruction. Late-occurring internal dislocations are caused by loosening of the prosthesis, associated with stem subsidence and/or tilting of the cup.

Hip dislocation after a total hip replacement is an alarming event both for the patient and surgeon. But what is the next step? Does the surgeon have to perform a revision procedure, or will conservative measures prove sufficient and, if so, what measures are indispensable? Is the remaining life of the implant affected by the dislocation, and what are the possible causes of dislocation? To help answer these questions we decided to investigate the corresponding data for our own patients.

6.1 Definitions, Impingement

6.1.1 Definitions

■ **Dislocation.** Complete loss of the articulating contact between two artificial joint components. Reduction without medical assistance is not usually possible.

The *main directions of dislocation* are posteriorly (in flexion - internal rotation - adduction movements) or anteriorly and laterally (in extension - adduction - external rotation movements). Although dislocations upwards (extension and substantial adduction with axial impact) and downwards (extension, abduction and traction on the leg) are possible in theory, these are rarely encountered in practice.

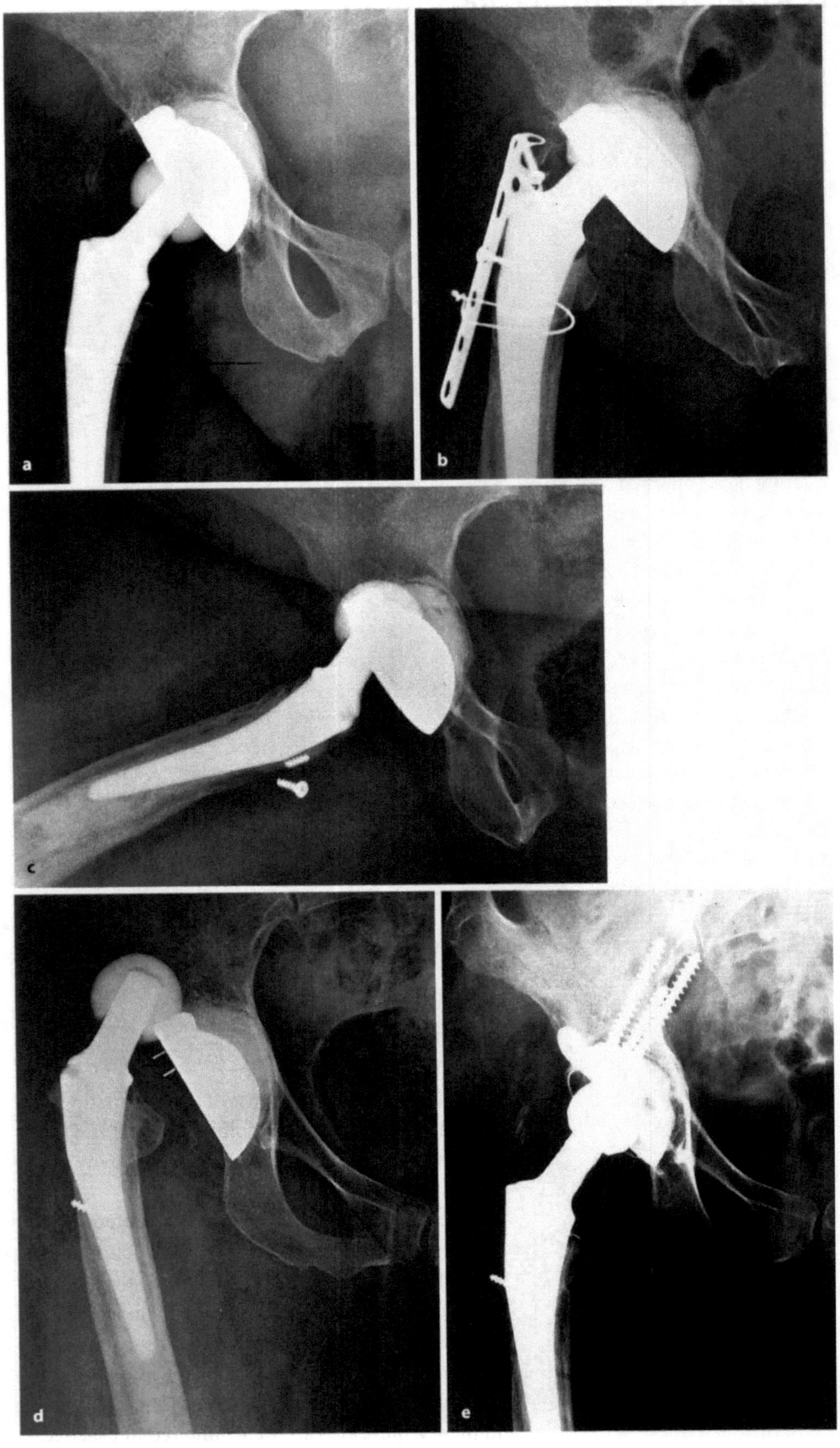
a
b
c
d
e

■ **Dislocation Mechanism.** By dislocation mechanism we mean the analysis of the dislocation event, e.g. dislocation dorsally when the patient stands up from a low chair, or dislocation ventrolaterally while lying in bed with an adducted, extended and externally rotated leg. A distinction has to be made as to whether the dislocation was traumatically induced or occurred without noticeable trauma. In deciding upon the therapeutic measures to be taken, the analysis of the dislocation mechanism is more important than the radiologically apparent dislocation position (Fig. 6.1). Consequently, careful eliciting of the sequence of events leading up to the dislocation is very important.

Unexpected dislocation mechanisms are increasingly encountered, e.g. a distraction of proximal femoral fragments after a transfemoral approach (Fig. 6.2), or an instability due to excessive stretching of the capsule in connection with a hip infection (Fig. 5.12).

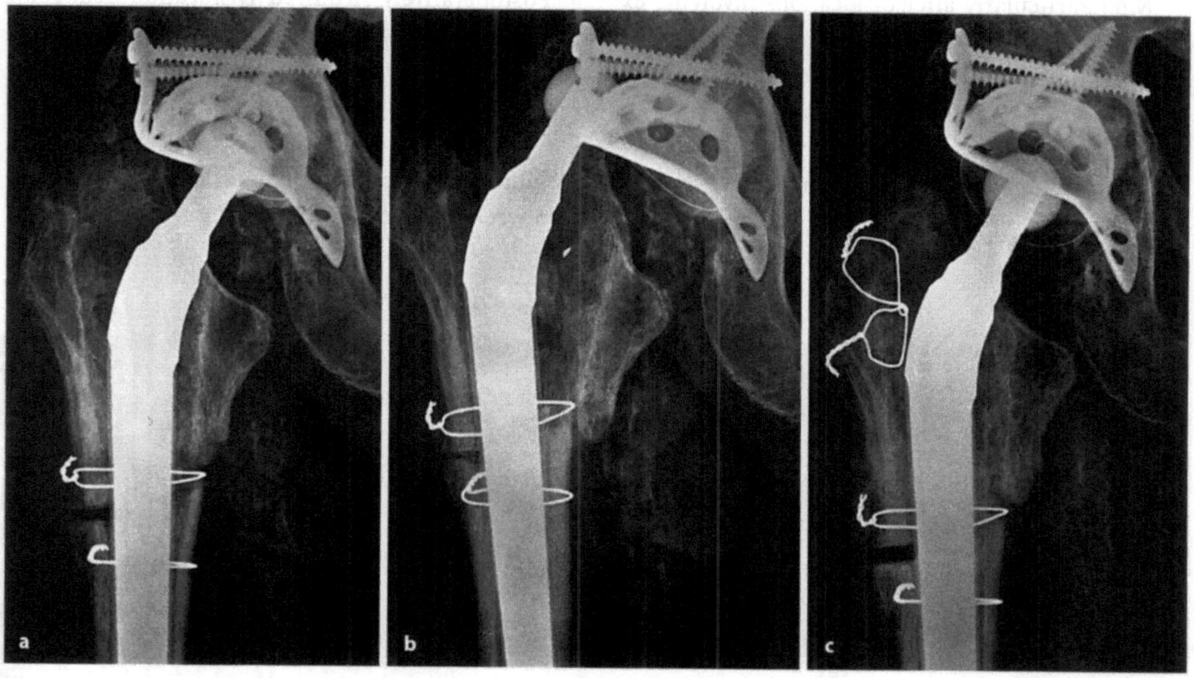

Fig. 6.2a-c. Dorsal dislocation in the presence of an unconsolidated transfemoral approach. B.A., male, 72 years (O.20239)
a Following two revisions for a chronically fistulating THR infection with a transfemoral approach, an antiprotrusio cage and SL revision prosthesis were inserted at reimplantation
b Two weeks postoperatively, the patient suffered a dorsal dislocation when standing up from a low chair. The radiograph shows substantial gaping of the proximal femoral fragments, leaving room for a dislocation despite the preserved dorsal capsule
c Because of repeated subsequent dislocations, a Brunswick cup was inserted during a revision procedure (Fig. 6.7) and cemented into the fixed antiprotrusio cage in a more anteverted position. The two main fragments of the proximal femur were secured together by wire cerclages. Radiograph after 3 months. No further dislocation during the course of the following 2 years

◄───

Fig. 6.1a–e. Differing head position after three dorsal dislocations. F.L., female, 60 years (O.15438). Patient with surgically stiffened lumbar spine
a Six and a half years after total hip replacement (PCA cup, standard straight stem). The cup is too sharply inclined and not anteverted. Internal fixation of the trochanter was subsequently performed to secure the avulsed trochanter
b Two years later a dorsal dislocation occurred following a fall over a cat. Dorsal dislocation position, leg in slight internal rotation and flexed
c Patient stumbles 6 years and 9 months after operation. Dorsocranial dislocation position with flexed, abducted leg
d Three months later. Third dislocation when getting out of bed. This time the head is dislocated in a ventrolateral position. The leg is adducted and externally rotated. Despite this dislocation position, the surgical revision confirmed the dorsal dislocation. The joint capsule was greatly overstretched
e The malposition is corrected by a cup replacement, thereby eliminating the dislocation tendency

■ **Dislocation Position.** The dislocation position describes the position of the head in relation to the cup after dislocation, and the position of the leg as presented on the radiograph. If the head is in a dorsal or dorsolateral position (Fig. 6.1), the leg is forced into an attitude of slight flexion and internal rotation, a position that is unpleasant for the patient and which calls for rapid reduction. If the head is in a ventrolateral position, the leg is loosely extended, shortened and externally rotated, as with a femoral neck fracture.

N.B.: Particularly after dislocations involving extensive capsule resection, the revision of major acetabular defects, or after several recurrences, dorsal dislocation positions become unstable and usually switch, immediately after dislocation, to a dorsolateral head position with external rotation and shortening (Fig. 6.1).

■ **Intraoperative Dislocation Tendency.** During the operation, the surgeon checks whether the hip dislocates during 90° flexion and internal rotation posteriorly, or during extension, adduction and external rotation to an anterolateral position. If such a dislocation tendency is present, certain routine precautions must be taken postoperatively. Since muscle tone is the main determining factor for this dislocation tendency, this test is not very predictive for dislocations occurring postoperatively.

■ **Postoperatively Acquired Dislocation Tendency.** In the case of loosening of the stem or cup, the implant can change to a position that might cause a late dislocation (Figs. 3.12, 6.3, 6.7, 14.2).

■ **Time of Dislocation.** Early dislocations occur up to 6 weeks after operation, during the period when

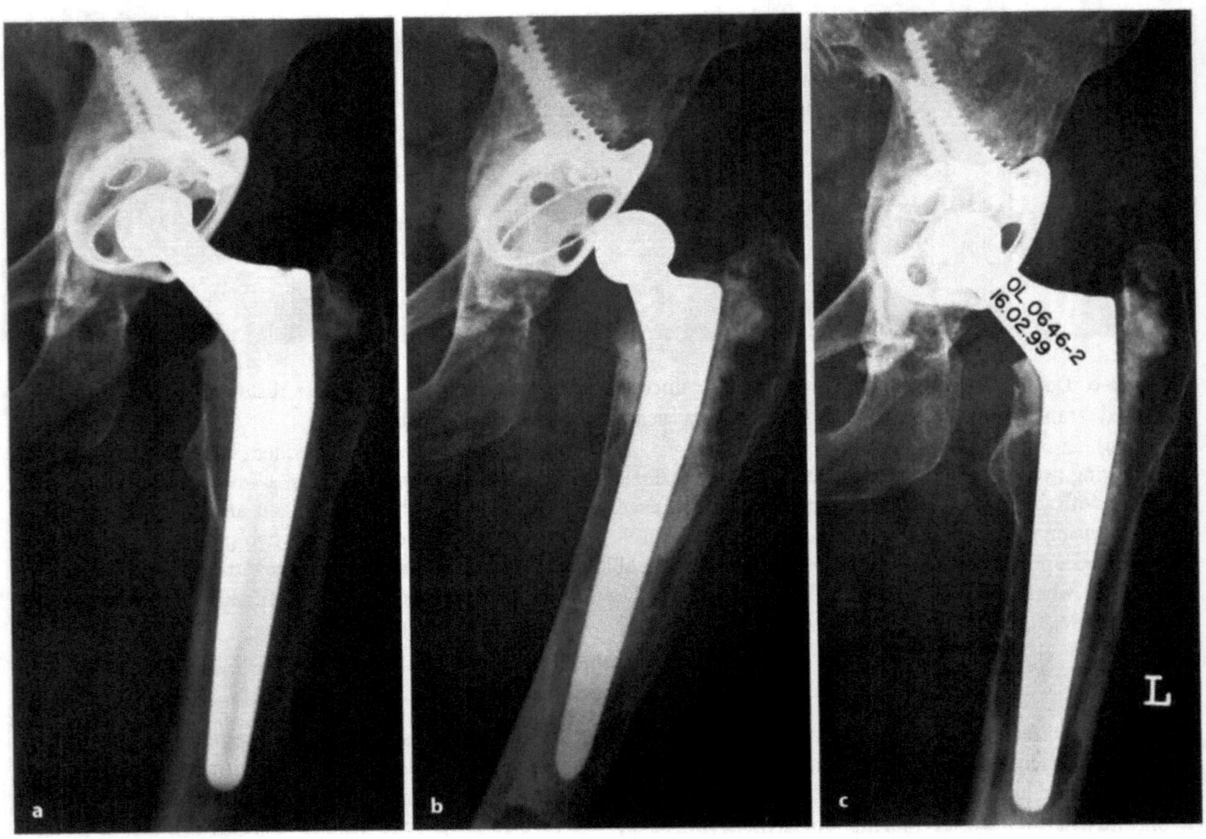

Fig. 6.3a–c. Internal dislocation with stem loosening and retrotorsion. R.A., female, 62 years (O.3904)
a Implantation of an acetabular reinforcement ring and a titanium alloy CDH stem
b Seven years later: patient admitted as an emergency following a dorsal dislocation
c Reduction, substantial stem loosening is discernible. Suspected significant retrotorsion with a very prominent lesser trochanter was confirmed at revision. Also apparent was a hip capsule that had become substantially expanded by granulation tissue

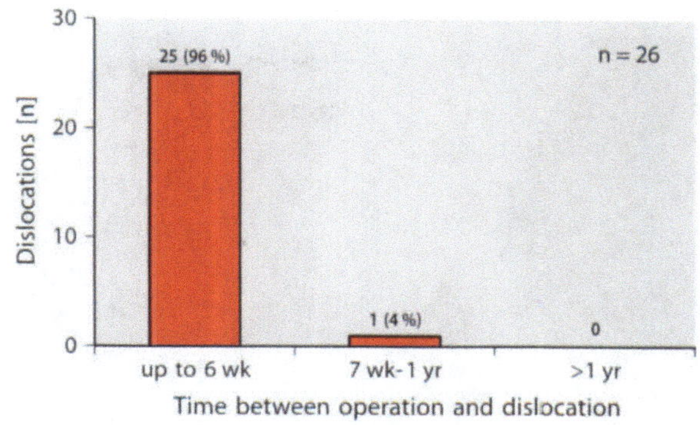

Fig. 6.4. Early and late dislocations. With the exception of one patient, all the dislocations in our population were early, occurring during the first 6 weeks

the new capsule has not yet formed, and late dislocations thereafter. The prognosis is much better for early dislocations than for late dislocations (Fig. 6.4). The former can occur even if the prosthesis is correctly positioned, whereas a faulty implant position is usually present if the latter occurs without any actual trauma. This may have arisen as a result of faulty placement during operation or secondary shifting due to implant loosening (Figs. 6.3, 6.7).

▪ **Subluxation.** During joint movement, the patient experiences a sudden jarring of the joint, occasionally accompanied by temporarily impaired mobility and frequently associated with shooting pains. The head knocks against the cup rim, but does not jump completely out of the cup. By performing a precisely described sequence of movements, the patient can sometimes put the joint back in place. Frequently, the joint reduces itself spontaneously (Fig. 6.5). Alternatively, if the cup is insufficiently anteverted or if retrotorsion occurs through stem loosening, the neck can strike against the cup rim (see also Impingement, Fig. 14.3).

▪ **Internal Implant Dislocation.** Subsidence of a femoral stem can cause the head to lose contact with the cup e.g. as a result of the greater trochanter

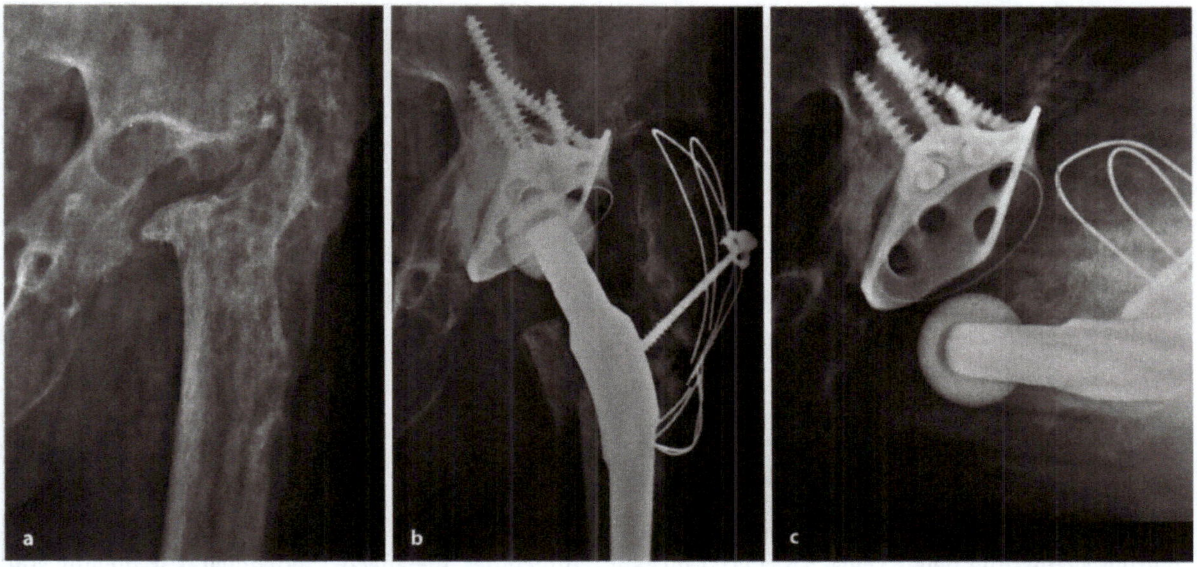

Fig. 6.5a–c. Subluxations after reimplantation 10 years after a Girdlestone hip. B.E., male, 85 years (O.580)
a Girdlestone situation 10 years after revision of an infected total hip replacement. Patient feels very unstable
b Reimplantation of a prosthesis with an acetabular reinforcement ring and SL revision stem. Onset of sciatic paresis with only partial subsequent recovery
c The patient regularly suffered subluxations, as documented in the axial view. Attempted treatment with a Hohmann support was only moderately successful

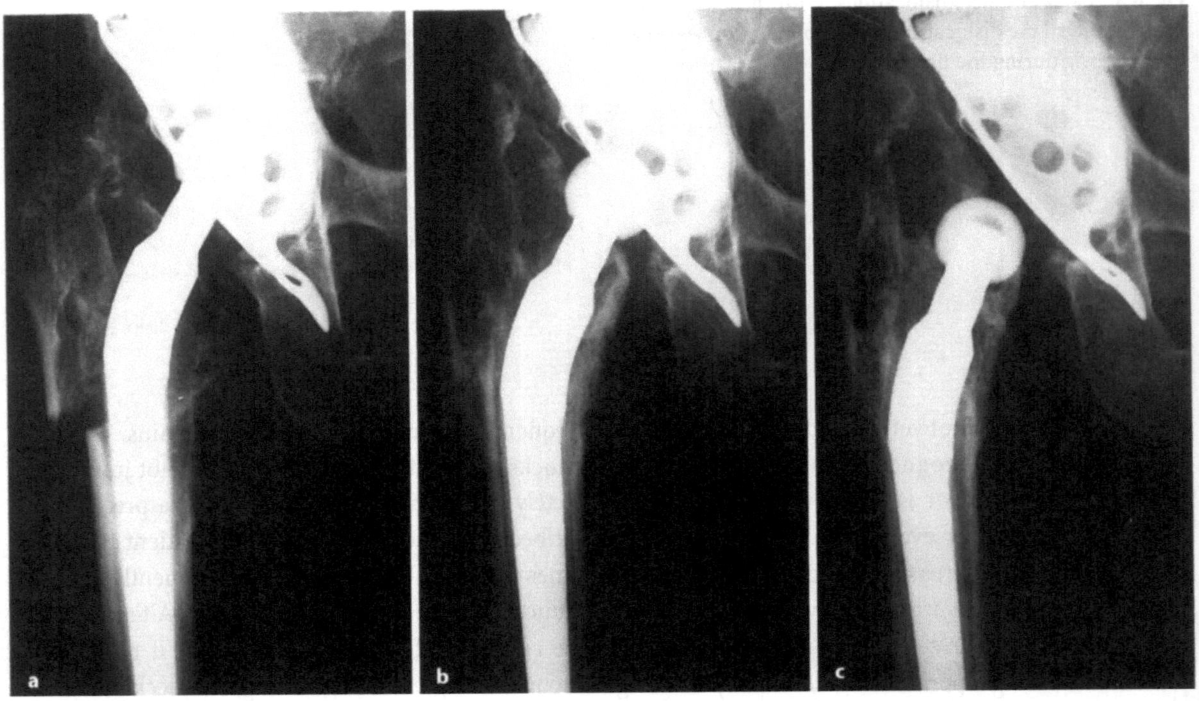

Fig. 6.6a–c. Internal dislocation due to subsidence of a revision stem. H.E., male, 78 years (O.4114)
a Mobility greatly impaired. Complete loss of contact between head and cup. Postoperative situation after replacement of THR with implanted antiprotrusio cage and SL revision stem. Subsequently increasing leg shortening and pains
b Distinct subsidence of the stem at the 1-year follow-up. The patient was walking with two sticks
c Just 4 years after the reimplantation, the patient decided to undergo a further revision because of considerably restricted mobility as a result of the greater trochanter butting against the pelvis following complete loss of contact between head and cup

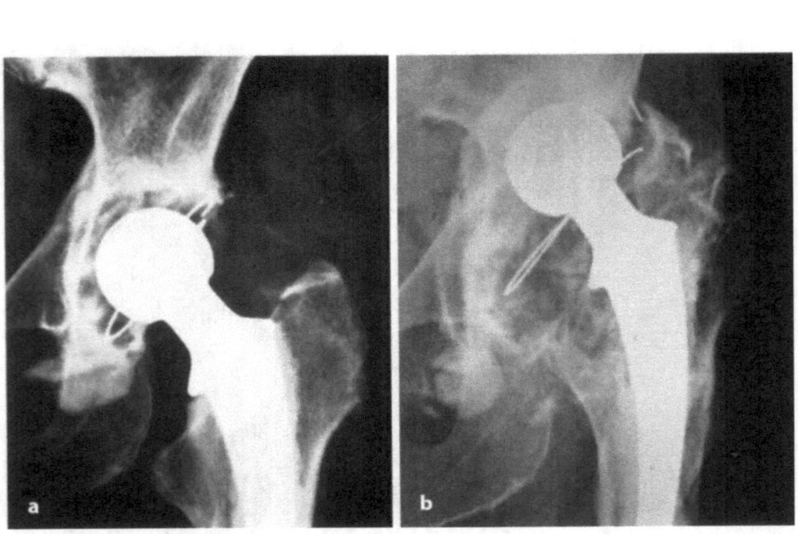

Fig. 6.7a, b. Permanent dislocation with loosened cup. W.N., female (O.266)
a Implantation of a total hip replacement on the left side at 68 years of age
b Ten years later, the patient returned for an implant change on the right following acute breakthrough of the cup into the lesser pelvis. A permanent dislocation of the prosthesis on the left side was already apparent at this point and was still present 13 years later (*photo*)

butting against the pelvis (Figs. 6.6, 3.12). Constant movement can cause a loosened cup to migrate sufficiently for it to be pushed aside by the head (Fig. 6.7). The head then articulates directly with the bone of the acetabulum. While this process is usually gradual and associated with pain, shortening and walking difficulties, the affected individual is frequently still able to walk. Only occasionally does a traumatic dislocation supervene, accompanied by a sudden inability to walk. We have only included loosening-induced dislocations in this study in those cases where the patient noticed a spontaneous traumatic event.

■ **Permanent Dislocation.** The artificial joint remains permanently dislocated. Nevertheless, in certain situations the patient is still able to walk, at least to a limited extent, e.g. if the implant head "rides up" against the cup rim (Fig. 3.12f), or if the dislocated head pushes the loose cup aside and articulates directly with the bony acetabular floor (Fig. 6.7).

6.1.2 Impingement and Dislocation

The maximum range of motion of a joint is determined on the one hand by the cup opening and, on the other, by the relationship between the head and neck diameters. The range of motion can be increased by selecting a larger head, a narrower neck diameter and a cup that encloses the head by less than 180° (Fig. 6.8a,b). An intelligently designed cup rim and taper can further extend the range of motion (Fig. 6.8c). The differing relationship between the taper and the head with differing neck lengths – for a given head diameter – likewise influences the range of motion (Fig. 6.8d).

The maximum possible range of motion in a standard artificial joint is around 110–120°. This figure is considered to be perfectly adequate if cup and stem are ideally positioned, i.e. if the cup was implanted at an inclination of 35–40° and with anteversion of approximately 15–20°, and the stem was implanted with antetorsion of 10–15°. If the inclination and anteversion of the cup are excessive, the head loses adequate ventrolateral covering during adduction and external rotation of the extended leg, with consequent anterolateral dislocation.

Anterolateral dislocation occurs not only as a result of inadequate covering, but also encroachment of the implant neck dorsomedially against the cup rim, i.e. impingement. Inadequate covering is the main reason for dislocation in cases where the joint bearing couple permits a very high range of motion, whereas impingement is the triggering factor for dislocations primarily in pairings offering an inadequate range of motion (Fig. 6.9). The site of impingement and the direction of the dislocation are determined by the combination of the maximum theoretical deflection, the position of the artificial joint and the patient's actual range of motion. The position of the joint components can change over time as a result of loosening, thereby modifying the dislocation risk and the direction of dislocation (Figs. 6.3, 6.7, 14.3).

Whereas impingement involving polyethylene cups can, at worst, lead to dislocations or subluxations, with hard bearing couples impingement can additionally result in clicks, and occasionally pain and cup loosening as well (see also Chap. 15).

In the hip, the naturally elastic limbus edges are imitated to a certain extent by the polyethylene of the artificial cup. This damping effect is lacking in hard bearing couples, such as ceramic to ceramic or metal to metal, potentially resulting in increased wear, clicking sounds and, ultimately, premature loosening of one or both components (Fig. 14.3).

Modifying the polyethylene cup design so as to deepen the acetabular hollow and make the opening angle slightly narrower will necessarily make the head more likely to snap into place. Although this design increases the resistance of the cup to dislocation, at the same time it also exposes the anchorage to increased mechanical loading and reduces the range of motion (Fig. 6.9). If the patient attempts to move the joint through a very wide range, this can readily lead to impingement. Nevertheless, such an implant can, in certain cases, be useful for reducing a dislocation tendency (Fig. 6.2).

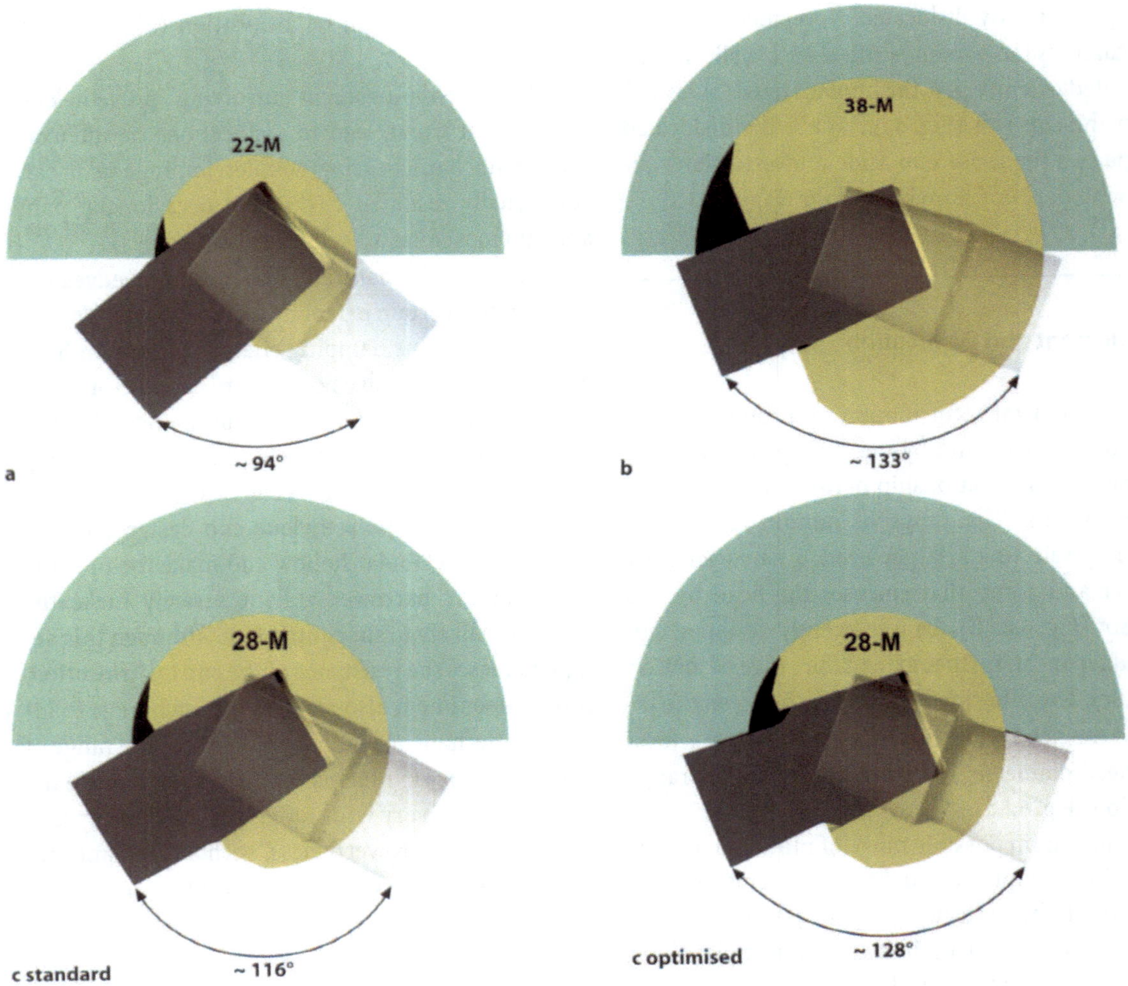

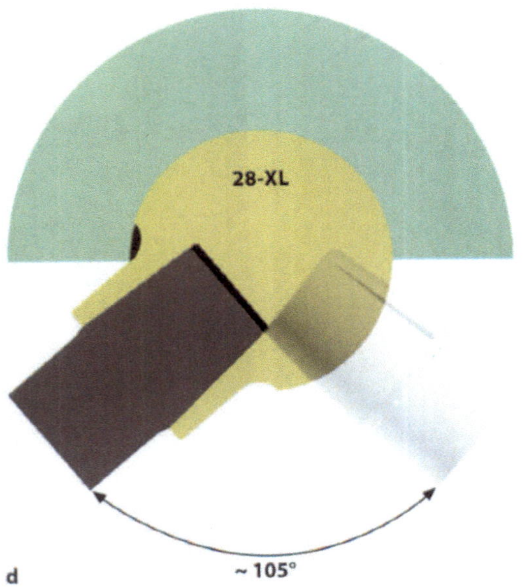

Fig. 6.8a–d. Factors influencing the range of motion
a The combination of a hemispherical cup (e.g. flat-profile polyethylene cup), a head diameter of 22 mm and a 12- to 14-mm taper produces a maximum range of motion of just 94°. This pairing is not usually used
b Simply increasing the head diameter to 38 mm can raise the range of motion to approximately 133°
c Under the same conditions, a range of motion of 116° is achievable with a 28-mm head and a medium neck length. By optimising the cup rims and taper, the range of motion with the 28-mm head can be increased up to 130°
d With an XL neck length, the chamfer behind the shortened taper cannot be exploited to increase the range of motion (see also Table 6.1)

Table 6.1. Optimisation of cup rim and taper in respect of the range of motion with differing neck lengths (S, M, L, XL). Example: 28-mm head

Neck length:	S	M	L	XL
Standard cup (28 mm)	115°	116°	114°	105°
Rim and stem neck optimisation (Fig. 6.7c)	124°	128°	130°	112°
Overall gain [Taper only opt.]	+9° [+2°]	+12° [+5°]	+16° [+9°]	+7° [+0°]

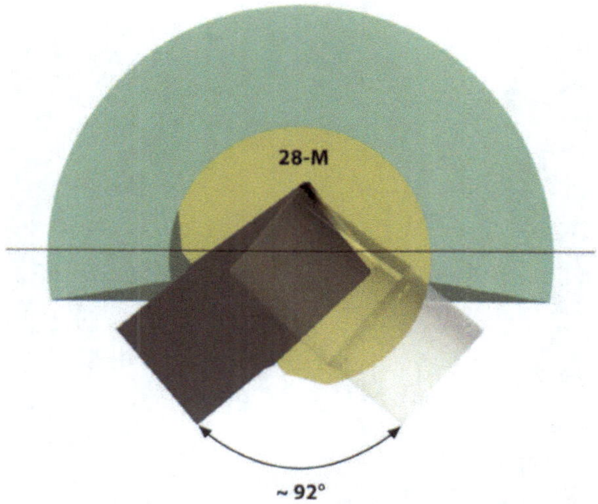

Fig. 6.9. Brunswick cup for revision in the event of recurrent dislocations. More of the prosthesis head is enclosed by the cup and the head is lightly held in place by a snap-fit mechanism. However, this results in a reduced range of motion of only 90°

6.2 Frequency

6.2.1 Frequency in Our Patient Population

In our patient population, dislocation was defined as an event involving a sudden and complete loss of articulation between the head and acetabular cup requiring reduction.

Among the 1098 primary implantations we observed an intraoperative dislocation tendency in 12 (1.1%) patients. Postoperative dislocation of a total hip replacement occurred in 23 (2.1%) patients. The intraoperative dislocation tendency subsequently resulted in an actual dislocation in just one patient. During the 330 revision procedures, an intraoperative dislocation tendency was apparent in seven (2.1%), although none of these patients subsequently suffered an actual dislocation. In three (0.9%) patients without an intraoperative dislocation tendency, dislocation subsequently occurred while they were still in hospital.

■ **Early Dislocations.** Twenty-five patients (93% of patients with a dislocation) suffered the first dislocation of their prosthesis within the first 6 weeks after operation, i.e. as an early dislocation (Fig. 6.4). Of these 25 patients, two suffered two further dislocations, one during the first 2 months after operation and the other during the first year after operation. Both patients required a revision procedure. Revision surgery was also required for another patient when the implant head slipped off the taper during a reduction attempt on the 2nd postoperative day (Fig. 6.10) (see also Sect. 6.5.1). Twenty-three patients remained free of recurrent dislocations following reduction under anaesthesia and conservative measures.

■ **Late Dislocation.** One female patient suffered a dislocation in the 7th week after implantation, necessitating surgical revision of the hip (see also Sect. 6.5.1, case 4).

■ **Dislocation Mechanism and Direction of Dislocation.** Twelve patients experienced their dislocation while lying in bed with their leg in a stretched, ex-

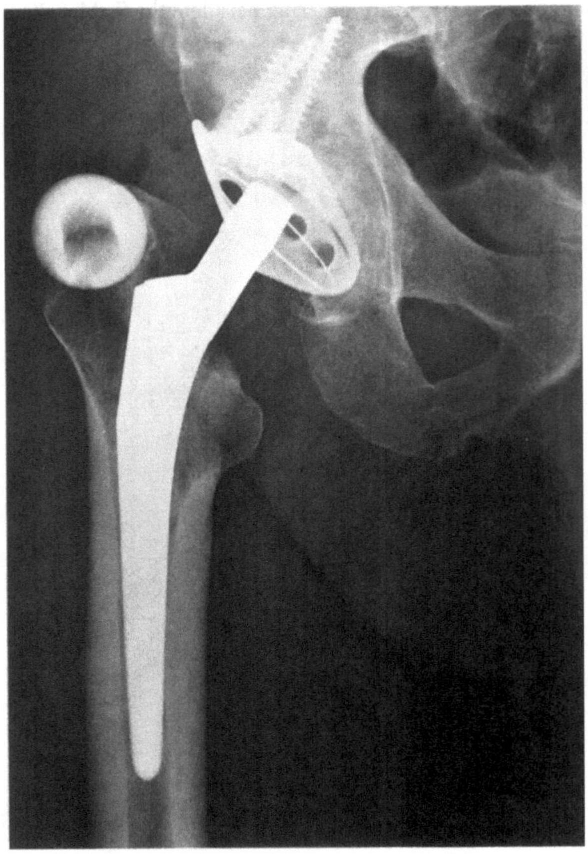

Fig. 6.10. Ceramic head that slipped off the taper during a reduction attempt under anaesthesia following dislocation. K.E., male, 49 years (O.4731). An open revision proved necessary

tended position. In six patients, the dislocation occurred with the hip in flexion, while sitting on a chair, on the toilet or on a bed. No specific information about the dislocation mechanism could be gleaned from the remaining eight patients, since either their dislocated hip was only discovered subsequently or else the patients were unable to provide precise details. Details concerning the direction of dislocation were available for 22 of the 26 patients: 13 dislocated anteriorly and nine posteriorly.

■ **Dislocation Position.** Following dislocation, the head was positioned dorsally in nine cases, cranially in four cases and ventrally in 13 cases. In three cases, a head that had dislocated dorsally shifted into a cranial position as a result of joint capsule laxity (Fig. 6.1). The direction of dislocation could not be ascertained in one patient.

■ **Profile of the Dislocation Rate Over Time.** The average dislocation rate was 1.8% (Fig. 6.11) and fluctuated over the years. Dislocations occurred slightly less frequently between 1992 and 1996, albeit not to any statistically significant extent ($p>0.05$). Nor was any significant difference apparent between the frequencies noted for different operators. Dislocations occurred 18 times (2.2%) in men and in 8 cases (1.4%) in women. The right side was affected in 12 and the left side in 14 cases.

■ **Preoperative Diagnosis.** A total hip replacement dislocated after being implanted for primary coxarthrosis in 15 cases (2% of operated patients) and for hip dysplasia in three cases (1.5%). In two cases the pre-existing condition was an inflammatory hip disorder (6.7%) and in three patients the sequelae of an accident (3.3%). The revision procedures involved two cases of aseptic loosening (0.7%) and one case of a Girdlestone hip (8%).

Implants:

- Cups: The following cups had been implanted: a cemented PE cup in four cases (1% of PE cups), an SLS cup in 11 cases (1.6%), an acetabular reinforce-

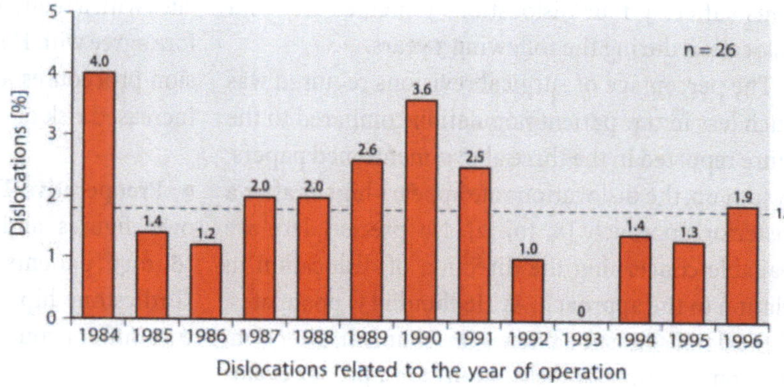

Fig. 6.11. Dislocation rates 1984–1996. Annual dislocation rates (%) in relation to implantations in the corresponding year. The *dotted line* shows the average dislocation rate (1.8 %). Throughout this period, all patients were placed in the supine position during surgery. Since 1992, a spirit level has been used to align the pelvis horizontally (Fig. 3.15)

ment ring in nine cases (2.7%) and an antiprotrusio cage in two cases (4.2%). Acetabular reinforcement rings and antiprotrusio cages were used primarily for larger defects. The outer diameter of the cup did not affect the frequency of dislocation.

- Head diameter: The head diameters of the dislocated prostheses were 1 × 22 mm (1.6% of implanted 22 mm heads), 16 × 28 mm (1.8%) and 9 × 32 mm (2%).
- Stems: The following stems were used: a standard straight stem in five cases (2.8%), a lateralising straight stem in nine cases (2.9%) and, in one case each, a CDH stem (1.6%), a Virtec stem (1.9%) and a Wagner revision stem (1.9%).

6.2.2 Frequency in the Literature

Hip dislocation rates of between 0.3% and 4.8% are reported in the literature [1–13]. Our own dislocation rate of 1.8% is therefore in the middle of this range.

In his population of 6774 patients, Ali Khan [1] observed 142 dislocations, corresponding to a dislocation rate of 2.1%; 44% of these hip dislocations remained stable after closed reduction. A surgical revision was performed in 34% of cases. The author highlights the absolute need for correction of any incorrectly placed implants. Stabilisation was not achieved in the remaining 22% of patients.

The chosen approach is significant. With a lateral surgical approach the dislocation rate was 1.9% (74 dislocations in 3935 prostheses), compared with 2.1% (53 dislocations in 2527 operations) using a posterior approach. With the Ollier procedure (patient in the lateral position, U-shaped skin incision, ventral approach between the tensor muscle of fascia lata and the middle gluteal muscle, osteotomy of the greater trochanter, exposure of the femur dorsally), the dislocation rate was as high as 4.8% (15 dislocations in 312 prostheses). In his study, the author describes 94 early (73% of dislocations) and 35 late dislocations; 81% of the early dislocations and 73% of the late dislocations were stable after reduction. The relapse rate was higher for late dislocations.

Woo [13] investigated a sample of 10,500 total hip replacements and found 331 dislocations (3.2%). In 735 operations involving a posterior surgical approach he observed a dislocation rate of 5.8% (radiologically observed dislocation positions: 77% dorsal, 20% cranial and 3% ventral). In 9765 operations with an antero-lateral approach he observed a dislocation rate of 2.3% (46% ventral, 46% dorsal and 8% cranial dislocation positions); 59% of the dislocations occurred during the first 3 months after the procedure, 77% within the first year and 94% within 5 years. In our own study, 145 and 698 patients have not yet reached the 1- and 5-year follow-up points, respectively, which explains why our figures appear slightly more favourable than those reported by Woo.

Woolson and Rahimtoola [14] observed 14 (4%) dislocations after 315 primary procedures involving a dorsolateral approach and complete resection of the dorsal capsule. Dislocations occurred more frequently, to a statistically significant extent, in patients with cerebral confusion of varying origin.

In his paper published in 1997, Hedlundh [6] reported a dislocation rate of 4% for 3685 primary and 823 revision implants. 65% of the patients with primary dislocations did not experience any recurrent dislocation during the subsequent 1–2 years. The prognosis deteriorated with each additional recurrent dislocation. Accordingly, just 13% of those patients suffering four dislocations remained free of a dislocation during the following 3 years.

The percentage of surgical revisions required was much less in our patient population compared to the figure reported in the three above-mentioned papers. To sum up, the dislocation rate appears higher after a posterior approach [8, 10, 12]. No precise data are available concerning the direction of dislocation in relation to the approach. As Hedlundh [3] postulates, all the details must be known (mechanism, direction, position and time of dislocation) for a proper evaluation of a dislocation situation. Repeated dislocations generally lead to a surgical revision.

6.3 Risk Factors

As noted by Ali Khan [1], various factors play a role in the frequency of dislocation.

▪ **General Condition.** Mentally confused and disoriented elderly individuals, alcoholics or patients suffering from epilepsy, hemiparesis, Parkinson's disease, the consequences of poliomyelitis or any other disorder affecting muscle tone, are more likely to suffer a dislocation [1, 14]. An intraoperative dislocation tendency, which is generally associated with pronounced muscle relaxation, does not appear to provide any indication of the probability of a subsequent dislocation.

▪ **Sex.** The dislocation rate was higher in men (2.2%) than in women (1.4%). The risk for men is therefore greater than that for women by a factor of 1.5, which corresponds with the figure reported by Hedlundh [6].

▪ **Revision Procedures.** Ali Khan [1] found that a third of his dislocations occurred after revision procedures. Woo [13] observed a doubling of the dislocation rate, from 2.4% to 4.8%, after revision operations. Our dislocation rate after revision procedures of 1% was only half as high as the figure observed after our primary procedures. To some extent, this favourable result is doubtless attributable to the fact that revision procedures in our hospital are performed only by experienced operators. As described in the literature [4, 5, 12], the increasing experience of the operator correlates with a reduction in the dislocation rate. We therefore agree with Hedlundh [6] when he states that revision procedures are not generally associated with an increased risk of dislocation.

▪ **Preoperative Diagnosis.** According to both our own figures and those reported in the literature [6,10,13], patients with a total hip replacement after a Girdlestone hip, rheumatoid arthritis or a hip fracture suffer a much higher dislocation rate.

▪ **Faulty Placement.** An incorrectly oriented cup or stem poses an increased risk of dislocation (Fig. 6.1). Lewinnek [9] shows that the dislocation rate with the desired anteversion of 15° increases if a deviation of more than ±10° is present. The dislocation rate is also higher if the cup deviates by more than 10° from the desired inclination of 40°.

▪ **Approach.** The dislocation rate is increased if a dorsal approach is employed, with the patient in a lateral position, and the dorsal capsule is sacrificed [1,13,14].

▪ **Other Factors.** Nolan [11] reports a correlation with concurrent cup loosening. Excessive ante- or retrotorsion of the stem or a trochanteric osteotomy also appear to raise the dislocation rate [1,13]. Overstretching of the capsule, whether in connection with an abscess (Fig. 5.12) or non-healing proximal femoral fragments (Fig. 6.2) can likewise result in dislocations. Subsidence of the stem can, understandably, be associated with an internal dislocation (Fig. 6.6).

6.4 Preventive Measures

With the aim of reducing the dislocation rate, we have sought to standardise the implantation technique and follow-up management.

▪ **Implantation Technique.** The patient is placed horizontally on the operating table under spirit level control (see also Chap. 3, Fig. 3.15a). With the spirit level suspended from the side of the operating table, near the anaesthetist, the patient's position is checked before the cup is inserted (Fig. 3.15b). The use of special bone levers designed by M.E. Müller (Figs. 3.17, 3.18) provides an accurate overview for cup adjustment. The cup inserter is fitted with special alignment rods that facilitate precise cup positioning (Fig. 3.19). We use the SL cup according to M.E. Müller, which possesses a lateral flange to prevent excessive inclination (Fig. 2.6). The corresponding polyethylene inlay has a raised rim covering a quarter of the circumference. The rim is usually positioned dorsally to prevent dorsal dislocations, although another position can be selected if there is a dislocation tendency in another direction. In one revision operation (case 3), stabilisation was achieved simply by rotating the inlay.

The use of computer-aided navigation for implant positioning is currently under discussion, although studies investigating their value compared to traditional methods are still pending.

■ **Follow-up Management.** To prevent early dislocations we routinely place the leg in a foam splint postoperatively after all total hip replacements. The legs are held in abduction using a chaff-filled pillow. Initial mobilisation with a physiotherapist starts on the 1st postoperative day. As soon as patients can achieve a flexion of 70° they are allowed to sit, with legs apart, on a coxarthrosis chair or on a toilet with an adapter. When a flexion of 90° is reached, they can then use normal, though fairly tall, chairs. A legs-apart position is still advisable and crossing of the legs is prohibited. Patients who are unable to sleep on their back can lie on their other side with a chaff-filled pillow between the legs.

6.5 Management of Dislocations

6.5.1 Our Own Measures

■ **Intraoperative Dislocation Tendency.** The patient, nursing staff and physiotherapist are briefed on the positions and movements to be avoided on the basis of the observed tendency. The management is essentially the same as that for a postoperative dislocation, with the exception that subsequent precautions are no longer necessary once normal muscle tone is achieved.

■ **First Dislocation.**

- Analysis: A detailed history of the dislocation event and a radiograph are recorded to determine the dislocation mechanism and the direction and position of dislocation.
- Reduction: The dislocation is reduced under short-term anaesthesia, during which a further careful check is made to determine the direction of any discernible dislocation tendency.
- General information on follow-up management: Bed rest is prescribed until the patient has received adequate instruction prior to renewed mobilisation. Plaster boots and hip spicas have not been used for more than 10 years.
- Follow-up management for ventrolateral dislocations: The patient is positioned with slightly flexed legs held in abduction by chaff-filled pads. The affected leg is held in a foam splint in a position of slight internal rotation. The dislocation mechanism is explained to the patient. Crossing of the legs, particularly when standing up, is avoided.
- Follow-up management for dorsal dislocations: The patient lies flat. A flexion limit of 70° is imposed for 3–4 weeks. While sitting down the patient must keep the legs apart. A toilet adapter and sitting on high chairs are recommended. An internal rotation movement in flexion should be avoided during physiotherapy.

■ **Recurrent Dislocations.** A further attempt at conservative management in accordance with the above-mentioned principles is usually made. Of the total of 26 patients with a hip dislocation during the investigation period, a revision was required in four cases as a result of the failure of conservative treatment.

Three revisions were performed after 25 early dislocations:

- K.E., male, 49 years (O.4731): provided with an acetabular reinforcement ring, an SL straight stem and a 28-mm ceramic head. The head slipped off the taper during the reduction under anaesthesia performed on the second day after implantation (Fig. 6.10). Seven years later, the prosthesis had to be changed because of a loose titanium stem. Dislocation also occurred after this revision, on the 4th day, though this stabilised after reduction under anaesthesia.

- G.W., male, 75 years (O.7072): provided with an uncemented SL cup, a lateralising straight stem and a 28-mm ceramic head. Following an initial dislocation in the ventrolateral direction after 4 weeks, two further dislocations occurred within the first 12 months. During the revision, the inlay was removed and, since the cup was excessively anteverted, a polyethylene cup was cemented in place in a less anteverted and inclined position. No further recurrences.

- M.E., male, 77 years (O.15220): provided with an uncemented SL cup, a standard straight stem and a 28-mm ceramic head. Three ventrocranial dislocations occurred during the first 2 months after replacement of a loosened titanium stem. The patient experienced the first dislocation 2 weeks after primary implantation. During the revision, the polyethylene inlay was rotated so that the projecting rim would prevent any further ventrolateral dislocation. A head with a long neck was also selected. No further complications noted since the revision 5 years ago.

One revision was done after the only late dislocation:

- N.E., female, 73 years (O.3722) was provided with a cemented polyethylene cup and a standard straight stem with a 32-mm head, supplemented by trochanter cerclage. Lengthening was apparent at operation, the cup was too steeply inclined and the stem showed excessive antetorsion. Following a dislocation in the 71st week, the implant was completely changed. No problems noted at the 13-year follow-up.

Two patients who underwent surgery after the documentation period and subsequently required a revision for a dislocation are described elsewhere (Figs. 6.2, 14.3h).

There are some general measures for recurrent dislocations and subluxations: If the patient is not willing to undergo surgery, or if the symptoms, as compared with the patient's general health, are not serious enough to warrant an operation, a stabilising Hohmann support may prove useful (Fig. 6.5).

6.5.2 Dislocation Management in the Literature

We were able to find only a small number of publications dealing with the issue of treatment. The management of dislocations as described in the literature is broadly similar to our own approach. Certain authors only start mobilising their patients on the 2nd postoperative day [1]. Positioning the patient in abduction using pillows or an abduction wedge is recommended. Reductions are generally performed under general anaesthesia with muscle relaxation. In his study, Woo [13] reports that 95% of the hip dislocations responded to closed reduction. Joshi [7] achieved a 97% success rate for closed reduction. Hedlundh [6] found that only 30% of first dislocations did not recur during the subsequent 2 years. After two dislocations this figure dropped to 29% and, after three dislocations, to 13%, irrespective of the therapeutic measures implemented. No obvious reason is apparent for these poor results.

Certain authors continue to recommend a follow-up strategy of bed rest with an internal rotation cast, a hip spica or an extension [1, 2, 13]. We do not consider this approach to be either necessary or useful.

All authors agree that recurrent dislocations and late dislocations require surgical correction. The following options are mentioned:

- Replacement of incorrectly oriented joint components
- Internal fixation for trochanteric fractures or pseudarthrosis
- Reorientation of the greater trochanter by osteotomy
- Tenotomy of the adductors
- Open reduction for an old dislocation

Hedlundh [6] replaced one or both components in 52 patients (1.15% of prostheses implanted in his patient population). The cup was revised in 28 cases, the stem in 13 cases, and both components in nine cases. In 11 cases the stem was simply removed, leaving a Girdlestone situation. Where an incorrect position could be corrected at operation, the dislocation problem was eliminated in two thirds of these patients. The overall picture for this series remains unfavourable, probably because of the excessively frequent faulty placement of the components.

6.5.3 Overview of the Therapeutic Options for Dislocations

To sum up, the following measures can be considered for the management of (recurrent) dislocations:

- *Acetabulum*: Removal of bone spurs that could cause impingement/dislocation

- *Cup:*
  - Reduction and physiotherapy
  - Rotation of an inlay with rim in an uncemented cup
  - Cementation of a new inlay or new cup in a shell (acetabular reinforcement ring, Burch–Schneider antiprotrusio cage, SL cup)
  - Reimplantation of the whole cup with reorientation of inclination and anteversion
    Use of a Brunswick cup (Fig. 6.9)
- *Stem:*
  - Neck extension. Lengthening of 9 mm is possible with neck lengths S to XL
  - Head with differently angled taper socket (e.g. "Batory head")
  - Change of stem and readjustment with a different length, antetorsion, lateralisation
- *Proximal femur:*
  - Fixation of loose proximal femoral fragments in connection with a pertrochanteric fracture or after a transfemoral approach
- *Other:*
  - Reinsertion of an avulsed greater trochanter
  - Reinsertion and tightening of incorrectly positioned muscles
  - Hohmann support if muscles are missing

6.6 Discussion

6.6.1 Early Dislocations

An analysis of our own data and those in the literature indicates that over two thirds of dislocations occur in the early phase, up to the 6th week after operation. During this period muscle tone is diminished and the joint is not protected by a neocapsule and is therefore more susceptible to dislocation. Depending on the surgical approach, the dislocations are more likely to be ventral (1/2 of the dislocations with a ventral approach) or dorsal (2/3 of the dislocations with a dorsal approach). Generally speaking, dislocations are more likely to occur after a dorsal approach. They are also encountered more frequently in patients with a Girdlestone hip, rheumatoid arthritis, fracture or diminished muscle tone, e.g. after a stroke.

A one-off dislocation can usually be reduced without any problems under short-term anaesthesia. A plaster cast is rarely needed these days during follow-up provided the patient is managed carefully by the physiotherapist. If no subsequent dislocations occur, then the potential survival of the prosthesis is not affected. If dislocations recur, however, the specific causes should be sought. The usual cause is an incorrectly oriented cup. The dislocation rate rises markedly even with a deviation of just ±10° from the correct position.

The most important prophylactic measures are, on the one hand, precise intraoperative positioning of the implant and, on the other, meticulous briefing and instruction of the patient, nursing staff, physiotherapists and the doctors responsible for follow-up.

The dislocation tendency observed at operation in our patient population was not associated with an increased frequency of postoperative dislocation. This may be attributable to the fact that the patients with a dislocation tendency are monitored and instructed with particular care, or that, provided the implant is correctly oriented, the subsequent resumption of normal muscle tone provides adequate protection for the joint.

6.6.2 Late Dislocations

If the starting point for a late dislocation is defined as 6 weeks or the formation of a resistant neocapsule, up to 33% of dislocations, depending on the author, can be said to be late. Late dislocations can also occasionally be managed by reduction alone. The literature reports figures of up to 70% stable prostheses after reduction during this phase. We consider this percentage to be very high. It contrasts with other reported figures [6].

Late dislocations are caused either by primary faulty placement or by a secondary reorientation of the prosthesis components as a result of loosening or subsidence. Recurrences are common and almost invariably end in a revision procedure. If the patient lacks motivation, stabilisation with a Hohmann support may be worth trying.

References

1. Ali Khan MAA, Brakenbury PH, Reynolds ISR (1981) Dislocation following total hip replacement. J Bone Joint Surg Br 63 B: 214–218
2. Elke R (1994) Operation und Nachbehandlung bei Hüftarthroplastik. Ars Medici 15: 981–986
3. Hedlundh U, Ahnfelt L, Fredin H (1992) Incidence of dislocation after hip arthroplasty. Comparison of different registration methods in 408 cases. Acta Orthop Scand 63: 403–406
4. Hedlundh U, Ahnfelt L, Hybbinette CH, Wallinder L, Weckestrom J, Fredin H (1996) Dislocations and the femoral head size in primary total hip arthroplasty. Clin Orthop 333: 226–233
5. Hedlundh U, Ahnfelt L, Hybbinette CH, Weckestrom J, Fredin H (1996) Surgical experience related to dislocations after total hip arthroplasty. J Bone Joint Surg Br 78: 206–209
6. Hedlundh U, Sanzén L, Fredin H (1997) The prognosis and treatment of dislocated total hip arthroplasties with a 22-mm head. J Bone Joint Surg Br 579-B: 374–378
7. Joshi A, Lee CM, Markovic MD, Vlatis G, Murphy JCM (1998) Prognosis of dislocation after total hip arthroplasty. Arthroplasty 13: 17–21
8. Kohn D, Ruhmann O, Wirth CJ (1997) Die Verrenkung der Hüfttotalendoprothese unter besonderer Beachtung verschiedener Zugangswege. Z Orthop 135: 40–44
9. Lewinnek GE, Lewis JL, Tarr R, Comper CL, Zimmermann JR (1978) Dislocations after total hip-replacement arthroplasties. J Bone Joint Surg Am 60-A: 217–220
10. Mallory TH, Lombardi AV, Fada RA, Herrinton SM, Eberle RW (1999) Dislocation after total hip arthroplasty using the anterolateral abductor split approach. Clin Orthop 358: 166–172
11. Nolan DR, Fitzgerald RH Jr, Beckenbaugh RD, Coventry MB (1975) Complications of total hip arthroplasty treated by reoperation. J Bone Joint Surg Am 57-A: 977–981
12. Unwin AJ, Thomas M (1994) Dislocation after hemiarthroplasty of the hip: a comparison of the dislocation rate after posterior and lateral approaches to the hip. Ann R Coll Surg Engl 76: 327–329
13. Woo RYG, Morrey BF (1982) Dislocations after total hip arthroplasty. J Bone Joint Surg Am 64-A: 1295–1306
14. Woolson ST, Rahimtoola ZO (1999) Risk factors for dislocation during the first 3 months after primary total hip replacement. J Arthroplasty 14:662–668

Periprosthetic Fissures, Fractures and Perforations of the Proximal Femoral Shaft

Thierry Münch

Periprosthetic fractures of the proximal femoral shaft are subdivided by Johannsson et al. into

- I. proximal fractures (trochanter and calcar area)
- II. fractures running in a proximal to distal direction
- III. fractures distal to the tip of the prosthesis

Further subdivision into cases with a stable prosthesis and those with a loose prosthesis determines whether the implant will need to be changed during the internal fixation procedure. The time of fracture diagnosis varies greatly: Fractures and fissures occurring during surgery may be noticed intraoperatively or postoperatively, or may be overlooked postoperatively. Fractures observed at a later date can be triggered by appropriate or inappropriate trauma. The number of fractures observed in our study with straight stem prostheses is either comparable with, or lower than, the figures cited in the literature. Our consistently pursued objective of stabilising every fracture or fissure at the time of diagnosis has enabled us to spare our patients prolonged stays in hospital and the risk of a further threatened fracture. In all cases, we achieved timely and uncomplicated bone healing after internal fixation. Two technical principles are particularly important in fracture management and fracture prevention:

- Remodelling of the bone is possible only if no cement enters the fracture clefts.
- Unstable areas must be bridged over a large area, ideally with a plate, in order to ensure uncomplicated mobilisation and bone ingrowth. Internal fixation with cerclage wiring is usually sufficient for fissures.

7.1 Introduction, Definitions

Periprosthetic fractures have become increasingly common in recent years, partly because of the increased number of prostheses used and partly because of the growing elderly population. Such fractures place considerable demands on the treating orthopaedic surgeons. Prosthesis stability must be ensured during fracture healing. If possible, the period of postoperative partial weight-bearing must be kept short.

In monitoring our patients with periprosthetic fractures, we seek to draw consequences from the treatment results so that we can then draw up an effective therapeutic management strategy.

Periprosthetic femoral shaft fractures are defined by their spatial relationship with a femoral implant. Corresponding fractures of the greater trochanter are dealt with in a separate chapter (see Chap. 8).

Fractures can be evaluated according to the following criteria:

- Fracture type
- Site
- Time of onset/time identified
- Stability of the prosthesis

7.1.1 Fracture Types

In this study we distinguish between hairline cracks, fissures, fractures and perforations.

- Hairline cracks: (n=4) Barely perceptible breaks in continuity with no gaping observed at any point during prosthesis implantation. During cementation they are not filled with cement. They are, in fact, clinically detectable only in the calcar area.

- Fissures: (n=24) Cracks in the bone that most commonly arise in the calcar or shaft area during rasping of the medullary canal. They gape open when the prosthesis is inserted (Figs. 7.1, 7.2, 7.4, 7.6). Fissures are particularly hazardous with cemented implants, since cement penetration in the fissures can permanently prevent the self-repair mechanism of remodelling from taking place in this area. Spontaneous healing can be expected to take place in patients with uncemented prostheses (Fig. 7.1).
- Fractures: (n=15) Complete breaks in continuity.
- Perforations: (n=4) Perforations arise when the medullary cavity is being widened with the rasp or during cement removal when a stem is being replaced. The site most commonly affected is the dorsolateral aspect of the femoral shaft. Leakage of cement will permanently prevent spontaneous closure of the perforation.

Hairline cracks, fissures and fractures are recorded with a high degree of reliability in our statistics since our standard practice is to manage the first two intraoperatively with cerclage wiring (Fig. 7.2) and to secure fractures by internal fixation. The number of

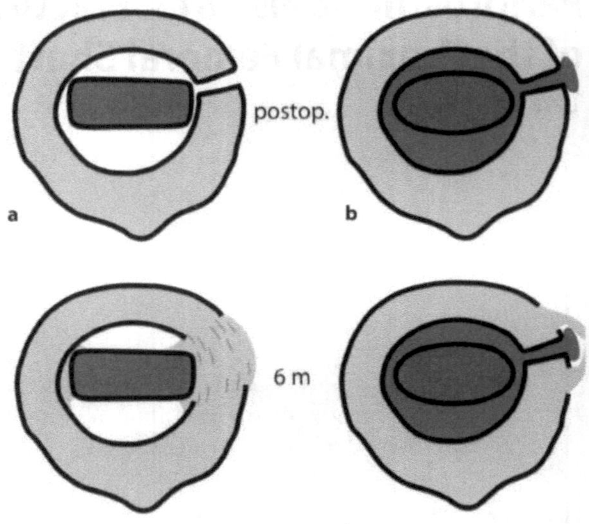

Figs. 7.1a, b. Effect of a fissure in cemented and uncemented prostheses
a Fissure in an uncemented stem: Following tight impaction of the prosthesis, the fissure gapes slightly postoperatively. Within the following 6 months, remodelling has occurred and securely closed the gap
b Fissure with a cemented stem: If the fissure is still gaping when the prosthesis is inserted into the cement-filled shaft, cement is pressed into the gap, permanently preventing any bone ingrowth into the gap. The body may attempt to form a bony bridge around the leaked cement (*green*), but this is unreliable and time consuming

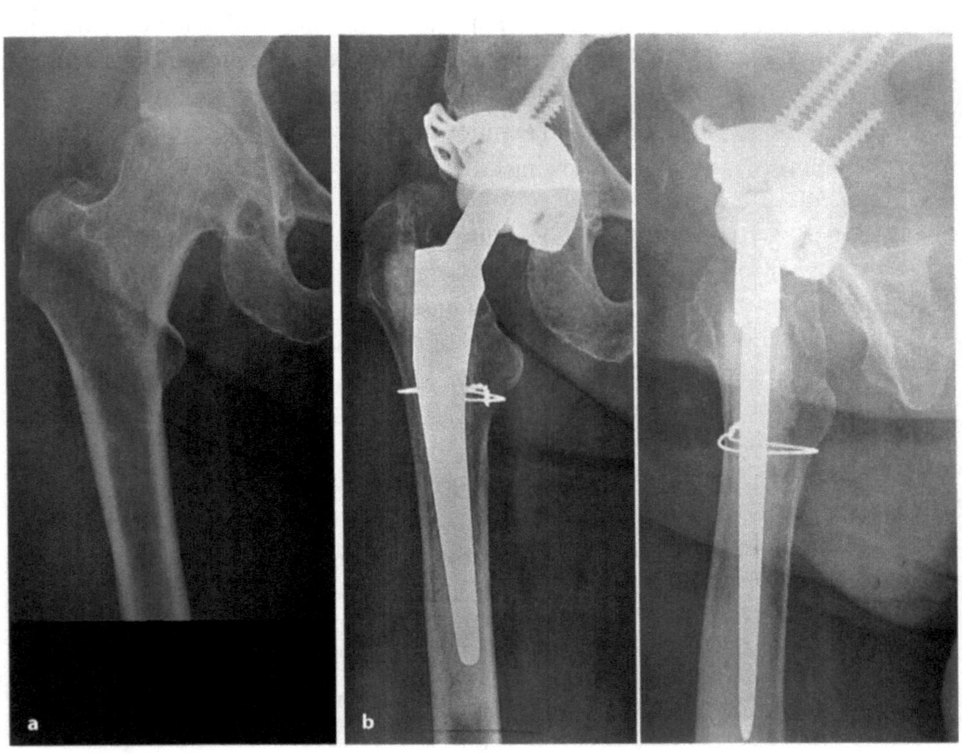

Figs. 7.2a, b. Cerclage wiring for a fissure detected at operation. B.E., female, 67 years (O. 13881)
a Coxarthrosis in a case of coxa valga. A fissure occurred intraoperatively on the medial side of the calcar and was managed with cerclage wiring (Fig. 7.6)
b Two-year follow-up: Patient can walk without sticks for 1 hour. Normal bone structure, no signs of loosening, no cortical remodelling problems in the fissure area

recorded perforations is too small since there is no reliable identifying sign, despite being recorded in the postoperative documentation sheet.

7.1.2 Site

Around ten classification systems of varying complexity are described in the literature [1, 3, 4, 10, 11, 14, 17]. Since it is easy to understand we have adopted the classification system proposed by Johannsson et al. (1981) to describe the sites (Fig. 7.3, Table 7.1). This classification allows a simple and reliable therapeutic strategy to be formulated. It is also regularly employed in the literature.

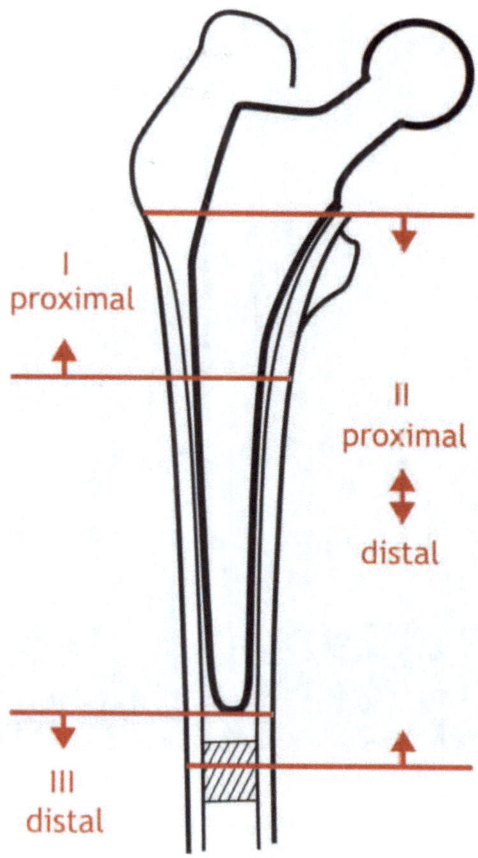

Fig. 7.3. Fracture classification. (After Johannssen et al. [7]; see also Table 7.1)

Table 7.1. Classification. (After Johannssen et al. [7])

Type I	Proximal fracture (trochanter – calcar area)
Type II	Fracture running in a proximal to distal direction (from the stem shoulder to below the stem tip)
Type III	Distal fracture (starting below the stem tip)

7.1.3 Time of Onset/Time Identified

As regards the time of onset and time identified, we distinguish between the following categories of fissures and fractures:

- Events observed intraoperatively
- Events overlooked intraoperatively/ observed only postoperatively
- Fractures occurring after trauma with a stable or loosened femoral stem

Combinations of these categories can occur. Thus, for example, a fissure missed postoperatively despite the detected leakage of cement can lead to a fracture when trauma subsequently occurs (Fig. 7.4).

Intraoperative detection and often prophylactic management are crucial factors in preventing a subsequent fracture (see also 7.5.1).

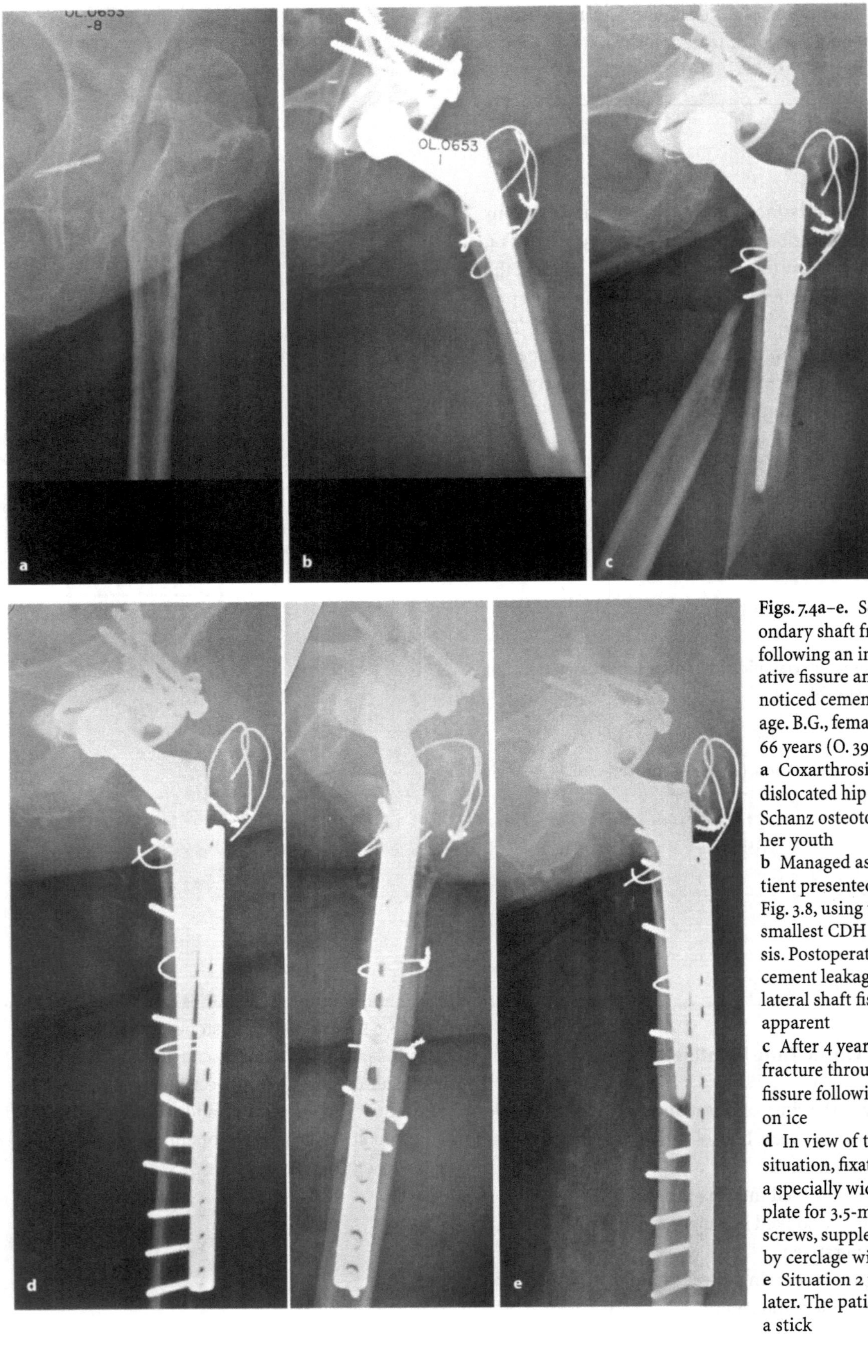

Figs. 7.4a–e. Secondary shaft fracture following an intraoperative fissure and unnoticed cement leakage. B.G., female, 66 years (O. 3953)
a Coxarthrosis with a dislocated hip after a Schanz osteotomy in her youth
b Managed as for patient presented in Fig. 3.8, using the smallest CDH prosthesis. Postoperatively, cement leakage from a lateral shaft fissure is apparent
c After 4 years, shaft fracture through the fissure following a slip on ice
d In view of the tight situation, fixation with a specially wide DC plate for 3.5-mm screws, supplemented by cerclage wiring
e Situation 2 years later. The patient uses a stick

7.1.4 Stability of the Prosthesis

If a prosthesis is firmly anchored in the main fracture fragment, internal fixation of the fracture is usually sufficient to remedy the situation (see also Sect. 7.5.1). If the prosthesis is loose or surrounded by osteolytic areas, then it will need to be replaced concurrently with the fracture repair procedure (see also Sect. 7.5.1). The prosthesis can be changed and the fracture secured by internal fixation or else the fracture can be bridged with a long-stem prosthesis.

7.2 Frequency

7.2.1 Frequency in Our Own Patients

■ **Frequency Over the Years.** Considerable year-on-year variations are apparent in the incidence of fractures (Fig. 7.5). On average, one to two fractures a year occur in connection with primary procedures (2.3%). In revision surgery, the period between 1993 and 1995 showed a transient increase in the number of fissures, fractures and perforations observed intraoperatively. Despite the increased use of a pneumatic rasp, the number of fractures has not declined in recent years. We have used this rasp ("woodpecker") for primary procedures since 1991 for the occasional case and since 1993 for most cases.

■ **Frequency in Relation to Site.** Primary prostheses: During the implantation of 1098 primary prostheses, 25 hairline cracks, fissures and fractures occurred intraoperatively. Seven fractures were subsequently triggered by trauma, in four cases combined with pre-existing loosening (Table 7.2). Usually, type I fissures and fractures were involved, less frequently types II and III. Men and women were equally affected. The average age of the patients was 72 years (45–92).

Revision prostheses: Eight fissures, nine fractures and three perforations were observed during 330 revisions, i.e. 20 in total, or 6% (Table 7.3). Most of these were fractures and fissures of types I and II. Men were slightly more frequently affected than women. The average age was 74 years (44–85), which roughly corresponds with the average age of the patients undergoing surgery (see also Chap. 2).

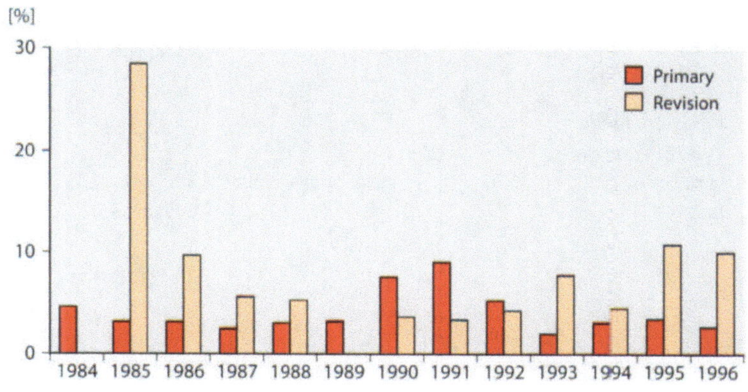

Fig. 7.5. Frequency of intraoperative fissures and fractures during primary and revision procedures between 1984 and 1996

Table 7.2. Frequency of periprosthetic femoral fractures associated with primary hip replacement

Fracture type (Johannssen)	Mechanism	Fracture type	Treatment	Follow-up
Primary THR Type I fracture (proximal) *n*=18	16 intra-operatively	3 hairline cracks 12 fissures 1 fracture	Cerclage: 16	3.8 years (1–7)
	2 trauma (postop) (1 loosening)	2 fractures	Plate: 1 (stable stem) Wagner+cerc.: 1 (revision)	(1 lost to follow-up) 2 patients † postop)
Primary THR Type II fracture (proximal-distal) *n*=7	5 intra-operatively	3 fissures	Plate: 2 Cerclage/screw: 1	5.7 years (4–8)
		1 fracture	Cerclage: 1	(2 lost to follow-up)
		1 perforation	Plate: 1	
	2 trauma (1 loosening)	2 fractures	Cerclage: 1 Plate: 1 (revision)	
Primary THR Type III fracture (distal) *n*=7	4 intra-operatively	1 fissure 3 fractures	Plate: 1 Plate: 3	4.4 years (2–12)
	3 trauma (postop)	3 fractures	Plates: 3 (2 revisions)	(1 lost to follow-up)

Table 7.3. Frequency of periprosthetic femoral fractures associated with revision THR

Fracture type (Johannssen)	Mechanism	Fracture type	Treatment	Follow-up
Revision THR Type I fracture (proximal) *n*=13	Intra-operatively	6 fissures	Cerclage: 4 Wagner stem: 2	3.7 years (1–10)
		7 fractures	Cerclage: 5 Wagner stem: 2	10 follow-ups (1 lost to follow-up)
Revision THR Type II fracture (proximal-distal) *n*=7	Intra-operatively	2 fissures 2 fractures	Plate: 2 Wagner stem: 1 Plate: 1	2 years (1–5) 7 follow-ups
		3 perforations	Cerclage: 1 Plate: 1 Wagner stem: 1	

7.2.2
Frequency in the Literature

Intraoperative fractures in connection with primarily implanted, cemented stems are suffered by between 0.1 and 6.3% of patients [4, 8, 10, 11, 14, 17]. Fractures are much more common during revision surgery. Risk factors such as previous revisions, osteolysis, osteoporosis, history of hemiparesis or alcoholism favour the onset of a fracture during operation. Figures as high as 17.6% are cited [3, 10, 14, 17]. The following problematic situations can represent predisposing factors for a postoperative fracture: ignored cement leakage [4, 6, 17], bone defects or shaft windowing for cement removal. A poor shaft blood supply resulting from overaggressive drilling can also lead to fractures [8, 17].

Another cause of an intraoperative fracture is the intraoperative dislocation of the femoral head from the acetabulum [4, 14, 17]. This is more likely to occur when the capsule is inadequately exposed and resected. No such incident has occurred in our series even though we routinely dislocate the hip before resecting the femoral head.

7.3
Risk Factors

Intraoperatively, calcar fissures occur particularly during the use of rasps. They are more common in connection with cementless systems, where a tight fit of the prosthesis is particularly important. On the other hand, they are much more hazardous when they occur in connection with cemented systems. If a fissure becomes filled with even a wafer-thin layer of cement, healing by remodelling is no longer possible and the fissure remains a possible starting point for a periprosthetic fracture (Fig. 7.1).

Calcar fissures probably occur more frequently in connection with an inexperienced operator and inadequate planning. Deeper seated fractures and fissures (types II/III) are not always avoidable, particularly with cementless systems or very tight medullary cavities (Fig. 7.4).

Revision operations are associated with a much higher risk of type I and II intraoperative fractures (Table 7.3), since the cortical bone has often already become much thinner.

Operators should particularly be aware of the following hazards:

Valgus hip:	Risk of calcar fissure (Fig. 7.2)
Tapering medullary cavity:	Risk of distal fissure (Fig. 7.4)
Stem loosening::	Bone defect, perforation

Certain diseases also involve an increased risk of fracture fissure (Table 7.4)

Table 7.4. Risk factors for a periprosthetic fracture

Intraoperative fractures	Postoperative fractures
Rheumatic disease	Weakened femur
Cementless systems	Predisposing factors:
Metabolic bone disease	Plate ends, screw holes, prosthesis tip too wide in relation to the tapered medullary cavity
Paget's disease	Perforation of the cortex
Osteogenesis imperfecta	Osteolysis
Femur deformities with dysplasia	Cement leakage
Coxa vara	Loose implants
Revision surgery	

7.4 Preventive Measures

The most important preventive measure is careful preoperative study of the standardised X-rays and detailed operation planning, as described in Chap. 3. During this process, the operator might, for example, be made aware of the risk of calcar splitting in a patient with a valgus hip or in a case where slight shortening is planned (Fig. 3.7).

7.5 Management of Complications

7.5.1 Fissures and Fractures Associated with Primary Prostheses

(Table 7.2)

■ **Intraoperatively Detected Fissures/Fractures.** We prefer to secure type I fissures observed intraoperatively with cerclage wiring rather than with other types of cables and bands that are more harmful to the periosteum [4, 5, 15, 18]. A fissure occurring during rasping or during the insertion of a trial prosthesis is secured with large-pronged reduction forceps so that the fracture cleft is no longer visible (Fig. 7.6). We then compress the fissure with cerclage wiring and reinsert the trial prosthesis. If the fissure starts gaping again, a prosthesis one size smaller should be used. With the reduction forceps still in place, the stem is now cemented in situ. Using this procedure we can avoid any penetration of cement in the fracture cleft (Fig. 7.1). Even if a hairline crack is suspected, we apply a cerclage as a precaution in order to keep the fracture closed during cementation.

We manage type II and III fractures with one or more cerclage wires or by plate fixation. The choice between cerclage wiring, a plate or a combination of the two will depend on the course of the fracture. For long spiral type II fractures, cerclage wiring alone may suffice in careful patients. But the most reliable way of stabilising the fracture is by plate fixation. We believe that maximum stability is achieved if as many screws as possible find purchase in the strong linea aspera (Fig. 7.7). Wherever possible we try to place the

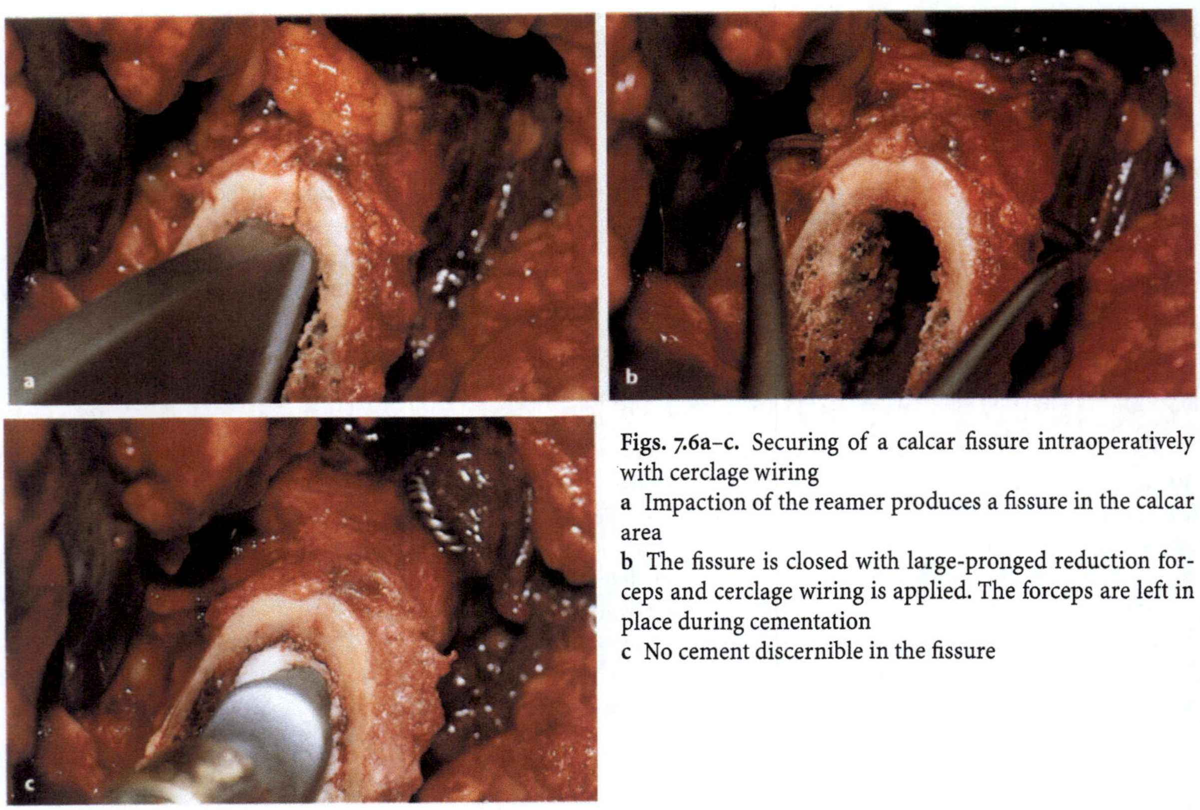

Figs. 7.6a–c. Securing of a calcar fissure intraoperatively with cerclage wiring
a Impaction of the reamer produces a fissure in the calcar area
b The fissure is closed with large-pronged reduction forceps and cerclage wiring is applied. The forceps are left in place during cementation
c No cement discernible in the fissure

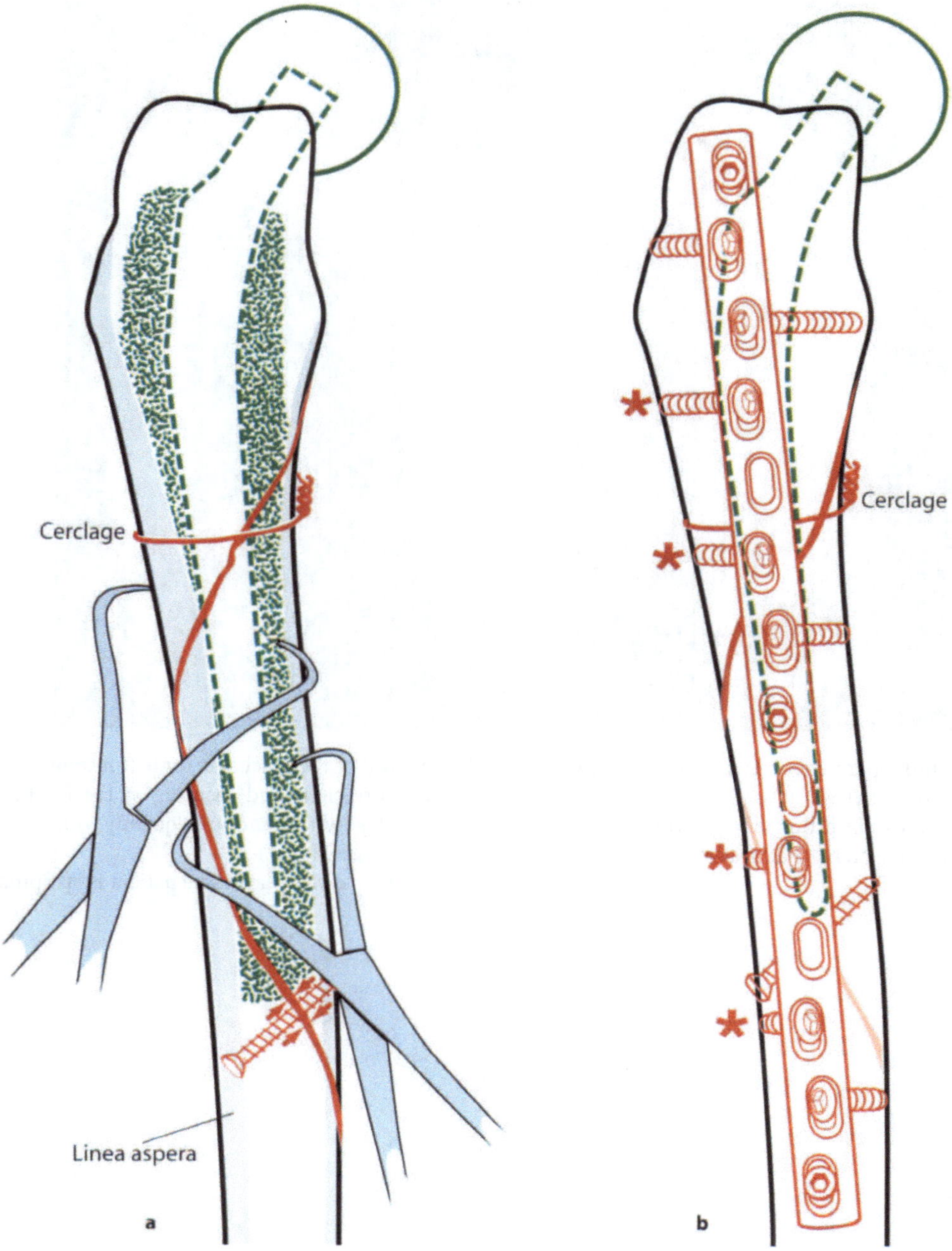

Figs. 7.7a, b. Plate fixation of a type II fracture. Sketch
a External and sectional view from the side. Reduction of the fracture transmuscularly with two reduction forceps with prongs, fixation proximally with cerclage wiring and distally with a lag screw. The strong cortical bone of the linea aspera can be seen dorsally
b A 16-hole plate is bent against the bone and positioned slightly dorsally. Fixation with screws alternately inserted dorsally and ventrally in relation to the prosthesis. The four screws inserted into the linea aspera are particularly important (*asterisks*)

screws alternately on the ventral and dorsal sides along the stem (Figs. 7.4, 7.8).

Type III fractures can occur in osteoporotic patients in the distal femoral metaphysis when a taper is reamed for an SL revision stem (Fig. 7.10). These complex situations can generally be managed with a forked or condylar plate.

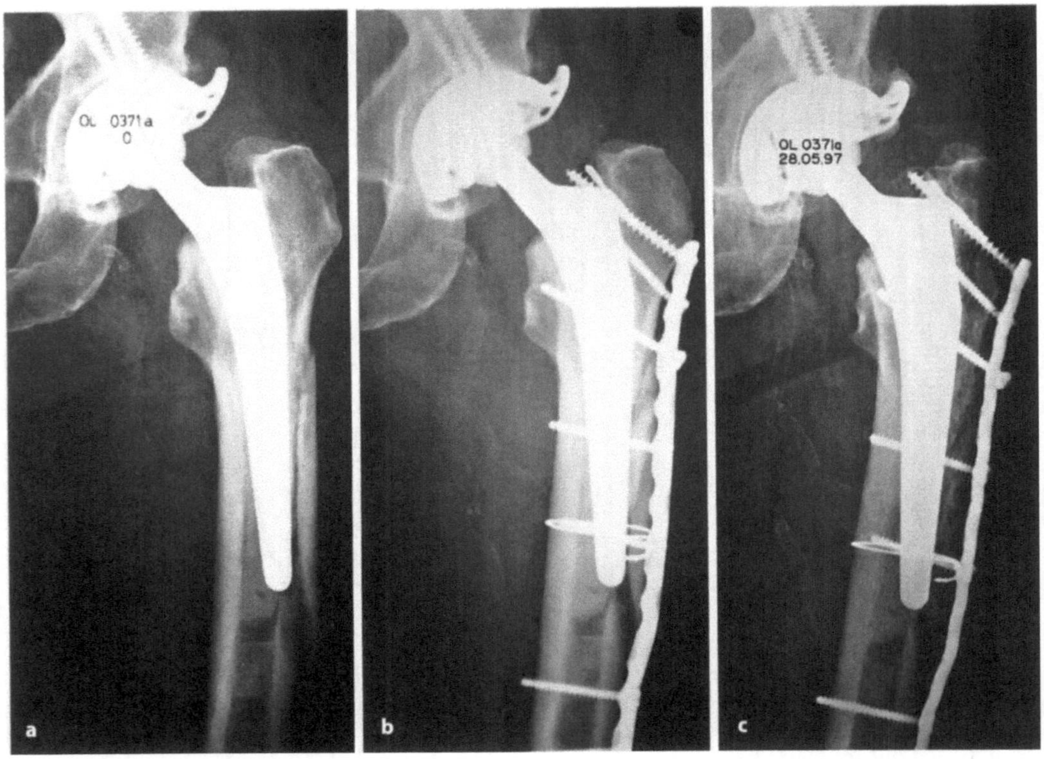

Figs. 7.8a–c. Intraoperatively noted type II fracture. F.A., male, 81 years (O. 1224)
a Excessively varus insertion of the prosthesis has produced splitting of a lateral shaft fragment
b Removal of the reachable cement intraoperatively from the fracture clefts and securing of the fracture, initially with cerclage wiring and subsequently with a long bridging plate (see also Fig. 7.7)
c Follow-up 6 years later. The patient is symptom free

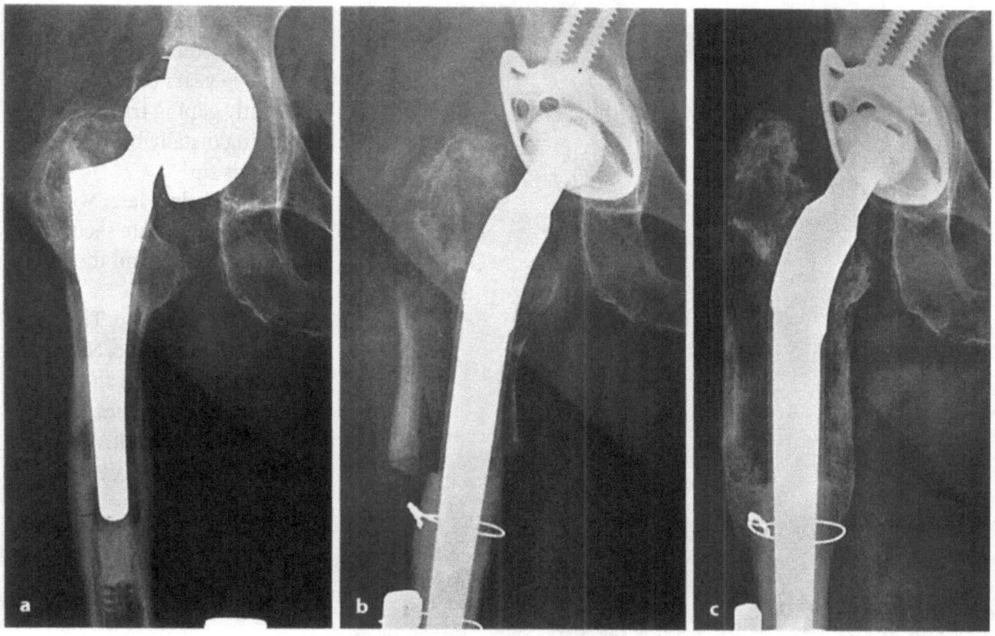

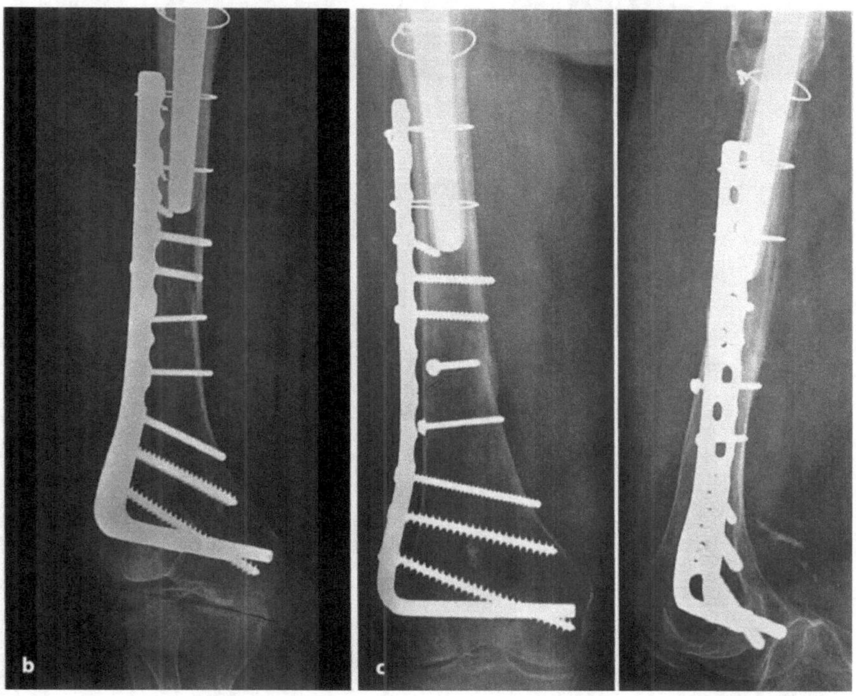

Figs. 7.9a–c. Intraoperative type III fracture of the distal femoral metaphysis. H.A., female, 74 years (O. 29339). Total hip replacement implanted 6 years ago, patient has been complaining of pain for a year
a Clinically, local inflammation with radiological evidence of cup dislocation and extensive areas of osteolysis and new subperiosteal bone growth in the femoral area. Aspirate: *Staphylococcus aureus*
b One-stage revision 2 weeks after the start of parenteral antibiotic therapy. A metaphyseal torsion fracture occurred distally during taper reaming, despite protection with cerclage wiring. The fracture was managed with two cerclage wires, two lag screws and a forked plate
c After 6 months, the transfemoral incision, distal shaft fracture and infection have healed completely in this patient, who has been fully weight-bearing for 3 months

■ **Postoperatively Detected Fractures and Perforations.** If fractures with cement leakage – generally near the tip of the prosthesis – are detected only postoperatively, we inform the patient straightaway about the possible risks and propose immediate stabilisation. We then attempt to remove the leaked cement and clean up the leakage site (Figs. 7.8, 7.9). The weakened zone is then bridged with a plate and reinforced so as to exclude any subsequent risk of fracture (see preceding section and Fig. 7.7 for details of the plate fixation technique.)

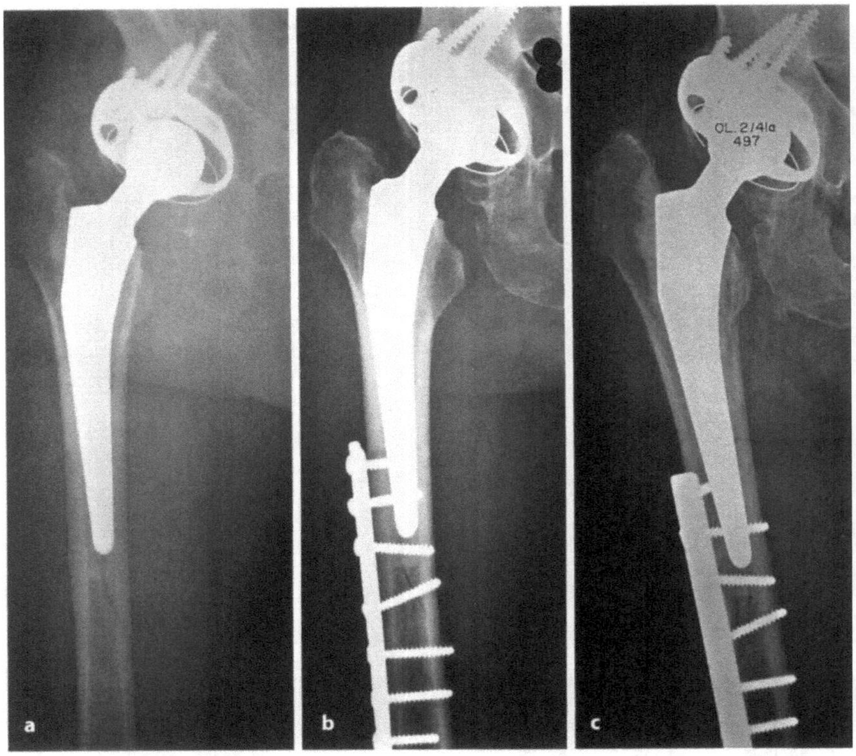

Figs. 7.10a–c. Postoperatively noted type II fracture at the level of the stem tip. L.N., female, 59 years (O. 2796)
a Slightly gaping fracture extending distally beyond the prosthesis tip
b Fixation 2 days later with a lag screw and a plate securing the transition around the prosthesis tip
c Ten-year follow-up. The patient is symptom free. No significant migration of the acetabular reinforcement ring measured by the EBRA method, even after 13 years

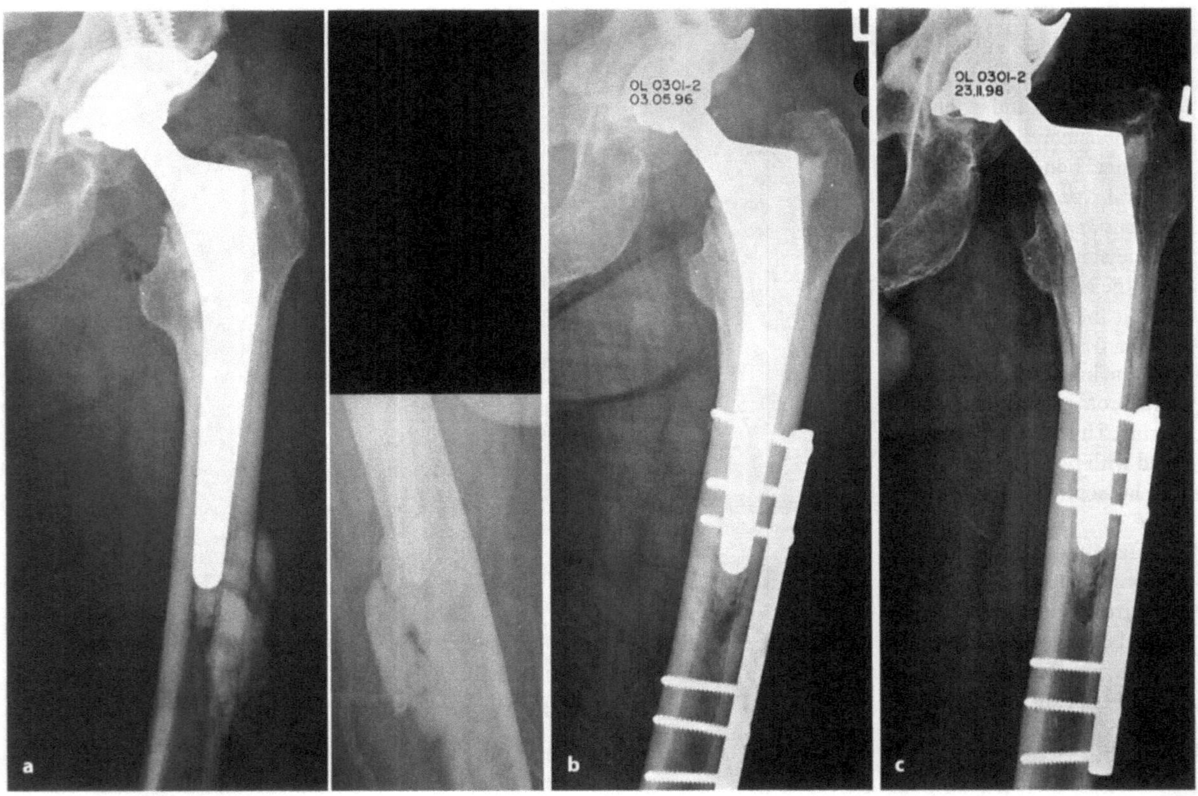

Figs. 7.11a–c. Shaft perforation with cement leakage. Fixation with a plate. L.J., male, 55 years (O. 3931)
a Following a stem replacement, a shaft perforation with cement leakage is only noted postoperatively
b After 4 days, the cement is removed and the area around the stem tip is secured with a plate
c Follow-up after 3 years. The patient is symptom free

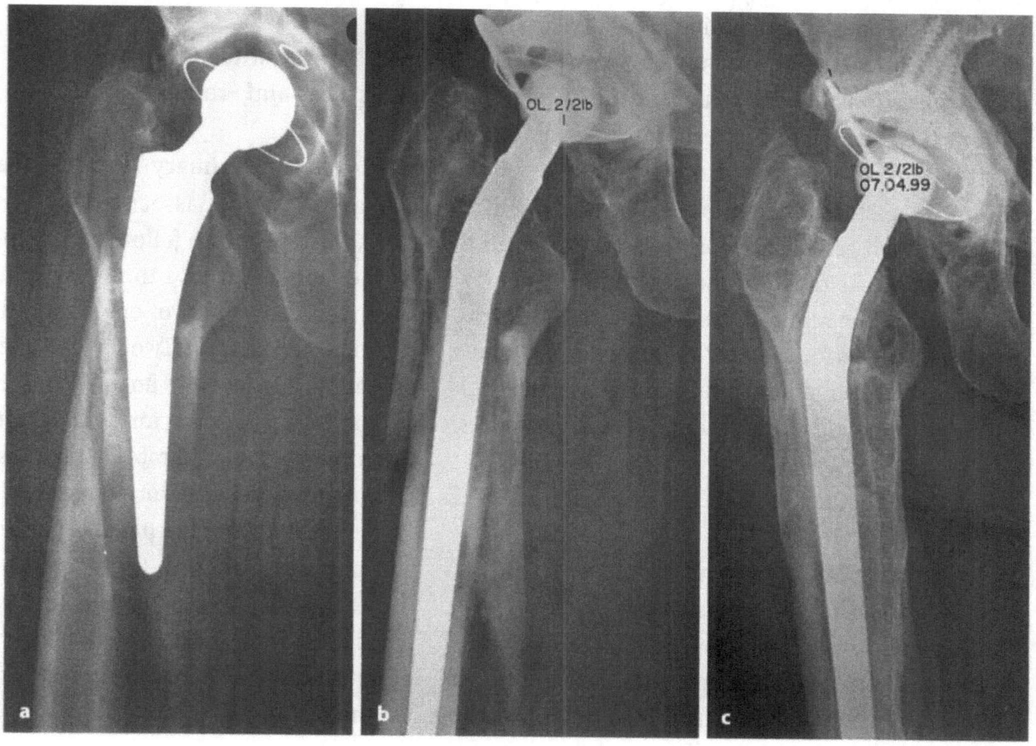

Figs. 7.12a–c. Stem replacement with a type II spiral fracture around a loosened shaft. B.R., male, 64 years (O. 5042)
a Fall 7 years after prosthesis implantation. The loose stem has already subsided by 5 mm and is surrounded by distinct areas of osteolysis. The cemented polyethylene cup has already been loose for several years
b To remove the prosthesis and cement, the proximal femoral fragment is split frontally via a transfemoral approach. Anchorage of a Wagner revision stem in the main distal fragment. Nowadays, we secure the distal fragment with cerclage wiring
c Follow-up after 8 years. The patient is still working part-time on a farm without experiencing any pain

Type III fractures, which usually occur as a result of perforation or appropriate trauma, are secured with a plate (Figs. 7.4, 7.11).

■ **Fractures Associated with Loose Prostheses.** If a periprosthetic fracture occurs around a loose femoral implant, then the stem will need to be replaced at the same time. For type I and II fractures (Fig. 7.3), a prosthesis with a long stem is generally more appropriate for the revision procedure. In cases involving a cementless revision prosthesis according to Wagner, we prefer to employ a transfemoral approach (Fig. 7.12). Cerclage wiring placed around the upper end of the distal shaft will help guard against splitting at this point. A cemented long-stem prosthesis is a very common option for elderly patients. In these cases, the cement must be applied over a distance of about 12 cm, calculated from the distal tip of the prosthesis (see also Fig. 3.12). It is not essential in every case to extend the cementation all the way up to the proximal end.

In type III fractures distal to the stem tip, a cemented short-stem prosthesis combined with plate fixation is one alternative option.

7.5.2 Fissures and Fractures Associated with Revision Prostheses (Table 7.3)

Fractures noted during operation involve splitting of the shaft and can occur both with cemented and cementless systems. Since the cortical bone is already weakened in most cases, the surgeon must proceed carefully. Preoperative planning is particularly valuable in such cases (Figs. 3.9–3.14). If we are prepared for the insertion of both a cemented and uncemented system, we then have the freedom to decide on the best strategy during the actual operation.

Type II fractures and perforations occurring in association with cemented prosthesis are managed by plate fixation. As much of the protruding cement as possible must be removed beforehand from the fracture cleft or perforation. With uncemented stems, cerclage wiring is generally sufficient for securing fissures, while a plate is reserved for genuine fractures.

7.5.3 Postoperative Management and Complications After Osteosyntheses

▪ **Postoperative Management.** With the exception of plate fixations and uncemented long-stem prostheses, the rehabilitation is no different from that after corresponding hip procedures without fractures. Patients undergo a 3- or 4-week phase of building up to full weight-bearing on two walking sticks, depending on the level of pain.

If a situation with a loose prosthesis is stabilised with an uncemented revision prosthesis, a 3-month period of partial weight-bearing is indicated in order to avoid subsequent implant subsidence. The fractures also heal during this period. In plate fixations, full weight-bearing can likewise only begin after 10–12 weeks.

▪ **Complications.** In our patient population, no delayed bone healing or refractures occurred following the correction of fissures and fractures. Nor were any problems attributable to the fracture consequences subsequently observed. The hospital stay was prolonged only slightly in cases of fractures detected at operation. In cases where the fracture was only noted postoperatively, stabilisation was completed during the following 4 days, extending the average duration of hospitalisation by a week. The treatment of fractures after revision procedures caused a hospital stay to be prolonged by an average of 1.5 weeks.

7.5.4 Results After Internal Fixation of Fissures and Fractures

▪ **Results with Primary Total Prostheses.** Of the 32 primary prostheses associated with fissures or fractures, we were able to follow up 26 patients (86%) for periods ranging from 1 to 12 years (Table 7.2). These were recorded as part of our standard hip follow-up regimen (see Chap. 1). Two patients died shortly after operation, and we were unable to trace four patients.

The clinical results for primary prostheses with fractures were comparable with those for patients with no fracture. After an average period of 4.3 years (1–12 years), 20% of the patients (6) described the result as very good, 57% (17) as good, while 10% (3) were satisfied. Of those patients that were merely satisfied, 2 had loosened cups (4 and 8 years) and the other a loosened stem (5 years), which may explain the modest results in these cases.

▪ **Results for Revision Procedures.** Ten of the patients (76%) with a type I fracture were followed up for 3.9 years (1–10 years) (Table 7.3). Four of these patients described the result as very good, five as good, while one with a possible loose stem was satisfied. Of the seven patients in the group with a type II fracture, six described the result after 2 years (1–5) as very good. The remaining patient was merely satisfied and showed radiologically stable implants.

7.5.5 Literature on the Management of Fissures and Fractures

In a literature review we were unable to find any prospective studies. The therapeutic strategies mentioned in the literature for dealing with periprosthetic fractures did not show any major differences.

As a rule, type I fractures are managed by cerclage. The cerclage should be fixed proximal to the lesser trochanter as this ensures significantly greater stability [19]. Compared with cemented systems, fewer problems are encountered with fissures around uncemented prostheses since there is no possibility of leaking cement interfering with fracture healing [5]. Consequently, these fractures are often considered to be stable and not in need of treatment [4, 5, 11, 13]. A wide variety of cerclage options is proposed: Multifilament cables, Parnham, nylon, Partridge or titanium bands in addition to the standard cerclage wiring. The Ogden plate and the Dall-Milles plate involve combinations of plate fixation and Parnham bands [4, 15]. Even careful reading of the relevant studies fails to elicit any clear advantages of these various materials over the simple cerclage wiring used by us.

There is widespread unanimity concerning the proposed management of type II and III fractures. Cerclage or internal fixation is recommended for stable prostheses. If the prosthesis is loose, authors recommend replacement with a long-stem prosthesis, cemented or uncemented [10, 11, 13]. Divergent opinions are expressed primarily in respect of fractures associated with revision surgery. Thus, some authors postulate that any revised cemented stem must be replaced by an uncemented one [8, 15, 16], claiming that this solution produces the best results. In one of the studies so many refractures were observed after internal fixations that the authors do not recommend this method [16]. On the other hand, the rotational stability produced in experimental trials with a cemented system in animal bone was impressive enough for the authors to recommend the more widespread use of such systems [17]. Opinion was unanimous concerning the detailed surgical technique for removing cement by windowing. In order to achieve adequate stability, a long-stem prosthesis must provide bridging of at least 2 shaft diameters below the window. Several authors describe the reintegration of the removed window after the edges are cleaned of cement residues, although this requires a good fit, cancellous bone grafting and securing with cerclage wiring.

If the bone quality is poor and the cortical bone has thinned out over long stretches, bridging by "bone impaction grafting" combined with a long-stem prosthesis is recommended. The aim of this technique is to rebuild the bone stock [7, 8, 10, 15, 16].

If the stability of an uncemented long-stem prosthesis is diminished in the lower section of the femoral shaft, the upper end of this section should be protected against splitting by cerclage [5].

The conservative contingent represents a minor curiosity. These authors describe special tractions and spica casts, which give uniformly poor results, in most cases ending in malposition or nonunion. Since the patients are confined to bed for the very prolonged treatment period, complications such as decubitus ulcers, venous thromboses, embolisms, pneumonia and other medical problems can occur. None of this is particularly conducive to the health of elderly patients with periprosthetic fractures [4].

To guard against the risk of periprosthetic fractures, some authors recommend avoiding fissures or windowing intraoperatively or bridging for any fractures that do occur. Cement should not be allowed to enter any defects to avoid hindering the remodelling process (Fig. 7.1). If the operator is not confident about the stability of the situation, cerclage or cancellous bone grafting should be employed too much rather than too little. If patients are consistently and rigorously followed up, revisions can be undertaken for fissures and perforations before any resulting periprosthetic fracture occurs [10].

7.6 Conclusions

In our treatise we have shown that the problems encountered to date can be effectively managed with the two standard methods of fixation (cerclage and plating). The following points can serve as guidelines:

1. Intraoperative fissures occurring in association with cemented stems must be identified before cementation and closed with a water-tight seal to prevent cement from penetrating the fissure.
2. Fissures detected only postoperatively should be rectified immediately, since bone healing is hindered by cement penetration in the fissure (Fig. 7.1), with a consequent major risk of a periprosthetic fracture.
3. Subsequent periprosthetic fractures require replacement of the prosthesis if stem loosening is found to be a contributory factor in causing the fracture.
4. The linea aspera is the best anchoring zone for plate fixations.

No refractures have been observed during our own follow-up examinations, which suggests that our therapeutic strategy is along the right lines. In contrast with some literature reports, we have not observed an increased incidence of fractures with the cemented straight-stem system. All fractures were managed surgically in the first instance. A conservative approach is no longer in keeping with the times, particularly since this involves prolonged bed rest with all its associated risks.

As regards instrumentation, our system can be applied universally without the need for special instruments or implants, since the fracture osteosyntheses are closely based on the most popular fixation systems. Planning ensures targeted management and optimises the therapeutic outcome. It also simplifies communication with the operating staff and gives the operator a clearer understanding precisely in those cases where unforeseen situations arise during surgery.

We have not observed any negative findings during the follow-up of patients with calcar fissures managed prophylactically with cerclage wiring. No infections occurred, and at no stage was metal removal required.

References

1. Adolphson P, Jonsson U, Kalén R (1987) Fractures of the ipsilateral femur after total hip arthroplasty. Arch Orthop Trauma Surg 106: 353–357
2. Beals RK, Toner ST (1996) Periprosthetic fractures of the femur. Clin Orthop 327: 238–246
3. Christensen CM, Seger BM, Schultz RB (1989) Management of intraoperative femur fractures associated with revision hip arthroplasty. Clin Orthop 248: 177–180
4. Duncan CP, Masri BA (1995) Fractures of the femur after hip replacement. In: Jackson DW (ed) Instructional course lectures. AAOS 44: 293–304
5. Fitzgerald RH, Brindley GW, Kavanagh BF (1988) The uncemented total hip arthroplasty. Clin Orthop 235: 61–66
6. Fredin H (1988) Late fracture of the femur following perforation during hip arthroplasty. Acta Orthop Scand 59: 331–332
7. Johannsson JE, McBroom R, Barrington TW, Hunter GA (1981) Fracture of the ipsilateral femur in patients with total hip replacement. A standard system of terminology for reporting results. J Bone Joint Surg Am 63: 1435–1442
8. Klein AH, Rubash HE (1993) Femoral windows in revision total hip arthroplasty. Clin Orthop 291: 164–170
9. Kolstad K (1994) Revision THR after periprosthetic femoral fractures. Acta Orthop Scand 65: 505–508
10. Lewallen DG, Berry DJ (1997) Periprosthetic fracture of the femur after total hip arthroplasty. J Bone Joint Surg Am 79: 1881–1890
11. McLauchlan GJ, Robinson CM, Singer BR, Christie J (1997) Results of an operative policy in the treatment of periprosthetic femoral fracture. J Orthop Trauma 11: 170–179
12. Missakian ML, Rand JA (1993) Fractures of the femoral shaft adjacent to long-stem femoral components of total hip arthroplasty. Orthopedics 16: 149–152
13. Moran MC (1996) Treatment of periprosthetic fractures around total hip arthroplasty with an extensively coated femoral component. J Arthroplasty 11: 981–988
14. Patterson BM, Lieberman JR, Salvati EA (1995) Intraoperative complications during total hip arthroplasty. Orthopedics 18: 1089–1095
15. Ogden WS, Rendall J (1978) Fractures beneath hip prosthesis: a special indication for Parham bands and plating. Orthop Trans 2: 70
16. Schmotzer H, Tchejeyan GH, Dall DM (1996) Surgical management of intra- and postoperative fractures of the femur about the tip of the stem in total hip arthroplasty. J Arthroplasty 11: 709–717
17. Schutzer SF, Grady-Benson J, Jasty M, O'Connor DO, Bragdon C, Harris WH (1995) Influence of intraoperative femoral fractures and cerclage wiring on bone ingrowth into canine porous-coated femoral components. J Arthroplasty 10: 823–829
18. Zenni EJ, Pommeroy DL, Claudle RJ (1988) Ogden plate and other fixation for fractures complicating endoprostheses. Clin Orthop 231: 83–90
19. Groh E, Wirtz DC, Weber M, Prescher A, Heller KD (1999) Experimental study concerning stabilization of fissures of the femoral shaft during total hip replacement. Presentation at the EFFORT congress, Brussels, 1999

Chapter 8

Trochanteric Problems

8

Martin Sarungi

Trochanteric osteotomies facilitate the approach to the hip, but involve the risk of nonunion and displacement of the fragments. In our patient population, osteotomies were performed in 0.9% of primary total hip replacements (THR) and in 13% of revision procedures (Figs. 8.4, 8.5). The preferred type of osteotomy in recent years has been the chevron osteotomy, subsequently fixed with a wire loop technique according to M.E. Müller (Fig. 8.1).

Trochanteric fractures occurred in 1.9% of primary THRs and 1.8% of revision THRs. A higher incidence was noted for women (2.5%) and for varus/protrusion hips. In our experience, fixation with a malleolar screw combined with a cerclage wire as a tension band has proved the most successful method (Fig. 8.6).

Trochanteric fractures and osteotomies have a negative influence on the outcome, especially after primary THR. Limping is more frequent, particularly in cases of nonunion. The management of nonunions is difficult, necessitating special revision techniques and fixation methods.

8.1 Introduction, Definitions

8.1.1 Introduction

During total hip replacement (THR), the greater trochanter may suffer an accidental fracture (FR). Occasionally, a trochanteric osteotomy (OT) is also required for technical reasons. Since the greater trochanter represents the most important attachment site for abductor muscles, the outcome of trochanteric union following an osteotomy or fracture has an important influence on the future function of the corresponding hip. It is no coincidence that trochanteric problems have been discussed by many authors [1, 14]. The aim of this chapter is to discuss the frequency, risk, prevention and treatment of trochanteric fractures and osteotomies.

8.1.2 Definitions

Trochanteric osteotomy. Surgical separation of the greater trochanter during THR to obtain better exposure of the hip in order to facilitate surgery.

- A *flat osteotomy* is a single-plane osteotomy performed using a chisel or oscillating saw.
- A *chevron osteotomy* is a biplanar V-shaped osteotomy, usually performed using an oscillating saw [3]. This shape facilitates stable osteosynthesis and prevents rotational movements during flexion (Fig. 8.1).
- A *transfemoral approach* involves exposure of the proximal femur via a transverse or oblique osteotomy distal to the lesser trochanter, supplemented by a frontal osteotomy proximally (Fig. 8.2). This

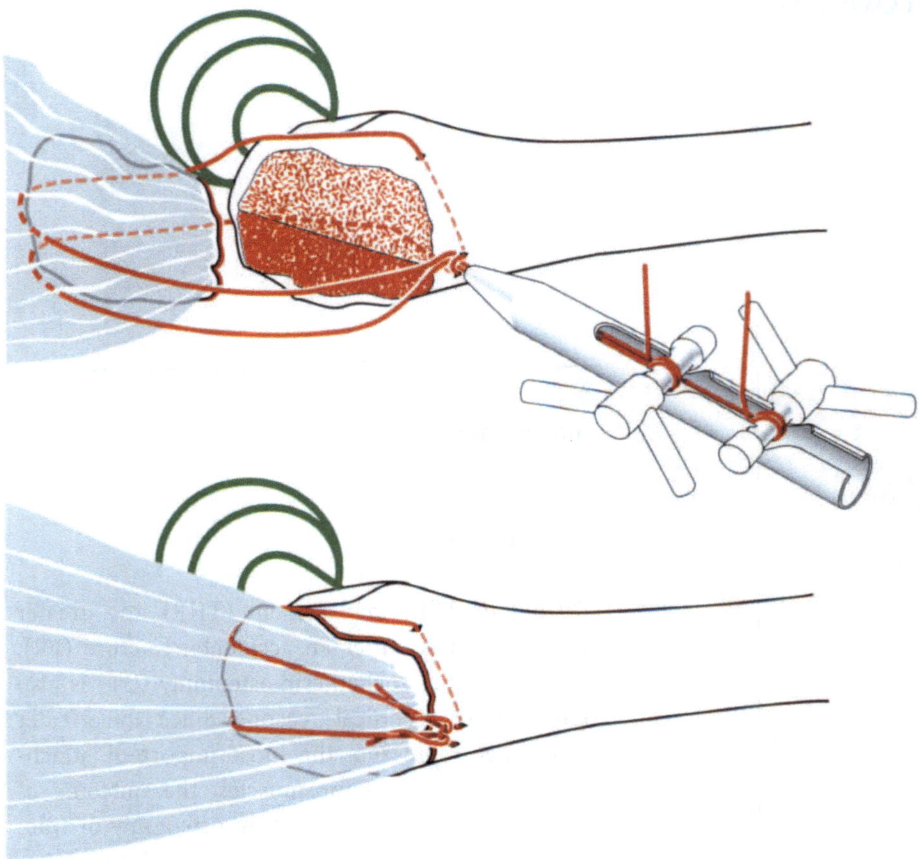

Fig. 8.1. Chevron-type osteotomy according to M.E. Müller. The V-shape of the osteotomy provides rotational stability. For fixation purposes, a wire loop is passed through a drilled hole dorsal and ventral to the prosthesis, the ends are pulled over the trochanter and through the loop and grasped with the tightener. The trochanter is reduced and the cerclage wires are tightened and bent back on themselves

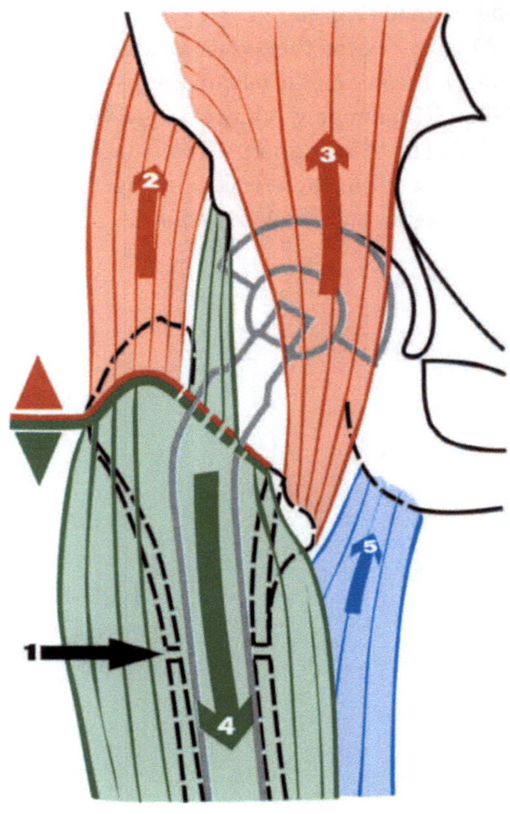

Fig. 8.2. Transfemoral approach. If a transverse osteotomy is performed distal to the lesser trochanter (*1*) and the proximal femoral section is split along the frontal plane, gaping of the fragments does not occur since the pelvitrochanteric muscles (*red*), which exert traction in a proximal direction, are counterbalanced by the quadriceps femoris and the adductors (*green*)

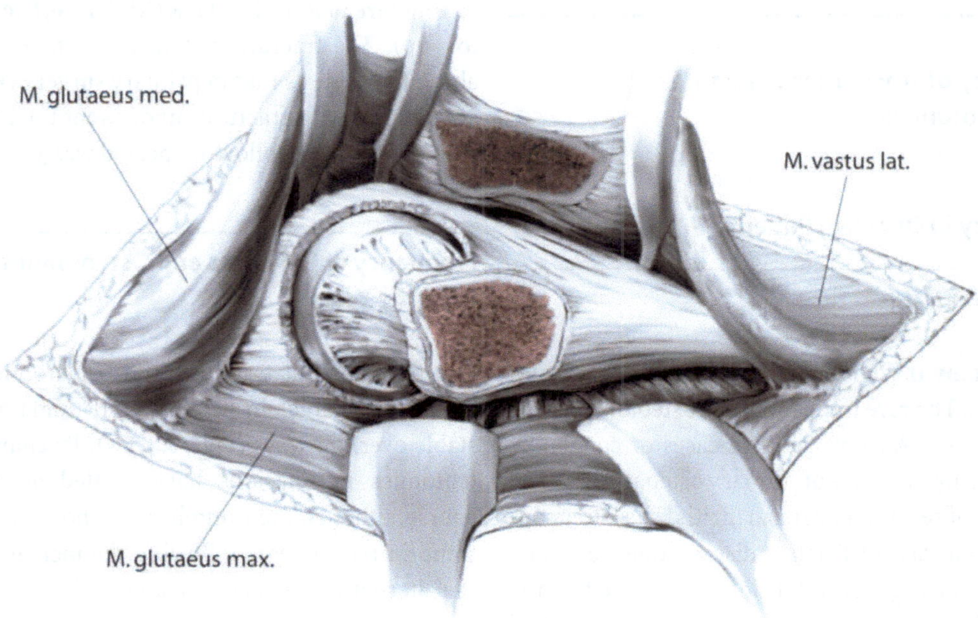

Fig. 8.3. Trochanteric flip osteotomy. With the patient in the lateral position, the trochanter is exposed and a flat osteotomy executed along the sagittal plane, starting from the dorsal side and preserving the dorsocranial capsule vessels. The dorsocranial muscle insertions are divided. The trochanter is then shifted ventrally, allowing the hip to be dislocated ventrally for prosthesis insertion

approach facilitates simple retrieval of the prosthesis, while still allowing the fragments to be held in check by the muscles. Particularly in cases where the greater trochanter is severely eroded by granulation tissue, healing can generally be achieved much more reliably after a transfemoral approach than after a trochanteric osteotomy.

- A *flip osteotomy* is a special form of a flat osteotomy that preserves the attachments of both the vastus lateralis and gluteus medius muscles (Fig. 8.3). Held in check proximally and distally, the greater trochanter can then be pushed to the ventral side and the hip dislocated to give the surgeon a good view of the operating field. At the end of the operation, the trochanter can be repositioned and held securely in place with an additional screw [13, 15, 16]. However, the tendency for the trochanter to migrate ventrally in unstable situations as a result of the lack of dorsal anchorage creates new problems (see also Sect. 8.5.2).

▪ **Trochanteric Fractures.** Accidental separation of the greater trochanter. This can be caused by an excessively distal or L-shaped femoral neck osteotomy. Distalisation and/or lateralisation of the greater trochanter occurring during a THR is associated with an increased risk of fracture (Fig. 8.6).

▪ **Fracture Classification.** In the Duncan-Masri classification of periprosthetic femoral fractures, trochanteric fractures are assigned to the Type AG subgroup [5]. These are not usually further subdivided into different groups.

8.2 Frequency of Trochanteric Fractures and Osteotomies

8.2.1 Frequency in Our Own Patients

Primary THR

▪ **Osteotomy in Primary THR (POT; n=10, all with follow-up).** The rare indications for osteotomy in primary THR (0.9%) involved five cases of congenital dislocated hip, one case of primary osteoarthritis and four cases of secondary osteoarthritis. The latter consisted of one case of Perthes' disease, one coxa vara, one situation after central dislocation of the femoral head and one severe deformity after a proximal femoral fracture. The mean follow-up period was 5 years (1–7).

▪ **Fractures in Primary THR (PFR; n=21, 20 patients with follow-up).** Fractures occurred in 1.9% of cases, affecting 2.4% of the female patients compared with just 1.5% of the male patients. This difference is probably attributable primarily to osteoporosis. There is some evidence to suggest that fractures occur more frequently in varus situations, such as protrusion hip. In these cases there is a special risk of intraoperative lengthening and lateralisation, with resulting increased tension on the greater trochanter. The mean follow-up period was 5 years (1–12).

Revision THR

▪ **Osteotomy in revision THR (ROT; n=42, 35 with follow-up).** Trochanteric osteotomy was performed more frequently in a total hip revision (16% of 153 cases) than in a stem or cup revision alone (10% of 176). Thirty-five patients were followed up for an average of 4 years (1–10), whereas four died and three were lost to follow-up.

▪ **Osteotomy in Revision THR with Previous History of Infection (RINFOT; n=5, all with follow-up).** All but one patient in this group underwent total hip revision. The mean follow-up period was 4.6 years (1–10).

▪ **Fracture in Revision THR (RFR; n=6, five with follow-up).** The fracture rate in revision surgery was about the same as that in primary surgery (1.8%). All six patients with fractures underwent total hip revision. The average follow-up period was 3 years (1–6).

Frequency of Fractures and Osteotomies Over the Years

The frequency of fractures and osteotomies of the greater trochanter in primary THR remained fairly stable over the years (Figs. 8.4, 8.5). Trochanteric osteotomies in revisions have plotted an irregular course, although their number has shown a declining trend in recent years following the increased use of the alternative transfemoral approach [7].

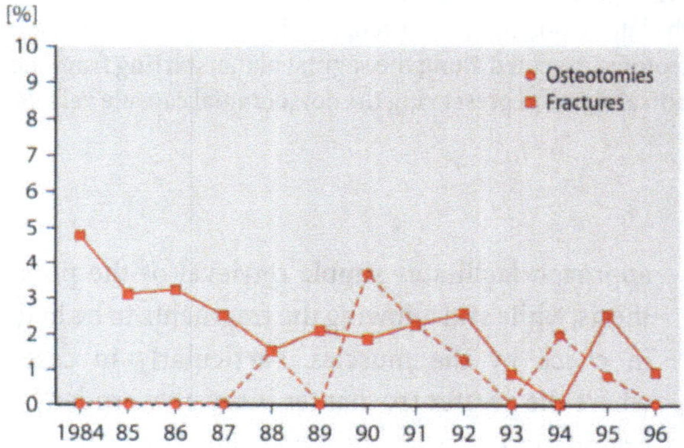

Fig. 8.4. Incidence of osteotomies and fractures of the greater trochanter during primary THR

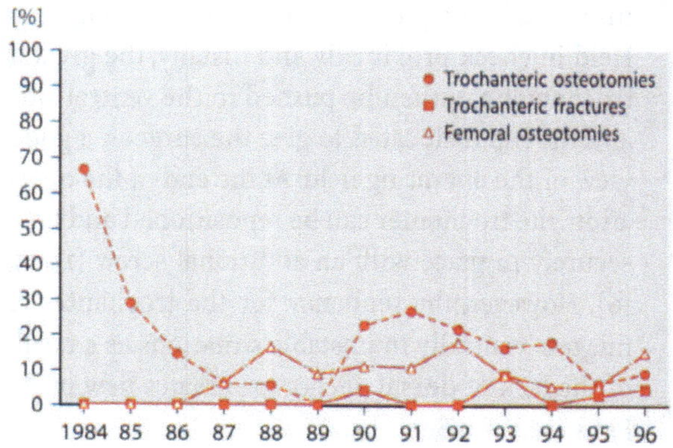

Fig. 8.5. Incidence of osteotomies and fractures of the greater trochanter during revision THR

8.2.2
Frequency in the Literature

Intraoperative femoral fractures have been reported with frequencies ranging from 0.4% for primary THR using cemented components to 17.6% for revision THR using uncemented femoral components [6]. Most figures, however, fluctuate between 1% and 2% [2, 5, 14].

8.3
Risk Factors for Trochanteric Fractures

A whole series of risk factors are known to favour a trochanteric fracture:

- Changes in bone structure due to systemic diseases (osteoporosis, rheumatoid arthritis, osteogenesis imperfecta, Paget's disease)
- Varus of the proximal femur (coxa vara congenita, hip protrusion, osteoarthritis after Perthes' disease)
- Difficulties with intraoperative hip mobilisation or hip dislocation (hip protrusion, pericapsular scarring, heterotopic ossification)
- Revision of the prosthesis, especially if the cup and stem have to be replaced
- Inadequate surgical exposure [11]

As regards our own patients, trochanteric fractures were most likely to occur during the preparation of the medullary cavity for the femoral component. Patients were particularly at risk if forced adduction of

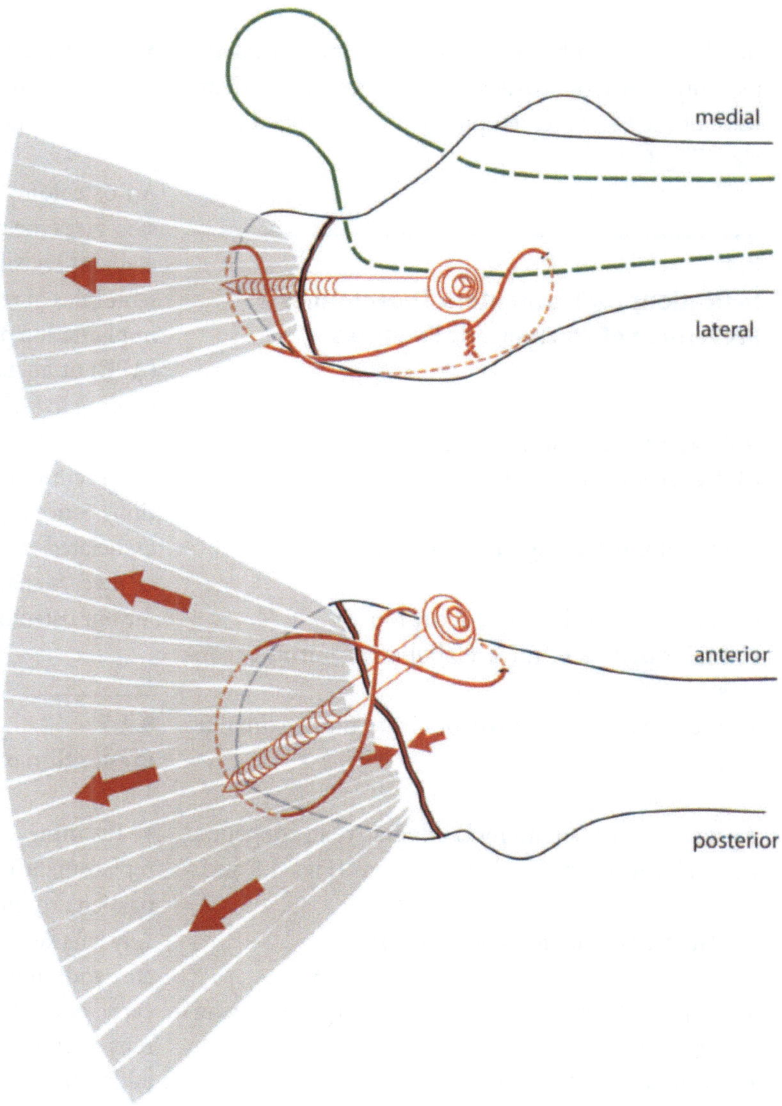

Figs. 8.6a,b. Fixation of a trochanteric fracture. B.H., female, 70 years (O. 4062)
a Drawing: A trochanteric fracture is particularly likely to occur during forced adduction and external rotation of the leg when the femur is being prepared for implantation of the stem. Traction exerted by the gluteus medius muscle (*arrows*) tears off the greater trochanter in the dorsocranial direction. The fracture is fixed by means of a malleolar screw inserted perpendicularly to the fracture plane and a tension band wire tightened around the screw. This arrangement compresses the fracture cleft perpendicularly to the fracture plane, providing resistance against the traction forces
b see p. 128

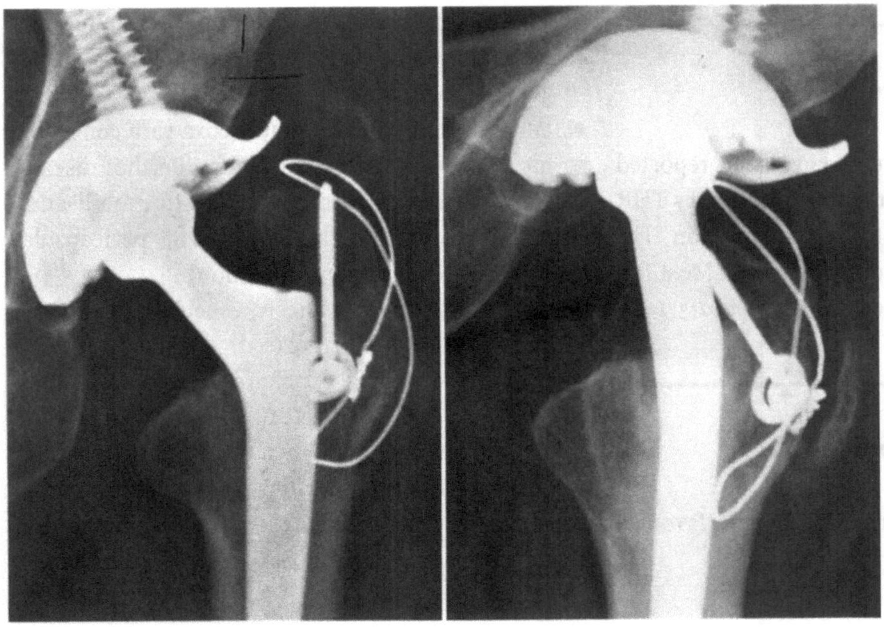

Fig. 8.6
b Radiograph. Despite particularly cautious management, a trochanteric fracture also occurred during a THR on the other side in this obese female patient with osteoporosis

the shaft was combined with a deep femoral neck osteotomy, if osteoporosis was present, if the patients were obese or possessed powerfully developed muscles (Fig. 8.6).

8.4 Indications for Trochanteric Osteotomies – Prevention of Trochanteric Fractures

8.4.1 Indications for Osteotomies of the Greater Trochanter

■ **Osteotomy During Primary THR**

- Congenital dislocation of the hip
- Major defects of the acetabulum requiring reconstruction
- Previous fracture or osteotomy of the proximal femur

A trochanteric osteotomy is imperative in congenital hip dislocation and similar situations (Figs. 3.8, 7.4).

■ **Osteotomy During Revision THR**

- Major defects of the acetabulum requiring reconstruction
- Pronounced stem subsidence
- Large quantities of cement to be removed from the femoral shaft
- Girdlestone situation (Fig. 6.5)

An osteotomy of the greater trochanter during revision gives the operator a clearer view, e.g. in major acetabular revisions. Over half (53% or 25 hips) of our osteotomies in revision surgery were associated with the implantation of a Burch-Schneider antiprotrusio cage (APC) or an acetabular reinforcement ring (ARR) according to M.E. Müller. The enhanced overview means that an osteotomy can also be performed during cement removal in order to avoid femoral shaft perforations. Since it provides an even better overview and is associated with a low risk of nonunion, we have in recent years changed over to the transfemoral approach for our osteotomies [8] (Fig. 8.2).

8.4.2 Prevention of Trochanteric Fractures

■ **Planning.** Careful preoperative planning of total hip replacement helps avoid unwanted leg lengthening, a particularly important risk factor in protrusion hips. Any lengthening proximal to the trochanteric area creates additional traction on the greater trochanter because of a relative shortening of the muscles. Concurrent lateralisation of the shaft is associated with an additional fracture risk (see also Chap. 3.4.3, Fig. 3.7).

■ **CDH Implant According to M.E. Müller.** This implant (Fig. 2.9a) was specially designed for patients with congenital dislocation of the hip (CDH) and prominent coxa vara. The specially shaped proximal end prevents any undesirable lengthening (Figs. 3.8, 7.4, 9.1).

■ **Femoral Neck Osteotomy.** Osteotomy of the femoral neck should be performed with an oblique rather than an L-shaped cut, particularly in patients with varus hips and osteoporosis. When exposing the femoral canal, the femur must be adducted and externally rotated continuously and slowly, without any jerking movements. Particular caution is indicated in fat patients and those with substantial muscle mass.

8.5 Techniques for Osteotomy and Fracture Osteosynthesis

8.5.1 Methods Used in Our Patients

■ **Osteotomies.** Whereas a flat osteotomy was the preferred technique in the early days, we have since abandoned this technique completely in favour of the chevron osteotomy. We are increasingly adopting the transfemoral approach, particularly for patients with advanced shaft defects.

■ **Osteosynthesis Techniques Used.** The osteosynthesis technique differs for osteotomies and fractures and has also changed between the start and end of the observation period. We use the following methods:

Method (Fig. 8.7)	(n)	Indication
Single cerclage wires (1CL)	18	Fractures – at the start
Multiple cerclages (MCL)	23	Osteotomies – at the start
Special plates (PLT)	5	Nonunions
Reabsorbable cord (PDS)	1	
Malleolar screw + cerclage (SCRCL)	14	Fractures and osteotomies
Single-wire loop Müller (MüCL)	13	Chevron osteotomies

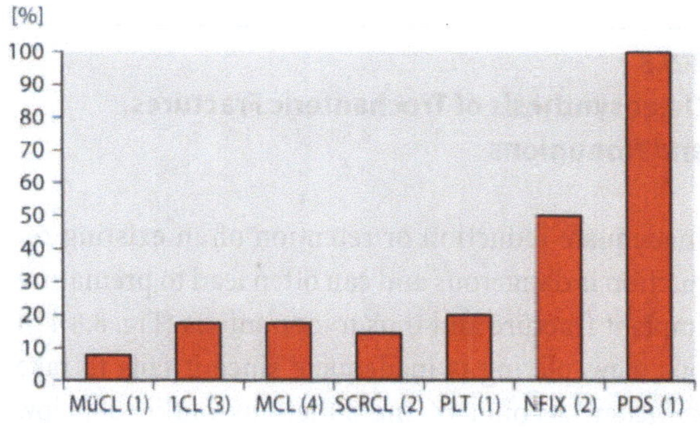

Fig. 8.7. Nonunions (n=14) in our patients after various fixation procedures for trochanteric fractures, osteotomies and nonunions. *MüCL*: single wire loop technique (Müller); *1CL*: single cerclage; *MCL*: multiple cerclages; *SCR CL*: malleolar screw + cerclage; *PLT*: special plates; *NFIX*: no initial fixation; *PDS*: PDS cerclage. The *y* axis shows the percentage of nonunions in each group

Four fractures not noticed during the operation were not fixed at all. Only those osteosynthesis methods still used by us are mentioned in the following sections.

8.5.2 Osteosynthesis of Trochanteric Osteotomies

■ **Osteotomy Technique.** We currently perform the chevron-type osteotomy since the procedure is simple and allows the surgeon to implement a subsequent fixation that is stable against rotational movements (Fig. 8.1). This technique has, however, largely been superseded in our hospital by the transfemoral approach, particularly for major defects of the greater trochanter (Fig. 8.2). We are rather sceptical about the technique of trochanteric flip osteotomy (Fig. 8.3).

■ **Osteosynthesis Technique.** The single, double-passed, wire loop technique using an AO wire tightener has proved an effective fixation method in our hospital (Figs. 3.8, 8.1). Alternatively, three separate cerclage wires can successively be passed through a hole 1 cm distal to the trochanteric osteotomy and over the trochanter through the muscle. Reabsorbable suture material is less suitable because of its elasticity and fairly low abrasion resistance.

8.5.3 Osteosynthesis of Trochanteric Fractures and Nonunions

Inadequate reduction or retention of an existing reduction is dangerous and can often lead to premature implant fracture and thus to nonunions (Fig. 8.8). In our view, plating is inadequate since it fails to take sufficient account of the situations outlined below (Fig. 8.9e).

In planning the osteosynthesis of a trochanteric fracture, it should be borne in mind that the fracture line is almost never oriented in a transverse plane. As a result of the traction exerted by the gluteus medius muscle in a dorsal and cranial direction, the fracture line almost invariably runs obliquely, in a ventrocranial to dorsodistal direction (Figs. 8.6, 8.10). Any tension banding procedure will need to take this situation into account.

■ **Osteosynthesis of Trochanteric Fractures.** Our best results have been achieved by combining a malleolar screw inserted perpendicularly to the fracture cleft with a tension band wire passed over the screw (Fig. 8.6).

■ **Osteosynthesis of Trochanteric Nonunions/ Pseudarthrosis.** Analysis of the situation: As long as functional tension banding of the gluteus medius muscle in relation to the femur is present, trochanteric nonunions may not even be noticed by the patients. Problems arise when a functional insufficiency is combined with pain. Management is especially difficult if there is a wide gap between the tip and base of the trochanter as a result of bone loss, shaft lengthening or distalisation of the head centre during cup revision. In such cases, it may not prove possible to secure the trochanteric tip at its original location, even under forced abduction of the leg. Bone grafts are not recommended as spacers to fill the gap because of the resulting risk of local instability. If major defects are present, a corresponding shortening on the femoral and/or acetabular side will occasionally need to be considered.

To prevent such hopeless situations, and particularly if leg length discrepancies are present preoperatively, the operator will need to carefully evaluate, at the planning stage, where lengthening proximal to the trochanteric area is permissible in specific cases and, if so, the extent of such lengthening (see Chap. 9.3.2).

Osteosynthesis of nonunion: Preoperatively, the patient must be made aware of the fact that a successful outcome can only be expected if the trochanteric tip can be fixed to its original insertion point with almost no tension, and that achieving this objective may call for additional measures. The first step is to remove the existing implants. Approach the

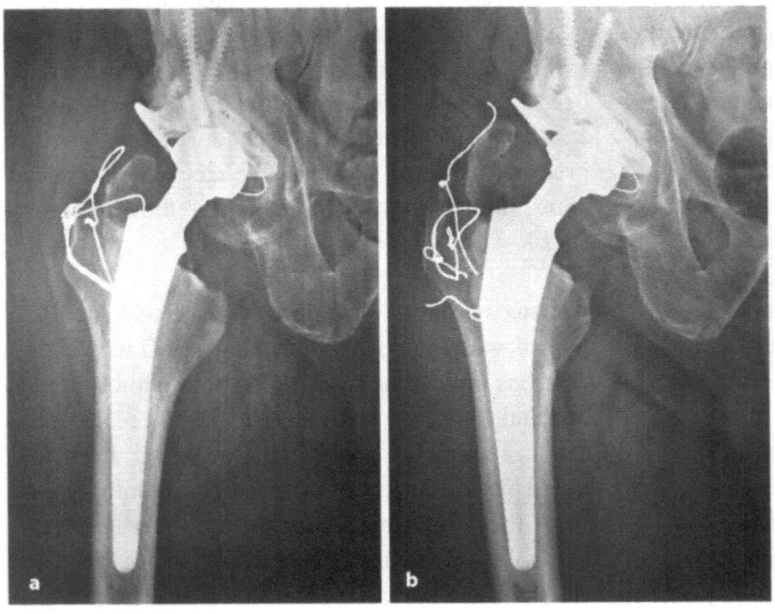

Figs. 8.8a,b. Inadequate fixation of a fractured greater trochanter. M.H., male, 70 years (O. 6922)
a Two cerclage wires were passed through a drilled hole at the base of the trochanter and tensioned without proper reduction of the trochanteric tip
b Four months later, one cerclage wire was broken and the greater trochanter displaced. Nevertheless, the patient was still able to walk without symptoms or a limp even 12 years after the operation.

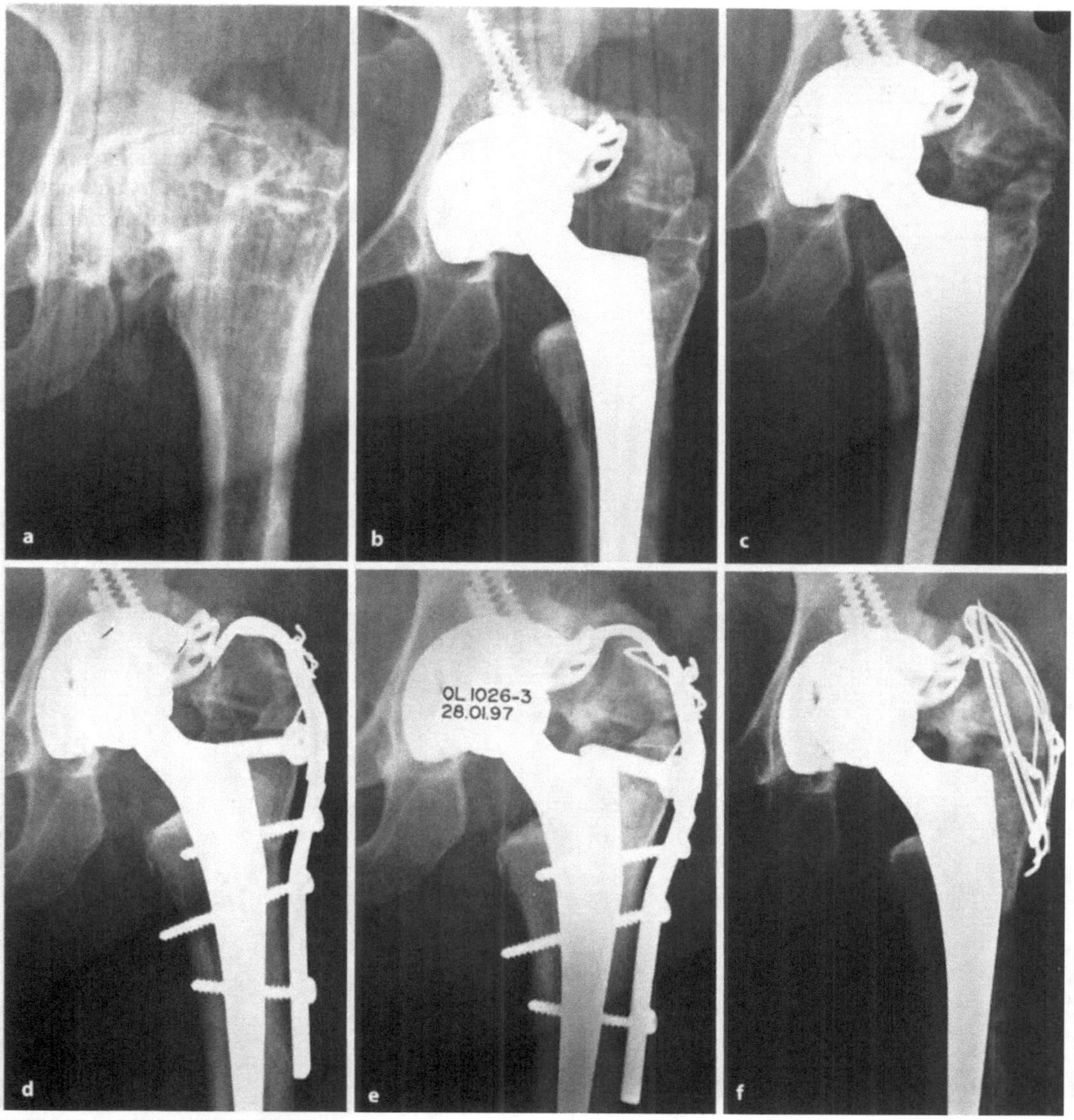

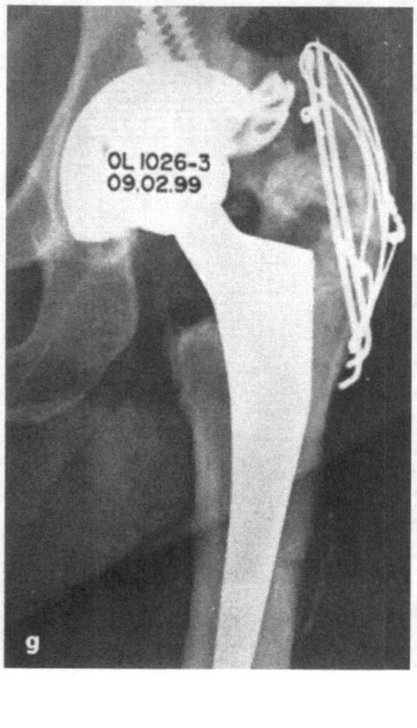

Figs. 8.9a–g. Problems with fixation of trochanteric nonunion. W.M., female, 45 years (O. 8556)
a History of osteoarthritis after a slipped capital femoral epiphysis in childhood and an intertrochanteric osteotomy
b Fracture of the greater trochanter noticed postoperatively
c Persistent pain and widening of the nonunion gap
d Attempted rectification with a trochanter plate
e Fatigue fracture of the plate as a sign of persisting nonunion
f The plate was removed and replaced by fixation with two 2.5-mm Kirschner wires. Two cerclage wires, one placed ventrally and one cranially, act as a double tension band (see also Fig. 8.10)
g Healing of the nonunion within 4 months.

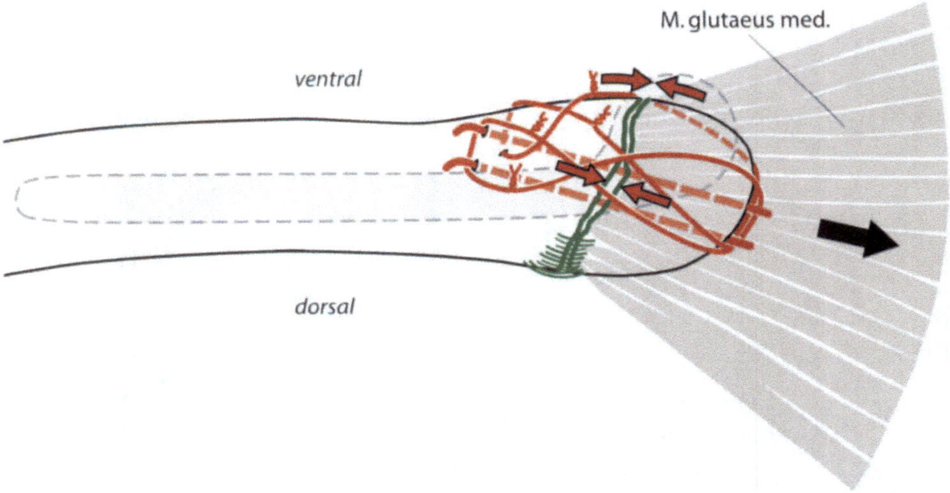

Fig. 8.10. Diagram illustrating the principle of tension band wiring in a trochanteric nonunion – lateral view. The nonunion remains closed. Connective scar tissue on the dorsal aspect of the nonunion is preserved in order to provide added stability

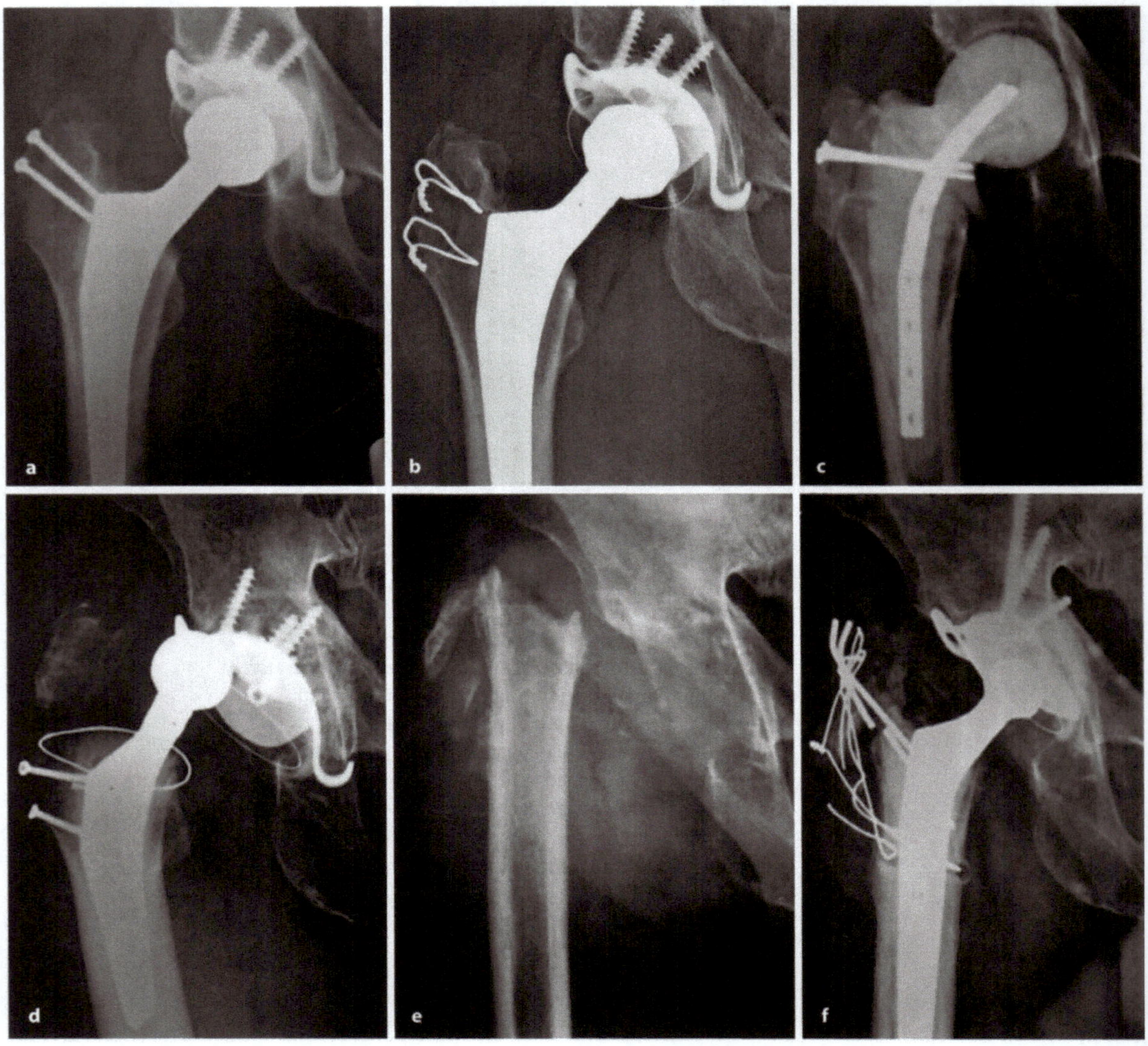

nonunion from the ventral side. Do not totally mobilise the nonunion area but try to preserve the dorsal tissue fibres bridging the nonunion (Fig. 8.10). Remove the scar tissue from the trochanteric tip and the gluteus medius, which may allow some lengthening, but spare the muscle and its innervation. Two additional measures may allow some shortening to be achieved without any major revision:

- Change to a shorter neck in a modular system
- If no threat of impingement exists, select a smaller cup inlay and fix with bone cement.

If these measures still fail to achieve proper adaptation of the trochanteric fragments, the stem and/or cup will need to be changed completely.

For the rerevision of persistent trochanteric nonunion, we have, in recent years, resorted to double tension banding with thick Kirschner wires (Figs. 8.9, 8.10), being a further development of previously employed methods [9, 17]. Autologous cancellous bone may be added on the medial side of the nonunion, between the base of the trochanter and the shoulder of the prosthetic stem. Postoperative management consists of an abduction position and limited flexion of about 70° for 6 weeks. Partial weight bearing of 30 kg is prescribed for a further 6 weeks, usually followed by full weight bearing.

Particular problems have been encountered recently as a result of the increasingly used technique elsewhere of trochanteric flip osteotomy (Fig. 8.11). Although the loosened trochanter remains securely held in place distally, it can occasionally become severely displaced ventrally, potentially causing great difficulties for subsequent reduction and effective fixation.

8.6 Outcome for Trochanteric Fractures and Osteotomies

8.6.1 Nonunion Rate

Our overall nonunion rate for trochanteric fixation is 16%. A similar rate has been observed for almost all the different fixation techniques, with the exception of the cerclage method according M.E. Müller, which is associated with a slightly lower rate, though the difference was not statistically significant because of the small sample and the shortage of comparable cases. Poor surgical technique is a real risk (Fig. 8.7).

Two of the four non-fixed trochanteric fractures ended in nonunion, both requiring more than one further operation (Fig. 8.9). We therefore recommend fixation of all trochanteric fractures as soon as they are identified.

Using the evaluation criteria recommended by the Hip Society [12], we have also evaluated the outcome of osteosyntheses in relation to the general situation (fracture versus osteotomy and primary versus revision THR) (Fig. 8.12). We analysed the rates of healing and displacement. The results were far better for fractures in revision surgery compared to primary surgery, whereas osteotomies in primary operations showed much better consolidation than those in revisions. Osteotomies in infected cases fared the worst.

Secondary fragment displacement was relatively common. Since this is a sign of instability it constitutes a risk for nonunion (Figs. 8.8, 8.12).

Figs. 8.11a–f. Serious infection sequelae after haematoma connected with a torn trochanter after a trochanteric flip osteotomy. M.H., male, 63 years (O. 22238)
a Elevated position of the greater trochanter after screw fixation of a trochanteric flip osteotomy
b Following fixation of the trochanter by two cerclage wires, a haematoma recurred six times. Colonisation with methicillin-resistant *Staphylococcus aureus* (MRSA)
c Nine months after the primary procedure and treatment with vancomycin, prosthesis removal and spacer implantation; 3.5 months later: reimplantation of a prosthesis
d Three and 3.5 weeks later: hip dislocation with torn greater trochanter, which is dislocated ventrocranially. Enterococci. After further dislocation, the prosthesis is replaced by a spacer
e Following the onset of sepsis, a Girdlestone procedure was performed 1 month later (leg shortening of over 10 cm). *Escherichia coli* and coagulase-negative staphylococci were identified as pathogens
f Reimplantation of total prosthesis after 1 year. The severely ventrally displaced greater trochanter was mobilised, put back and reinforced with a cancellous bone graft. Trochanter remains stable despite the breakage of one Kirschner and one cerclage wire (photo). Nine months postoperatively, the patient was almost pain free, could flex the hip through 100° and walk for up to 6 h with two sticks despite a shortening of 6 cm

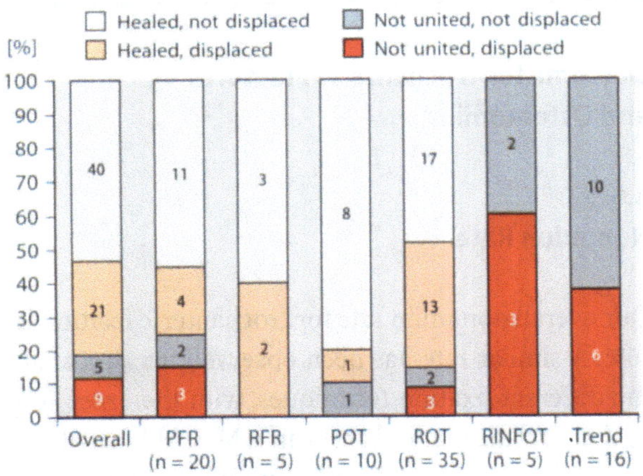

Fig. 8.12. Healing of the greater trochanter in relation to the local situation. *PFR:* primary THR and fracture; *RFR:* revision THR and fracture; *POT:* primary THR and osteotomy; *ROT:* revision THR and osteotomy; *RINFOT:* revision THR, infection and osteotomy; *Trend:* all the patients with positive Trendelenburg sign; *Troch:* all patients with trochanteric nonunion

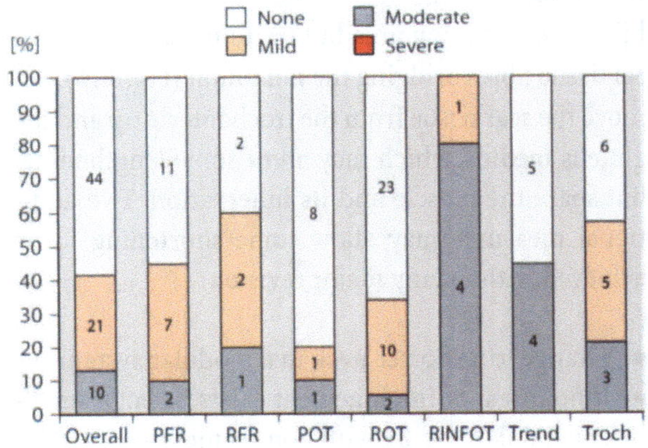

Fig. 8.13. Pain in relation to the local situation. Abbreviations: see Fig. 8.12

Several well-known authors have focused on trochanteric problems [3, 4, 9]. Frequencies cited for trochanteric nonunion range from 0% [9] to 20% [17]. Our nonunion rate is towards the upper end of this range and can be explained by the fairly negative selection of our cases.

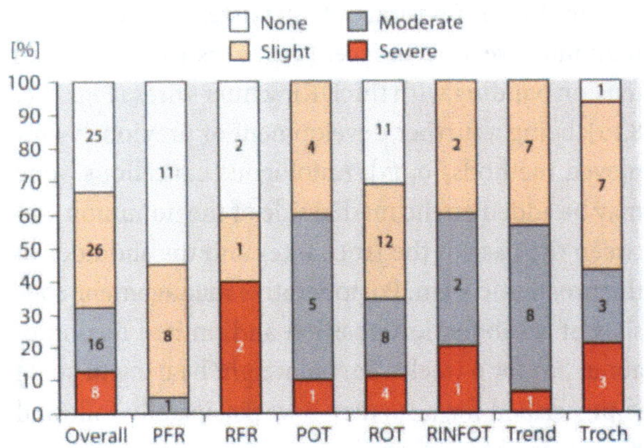

Fig. 8.14. Limping in relation to the local situation. Abbreviations: see Fig. 8.12

8.6.2 Clinical Outcome

■ **Pain.** Pain is the most serious consequence of a trochanteric problem(Fig. 8.13). Fifty-nine percent of patients with trochanteric problems were pain free when last seen. Mild (28%) and moderate (13%) pain was particularly frequent after trochanteric fractures, less so after osteotomies. As might be expected, pain is experienced much more frequently in patients with a positive Trendelenburg sign and/or trochanteric nonunion. Pain is occasionally caused by a trochanteric bursitis. In three instances of bursitis that failed to respond to conservative measures, partial improvement was achieved by removing the metal.

■ **Limping.** On cursory examination, a distinct relationship appears to exist between osteosynthesis of the greater trochanter and limping (Fig. 8.14). Closer analysis, however, reveals that this relationship is only statistically proven for primary hip replacement (Figs. 10.1, 10.2). In revision surgery, limping is equally frequent in patients with and without trochanteric fixation. It is not surprising to discover that limping is almost always present in cases with a positive Trendelenburg sign and in trochanteric nonunion.

■ **Evaluation by the Patients.** Only 14% of patients with a trochanteric problem described the result of their treatment as "very good" (Fig. 8.15). A further 69% rated the results as "good", and 17% as "fair" or "poor". These results do not match those normally achieved after a primary or revision THR. Limping and nonunion have an additional negative impact on the evaluation.

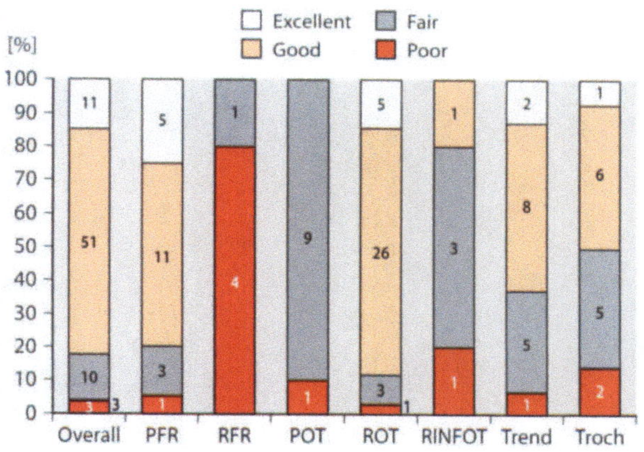

Fig. 8.15. Evaluation of the results by patients in relation to the local situation. Abbreviations: see Fig. 8.12

References

1. Amstutz HC (1978) Complications of trochanteric osteotomy in total hip replacement. J Bone Joint Surg Br 60: 214–216
2. Beals RK, Tower ST (1996) Periprosthetic fractures of the femur. An analysis of 93 fractures. Clin Orthop 327: 238–246
3. Berry DJ, Müller ME (1993) Chevron osteotomy and single wire reattachment of the greater trochanter in primary and revision total hip replacement. Clin Orthop 294: 155–161
4. Charnley J (1972) Long term results of low friction arthroplasty of the hip performed as a primary intervention. J Bone Joint Surg Br 50: 61–76
5. Duncan CP, Masri BA (1995) Fractures of the femur after hip replacement. Instr Course Lect 44: 293–305
6. Fitzgerald RH, Brindley GW, Kavanagh BF (1988) The uncemented total hip arthroplasty. Intraoperative femoral fractures. Clin Orthop 235: 61–66
7. Frankel A, Booth RE, Balderston RA, Cohn J, Rothman RH (1990) Complications of trochanteric osteotomy. Clin Orthop 288: 209–213
8. Grünig R, Morscher E, Ochsner PE (1996) Three- to 7-year results with the uncemented SL femoral revision prosthesis. Arch Orthop Trauma Surg 116: 187–197
9. Harris WH, Crothers OD (1978) Reattachment of the greater trochanter in total hip arthroplasty. J Bone Joint Surg Am 60: 211–213
10. Haentjens P, Casteleyn PP, Opdecam P (1995) Hip arthroplasty for failed internal fixation of intertrochanteric and subtrochanteric fractures in elderly patients. Arch Orthop Trauma Surg 113: 222–227
11. Johansson JE, McBroom R, Barrington TW, Hunter GA (1981) Fracture of the ipsilateral femur in patients with total hip replacement. J Bone Joint Surg Am 63: 1435–1442
12. Johnston RC, Fitzgerald RH, Harris WH, Müller ME, Sledge CB (1990) Clinical and radiologic evaluation of total hip replacement. A standard system of terminology for reporting results. J Bone Joint Surg Am 72: 161–168
13. Lindgren U, Svenson O (1988) A new transtrochanteric approach to the hip. Int Orthop (SICOT) 12: 37–41
14. Patterson BM, Liebermann JR, Salvati EA (1995) Intraoperative complications during total hip arthroplasty. Orthopaedics 11: 1089–1095
15. Schneeberger AG, Murphy SB, Ganz R (1997) Die digastrische Trochanterosteotomie. Operat Orthop Traumatol 9: 1–15
16. Siebenrock KA, Gautier E, Ziran BH, Ganz R (1998) Trochanteric flip osteotomy for cranial extension and muscle protection in acetabular fracture fixation using a Kocher-Langenbeck approach. J Orthop Trauma 12 (6): 387–391
17. Simank HG, Chatzipanagoitis C, Kaps HP (1996) Die Komplikationsrate nach Trochanterosteotomie bei Hüfttotalendoprothesen. Z Orthop 134: 457–464
18. Wiesman HJ, Simon SR, Ewald FC, Thomas WH, Sledge CB (1973) Total hip replacement with and without osteotomy of the greater trochanter. J Bone Joint Surg Am 60: 203–210

Leg Length Discrepancies

ANJA S. PIRWITZ

In describing true leg length discrepancies we make a distinction between discrepancies near the hip and those elsewhere in the skeleton. Functional leg length discrepancies are usually caused by contractures.

Leg length discrepancies of up to 1 cm are common after total hip replacements and are usually within the margins of error of the implantation method. If the legs were equal in length before the operation then the patient's satisfaction with the outcome can be diminished even in the presence of only one centimetre of difference. Refining the surgical technique is therefore worthwhile. Careful planning is the first requirement (Chap. 3). Achieving equal leg lengths is simplified through the use of cemented stems. Measurement of the distance between the edge of the cone and the femoral neck osteotomy or lesser trochanter is a simple way of checking the position of the prosthesis during the operation. Full correction of hip-related discrepancies in leg length is most appropriate in cases where these have developed at a late stage. Longstanding and particularly pronounced differences should be corrected carefully, in some cases without full correction, particularly if the true length discrepancy exceeds 4 cm. The compensation of leg length discrepancies in the hip area with a non-hip-related origin can lead to functional problems in the hip joint.

Postoperatively detected leg length discrepancies should initially be observed for 3 months to assess their impact and only then corrected by adaptation of the footwear. Slight undercorrection is the norm.

Maintaining or restoring equal leg length in hip replacement is important for the success of the operation. This particularly applies to the implantation of primary prostheses, whereas compromises often have to be accepted during revision procedures.

9.1 Definitions, Classification

9.1.1 True Leg Length Discrepancy

True leg length discrepancy is a reflection of unequal bone configurations that can arise as a result of a growth disorder or posttraumatically. The origin of true leg length discrepancy may lie in the hip area or elsewhere in the skeleton.

■ **In the Hip Area.** Leg length discrepancies in the hip area originate in a disturbance of the functional triangle formed by the femoral head centre, the greater trochanter and the iliac crest. If the distances between these three structures change, then the muscular lever arms and leg lengths are also affected (Figs. 9.1–9.4).

■ **Shortening.** "Simple" shortening originates from wear of the joint cartilage, and in some cases the adjacent bone substance as well, and a certain degree of subluxation. It represents the typical feature of advanced osteoarthritis (Fig. 3.2). "Complex" shortening is usually associated with a long history. A cranially displaced head centre, an absent femoral neck and an adduction contracture can occur in combination (Fig. 9.1). Severe femoral head necrosis can also lead secondarily to wear of the acetabulum (Fig. 9.2). A Girdlestone situation causes substantial and unsta-

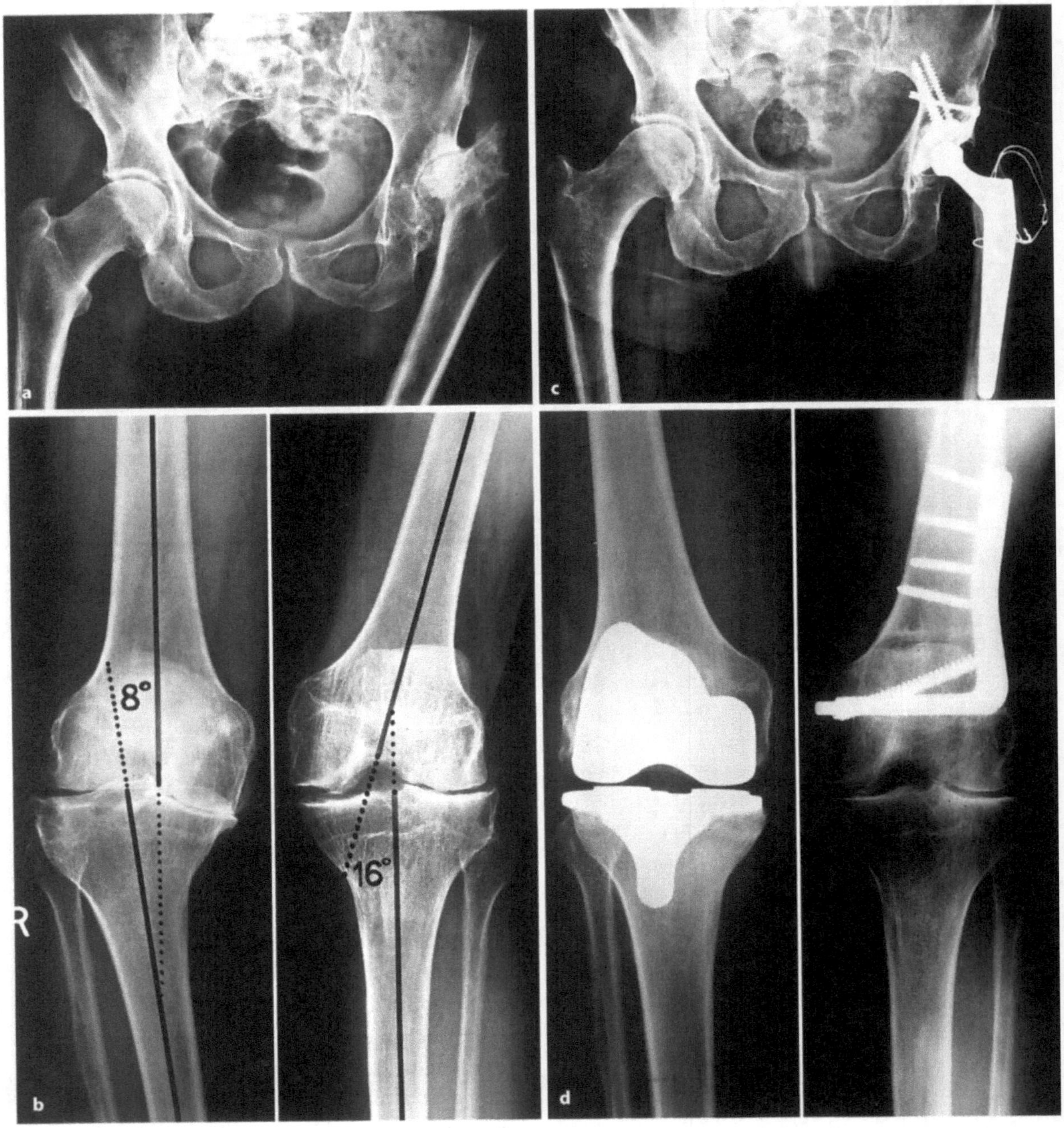

Fig. 9.1a–d. Substantial leg length discrepancy due to functional coxa vara, subluxation and adduction contraction. G.H., male, 64 years (O. 3095)

a Functional left leg shortening of 12 cm

b Radiographs of patient standing on one leg: valgus gonarthrosis on left of 16°, varus gonarthrosis on right of 8°. Combined total hip replacement on the left (see Fig. 3.8 for planning) with supracondylar axial correction on the left with a forked plate

c Three years after total hip replacement and supracondylar varisation osteotomy: shortening of 3.5 cm still remains on the left. No migration of the acetabular reinforcement ring measured by the EBRA method

d Because of increasing pain, a total right knee replacement with concurrent axial correction is performed secondarily

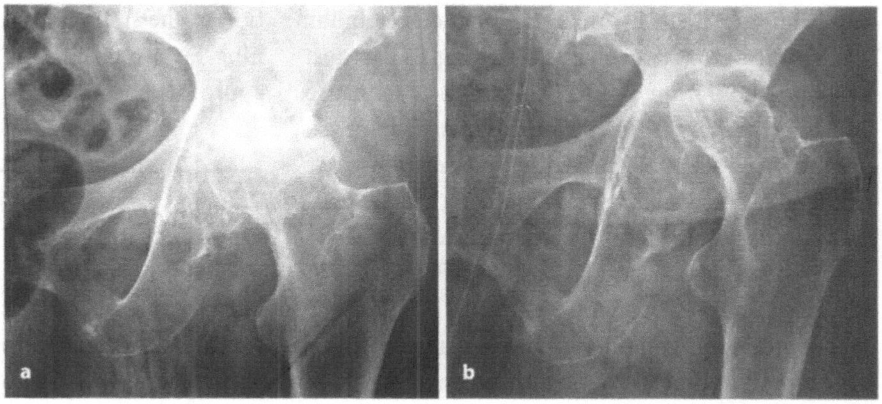

Fig. 9.2a,b. Leg shortening in the hip area due to femoral head necrosis, acetabular wear and slight adduction position. C.E., female, 85 years
a First examination
b Three and a half years later, cranial migration of the head centre due to head collapse and acetabular wear. Equal leg lengths restored after total hip replacement

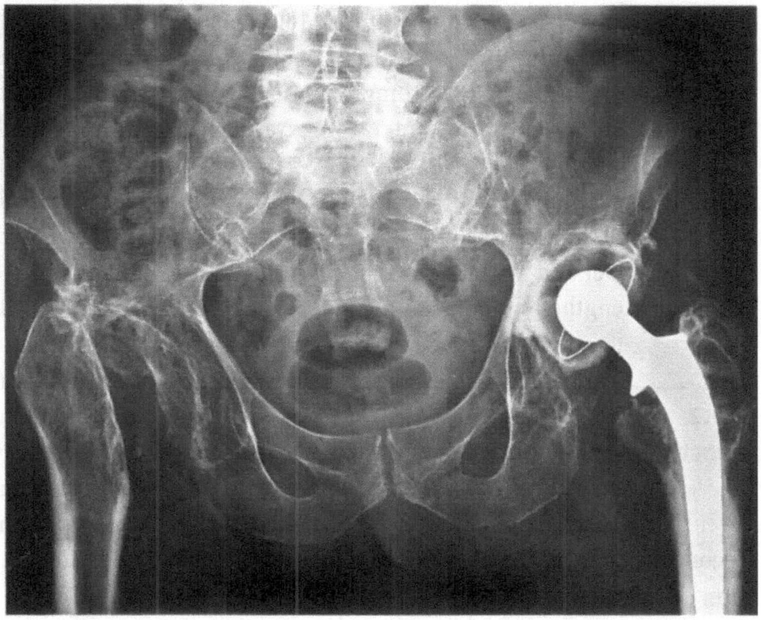

Fig. 9.3. Leg shortening with a Girdlestone hip despite cranial placement of the cup during a total hip replacement on the other side. W.A., male, 77 years. The patient wanted a total hip prosthesis primarily because of the instability, rather than the difference in leg length. No attempt was made at full correction of the length inequality

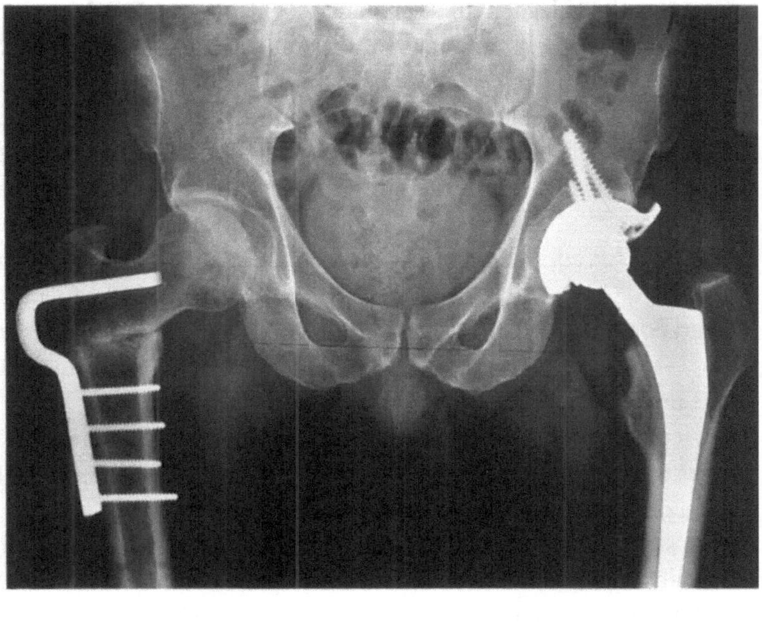

Fig. 9.4. Leg length discrepancy after varisation osteotomy and adduction position of the leg on the right side and total hip replacement on the left with slight lengthening. S.P., male, 51 years (O. 11786). After the varisation osteotomy and the total hip replacement, the patient felt severely hampered by an actual leg shortening of 2.5–3 cm. This feeling was aggravated by an adduction position. The patient is taking legal action

ble shortening, which increases during weight bearing (Fig. 9.3). Excessive reaming of the acetabulum can also lead to (iatrogenic) shortening, as can postoperative migration of a loosened cup. Other causes include coxa vara, slipped capital femoral epiphysis, Perthes' disease, posttraumatic fragment displacement after acetabular or proximal femoral fractures. In many cases, shortening can also result from an intertrochanteric varisation osteotomy (Fig. 9.4).

▪ **Lengthening.** Lengthening occurs almost invariably at operation (Fig. 9.4), more frequently as a result of the use of uncemented femoral implants, less frequently as a result of lengthening on the acetabular side. Lengthening also occurs occasionally as a result of a previous pelvic osteotomy, e.g. after a Salter osteotomy or an intertrochanteric valgisation osteotomy (Figs. 9.1-4).

▪ **Elsewhere in the Skeleton.** Asymmetry of the pelvis or upper and lower legs can lead to both shortening and lengthening.

9.1.2 Functional Leg Length Discrepancy

Even if the bone configurations are well balanced, secondary changes to soft tissues (abduction, adduction or flexion contractures), the joints or the spine (fixed scoliosis) can produce a pelvic tilt with consequent functional leg length discrepancy.

In clinical respects, and thus for the surgical procedure as well, it is important to make the distinction between a correctable (ligament contractures) and an uncorrectable (e.g. fixed scoliosis) leg length discrepancy.

9.1.3 Mixed Form

In its mixed form, a leg length discrepancy is caused by a combination of bone-related and functional causes of differing degree (Figs. 9.1, 9.3).

If a difference in leg length is noted preoperatively, the surgeon will need to ascertain whether this is clinically asymptomatic, or whether the patient is complaining of secondary problems such as back pain. In any case, clinical and radiological examination of the spine is an essential part of careful planning for a total hip replacement. The same criteria apply to a postoperative length discrepancy.

9.2 Frequency in Our Own Patients

9.2.1 Material and Methods

In the immediate pre- and postoperative period and 1 year postoperatively, the figures for the leg length discrepancies were recorded prospectively on evaluation sheets by the investigator, on the basis of clinical and radiological investigations. The sheets included a section headed "functional leg lengths", with no further details concerning the methodology. Since this led to a degree of ambiguity among some investigators, the data had to be checked retrospectively. To this end, the patients with preoperatively equal leg lengths (group 1) were checked again if the postoperative evaluation forms reported length discrepancies of more than 2 cm. In most cases, these figures were incorrect and had to be reassessed. Consequently, all extreme values were checked once again and compared with the figures recorded at subsequent follow-ups and in the patient's case notes.

9.2.2 Analysis of the Patient Population

A total of 1428 patients undergoing a total hip replacement between 1984 and 1996 were investigated (Table 2.1). Based on the documents available at the 1-year follow-up, leg lengths were compared and evaluated in 1171 patients (903 patients with primary and 268 patients with revision prostheses).

In accordance with our main objective, we made a basic distinction between two groups of patients:

Group 1	Preoperatively equal leg lengths
Group 2	Preoperative leg length discrepancy

Table 9.1. Pre- and postoperative leg length discrepancy in primary hip arthroplasty in patients with preoperatively unequal leg lengths

postop/preop	≤2 cm	−1 cm	0	+1 cm	≥2 cm
≤2 cm (n=124)	17	40	61	6	0
−1 cm (n=280)	8	78	163	30	1
+1 cm (n=90)	1	10	55	23	1
≥2 cm (n=18)	0	2	3	6	7
(n=512)	26	130	282	65	9

Our objective was to ascertain the percentages in both groups for postoperatively equal leg lengths at the 1-year follow-up. The primary procedures and revisions were analysed separately.

▪ **Primary Procedures.** Of those patients with preoperatively equal leg lengths, almost one third showed different leg lengths 1 year after operation (Fig. 9.5), although the maximum change was just 1 cm (Fig. 9.6). Of those patients with preoperatively unequal leg lengths, over half (55%) showed equal leg lengths 1 year after the operation (Fig. 9.5). The leg length difference diminished in 11% of patients, remained the same in 32% and increased in 2% (Table 9.1).

▪ **Revisions.** In patients with equal leg lengths prior to the revision procedures, a third also showed unequal leg lengths 1 year postoperatively (Fig. 9.7). Here too, the maximum change was one centimetre (Fig. 9.8). In patients with a discrepancy preoperatively, almost half (45%) of the patients showed equal leg lengths 1 year after operation (Fig. 9.7). In evaluating this result, it should be remembered that complete leg length equalisation had not always been planned (see also Sect. 2.2). Of the 185 patients with a residual difference, the discrepancy compared to the other leg was greater than the preoperative figure in just three cases (Table 9.2).

▪ **Subjective Patient Satisfaction.** We investigated whether the subjective satisfaction of the patients correlated with equal leg lengths. We described patients as "satisfied" if they considered the surgical result to be good or very good. Patients who considered their result to be fair or poor were classed as "dissatisfied".

A clear trend emerged (Table 9.3). Of the four subgroups, patients experiencing a leg length discrepancy for the first time were the least satisfied. The highest level of satisfaction was expressed by patients whose leg length discrepancy was corrected by the operation. "Equal to Equal" is accepted as a matter of course, while "Unequal to Unequal" is tolerated. Surprisingly, patients with a primary prosthesis were more tolerant of differences than those undergoing a revision procedure.

▪ **Limping.** The subjectively noticed leg length discrepancy is usually perceived by the patient as limp-

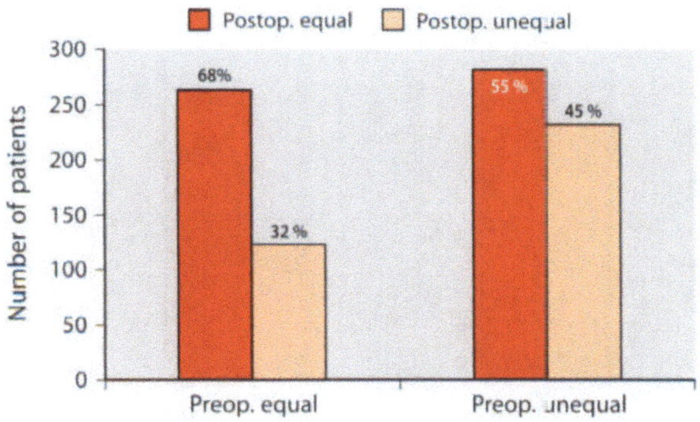

Fig. 9.5. Pre- and postoperative leg length in primary hip arthroplasty

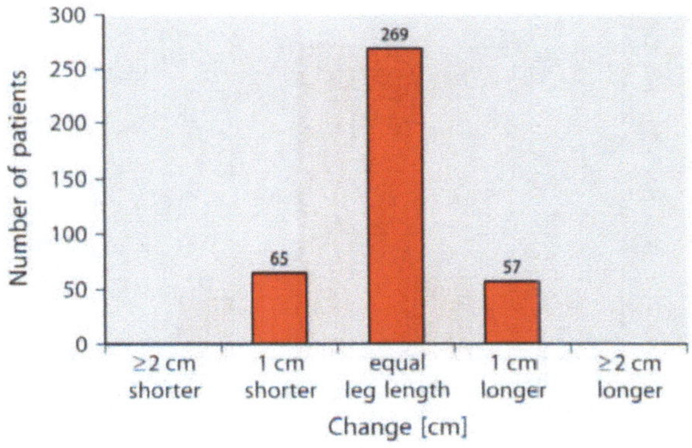

Fig. 9.6. Postoperative change in leg length after primary hip arthroplasty with equal lengths preoperatively

Table 9.2. Pre- and postoperative leg length discrepancy in revision hip arthroplasty in patients with preoperatively unequal leg lengths

postop/preop	≤2 cm	-1 cm	0	+1 cm	≥2 cm
≤2 cm (n=63)	16	26	16	5	0
-1 cm (n=89)	1	24	49	13	2
+1 cm (n=23)	0	3	14	6	0
≥2 cm (n=10)	0	1	4	3	2
(n=185)	17	54	83	27	4

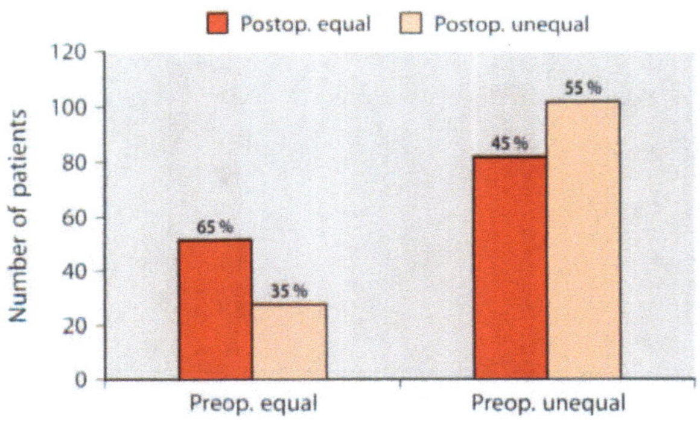

Fig. 9.7. Pre- and postoperative leg length in revision arthroplasty

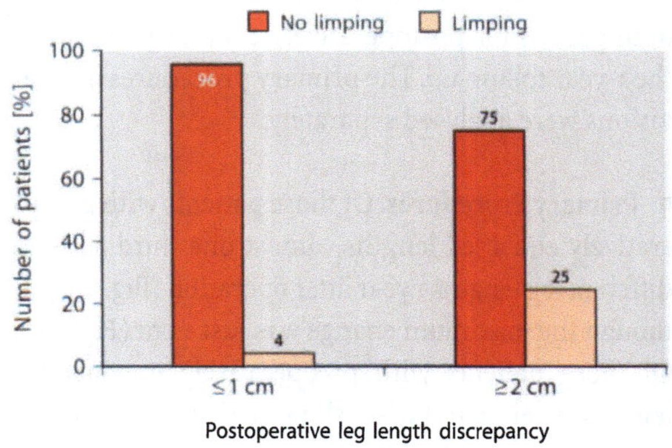

Fig. 9.9. Postoperative limping after primary procedures in relation to an existing leg length discrepancy

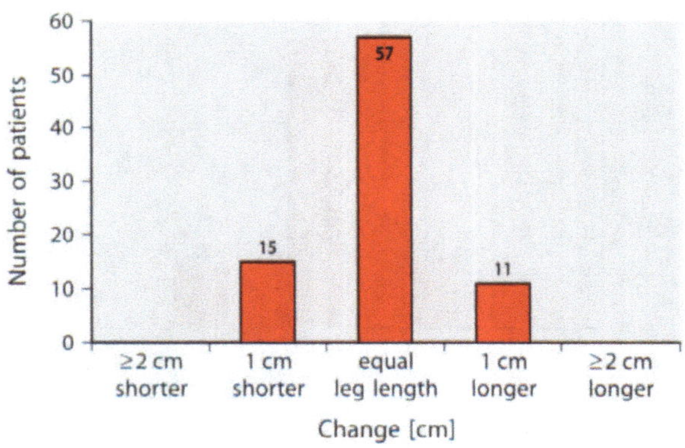

Fig. 9.8. Postoperative change in leg length after revision hip arthroplasty with equal lengths preoperatively

ing. We therefore also investigated the correlation between the various leg lengths and any resulting limping. We subdivided the patients into two groups:

Group 1 Postoperative leg length difference of 1 cm or less

Group 2 Postoperative leg length difference of 2 cm or more

Following the *primary procedures*, 94% of all patients had a leg length discrepancy of 1 cm or less (group 1). Most of these walked without a limp (Fig. 9.9). Six percent of all patients showed a leg length discrepancy of 2 cm or more (group 2). Only 3/4 of these patients walked without a limp (Fig. 9.9).

Following the *revision procedures*, 89% of the patients showed a leg length discrepancy of ≤1 cm (group 1). Five of six remained without a limp 1 year postoperatively (Fig. 9.10). Of the 11% of patients with a postoperative leg length discrepancy of ≥2 cm (group 2), almost half walked with a limp.

9.3 Frequency in the Literature

■ **Idiopathic Leg Length Discrepancies.** In 1972, Morscher et al. [12] reported incidences ranging from 15% to 87% for idiopathic leg length discrepancies of up to 2 cm in investigated patient populations not undergoing a total hip replacement. Most congenital differences or those developing over a prolonged pe-

Table 9.3. Percentage of patients satisfied in relation to postoperative leg length

	Preoperatively	Postoperatively	Satisfied patients [%]
Primary hips	Unequal	Equal	96
	Equal	Equal	91
	Unequal	Unequal	94
	Equal	Unequal	89
Revision hips	Unequal	Equal	95
	Equal	Equal	81
	Unequal	Unequal	84
	Equal	Unequal	78

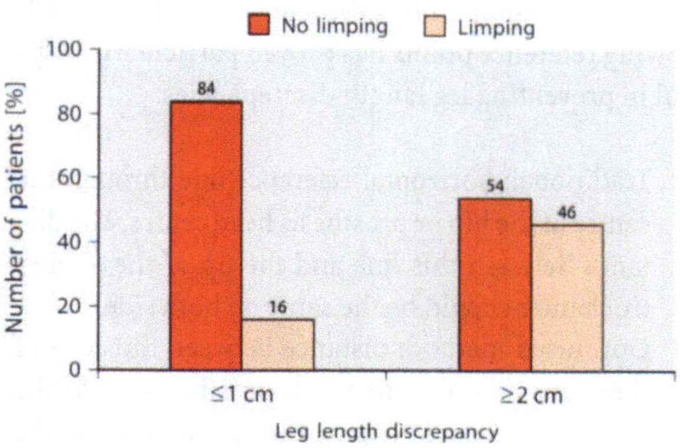

Fig. 9.10. Postoperative limping after revision procedures in relation to postoperative leg length

riod are often not perceived subjectively and are therefore neither noticed nor treated. While discrepancies in leg length are likewise a not infrequent occurrence after hip replacements, they are experienced more strongly because of their sudden onset [4, 5, 10, 15, 16]. Few reports are available in the literature up to 1978 regarding the frequency of leg length discrepancies after prosthetic implantation, possibly owing to the difficulty of measurement, but also to the lower expectations still prevailing among patients at that time.

▪ **Consequences of Leg Length Discrepancy.** A variety of consequences potentially arise from a leg length discrepancy after a total hip replacement.

• *Dissatisfaction.* The subjective dissatisfaction of the patient is the most important consequence. Various authors have remarked that it is the sudden change in leg length that is particularly perceived as uncomfortable [8, 14].

• *Clinical Symptoms.* Patients complain particularly of limping and back pain [5]. Nerve lesions caused by overstretching are rare and are only likely to occur in cases of substantial lengthening (Sect. 11.3). Nercessian et al. [13] did not find any nerve lesions in 1284 prosthetic implantations (1152 primary and 135 revision procedures) with lengthenings ranging from 0.4 to 5.8 cm. This was also confirmed by Cameron et al. [3], who stated that neurological problems are only likely to be expected in patients with lengthening of over 4 cm.

• *Legal Consequences.* Higher expectations are also associated with legal claims by patients with leg length discrepancies [5]. However, most patients are satisfied if the difference does not exceed 1 cm [4].

▪ **Preoperative Determination of Leg Length Discrepancies.** Most authors rely on the direct measurement of the leg lengths or blocking up the shorter leg with boards of known thickness until the pelvis is correctly aligned [1, 2, 5, 14]. A precision of ±0.5–1 cm is considered sufficient.

For radiological measurement, most authors recommend a pelvic overview in the standing position. Leg lengths can then be measured indirectly by this method, which is likewise associated with an error rate of 0.5–1 cm [5].

▪ **Intraoperative Determination of Leg Length.** The tip of the greater trochanter usually serves as a reference point. A wide variety of measuring instruments have been suggested for precise intraoperative measurement [5, 7, 9, 11], although the accuracy of these instruments is highly dependent on the extent to which the surgeon can reproduce the exact leg position before each measurement. The operator can often be lulled into a false sense of security in this respect [2]. According to Engelbrecht [5], the precision of such instruments is within the range of ±0.5–1 cm, i.e. no higher than the level of precision achievable through careful preoperative planning alone (Chap. 3.4).

9.4 Preventive Measures

9.4.1 Clinical and Radiological Recording

The patient's medical history will reveal whether any congenital or acquired problem is present.

▪ **Determination of Leg Length Discrepancy.** The patient stands fully erect with knees together while the examiner palpates both posterior superior iliac spines and the two iliac crests from behind. In the presence of a pelvic tilt, boards of known thickness are placed under the shorter leg until the pelvis is correctly aligned. If the legs are assumed to be equal, the patient is asked to bend forward so that the examiner can check whether the spine is also balanced. A flexion contracture should be suspected if the patient is unable to straighten his knee fully without forward inclination of the spine. If a fixed hip contracture (adduction or abduction contracture) is present, it will not be possible to align the pelvis by blocking up the apparently shorter leg. In such cases, the leg length is measured with the patient in a supine position, the functional leg length discrepancy being compared with the distance between the anterior superior iliac spine and the medial malleolus. Any flexion contracture is also determined by means of the Thomas manoeuvre.

Since it is difficult to measure leg length with millimetre accuracy, all measurements involve a source of error of varying degree. Even at the clinical examination stage, the experience of the examiner plays a crucial role, particularly when a complex clinical picture is present.

We routinely limit our radiographic investigations to standard X-rays (pelvis ap centred on the symphysis with legs hanging down and a "faux profil" hip – see also Chap. 3.4.1, Figs. 3.5, 3.6). If the history or clinical examination provides any indication of congenital or acquired deformities or shortening, full-leg radiographs are recommended so as to allow a more detailed analysis. Measurement of length or rotation by computer tomography is only required in exceptional cases.

9.4.2 Preoperative Planning in Cases of Leg Length Discrepancy

During the preoperative planning on the radiograph with the help of prosthesis-specific templates, the surgeon is guided by bony landmarks and seeks to achieve the most accurate fit for the implant. For standard planning (Fig. 3.6), determination of the following reference points has proved particularly helpful in preventing leg length discrepancies:

- Traditional: horizontal reference line through the centre of the hip or prosthesis head centre. The distance between this line and the tip of the greater trochanter should be the same on both sides.
- Optimised method: distance between the edge of the cone on the femoral prosthesis and the femoral neck osteotomy or the upper border of the lesser trochanter (Fig. 3.6f)

▪ **Correction of True Leg Length Discrepancies.** Whether an intraoperative leg length correction is advisable or not will depend on the site of the leg length discrepancy (see also Sect. 9.1):

- *Shortening in the hip area, other side normal:* Correction should be attempted if "simple" shortening is involved (see above). If "complex" shortening is present, correction should generally be attempted if a functional force triangle can be restored. If this is not a likely outcome, a certain degree of undercorrection can be beneficial (Fig. 9.1). Lengthening of more than 4 cm also involves the risk of overstretching of the sciatic nerve if the shortening is not of recent onset [2].
- *Bilateral shortening in the hip area*: In the event of bilateral osteoarthritis it may be worth accepting a leg length discrepancy temporarily, which can subsequently be corrected during surgery to the other side.
- *Iatrogenic lengthening in the hip area:* Correction during surgery to the other side is only recom-

mended if the lengthening is tolerated without any problems.

- *Lengthening or shortening elsewhere in the skeleton*: Corrections close to the hip should only be undertaken if the discrepancies are minor. Excessive alteration of the length relationships in the hip region can lead to limping as a result of muscle insufficiency. If the patients have become used to such pre-existing leg length discrepancies and are free of symptoms, correction is probably not advisable. If bilateral osteoarthritis is present, it may be appropriate to divide the correction between the two sides.

As a rule, measures for modifying leg lengths should be planned individually, and the strategy outlined here can serve only as a guide.

▪ **Correction of Functional Leg Length Discrepancies/Contractures.** Correction of contractures should always be attempted if the patient will be able to maintain the correction postoperatively by his own muscle control. Rectification of a contracture, particularly in the hip area, will often affect the leg length compensation to a greater extent than the actual leg lengthening procedure. Above all, rectification of a flexion contracture will allow the patient to stand up straight with a balanced lumbar lordosis (Fig. 9.1). If a fixed scoliosis or substantial leg length discrepancy is present, e.g. in connection with poliomyelitis, a functional length difference can occasionally be helpful in avoiding any additional overhang or excessive shoe compensation. Occasionally, an attempt to correct a contracture will fail, e.g. if an abnormal posture has been present for a very long time (Fig. 14.8).

9.4.3 Intraoperative Reference Points

The most important reference points for intraoperative checking of correct prosthesis fit are, on the acetabular side, the lower edge of Köhler's radiographic teardrop and, on the femoral side, the two trochanters.

The upper edge of the lesser trochanter should always be exposed at operation, as this allows the surgeon constantly to check the insertion depth during implantation of the stem. The upper edge of the greater trochanter is less easy to locate since it remains covered by muscles and is only suitable for positional checking after the (trial) reduction of the hip. Fairly minor leg length discrepancies of the order of 3–6 mm can be corrected by selecting differing neck lengths for the prosthesis head. This is particularly important with uncemented implants, since the femoral components have to be hammered in to achieve a firm fit, which does not always result in the ideal length.

9.5 Management of Postoperative Leg Length Discrepancy

9.5.1 Leg Length Discrepancy in the Immediate Postoperative Period

Correction is indicated in the following situations: abnormally sensitive patient; limping due to shortening or lengthening (see also Chap. 10); back pain.

We recommend a wait-and-see approach for the first 3 months with comprehensive briefing of the patient. If residual contractures are present, adaptation of the leg lengths during the first few months is contraindicated since there is still a chance of correction by means of physiotherapy.

Shoe adaptation is indicated if symptoms persist. We generally aim for a slight undercorrection of about 0.5 cm. An exception is the provision of shoe inserts for patients with back pain, in which the correction is determined on the basis of the alleviation of symptoms. If a leg length discrepancy was tolerated without symptoms before operation, undercorrection is often advisable.

Technically speaking, shoe adaptation with an insert is appropriate for differences up to 0.5 cm, a heel wedge combined with an insert for differences between 1 and 1.5 cm and a combined heel and sole wedge for corrections exceeding 1.5 cm.

9.5.2 Leg Length Discrepancy of Gradual Onset Postoperatively

A discrepancy of gradual onset can be caused by migration of a loosened acetabular or femoral component. Subsequent correction will be based on the extent of the resulting problems.

9.5.3 Management of Leg Length Discrepancy in the Literature

Most authors recommend a wait-and-see approach during the first 3 postoperative months. Patients can become accustomed to new, distinctly perceived differences if these are no more than 1.5 cm [2]. The correction of a preoperative functional leg length discrepancy can also bother the patient initially [2, 14]. After 3 months, the leg length discrepancy should be established definitively and (in some cases) corrected. For discrepancies of at least 2 cm, Cameron recommends a heel wedge [2]. Surgical revisions are considered in only the very rarest of cases.

9.6 Conclusions

The analysis of leg length discrepancies is limited primarily by the relative imprecision of the prospective documentation used. If we wish to investigate the impact of new planning methods we need to formulate more specific questions.

If a length correction near the hip is to be planned, the force triangle of greater trochanter, lesser trochanter and head centre should be preserved or, if possible, restored.

The subjective satisfaction of patients shows a definite correlation with the presence of postoperative leg length discrepancies. A patient is particularly satisfied if unequal leg lengths are subsequently corrected (Table 9.3). Patients expect to maintain existing equal leg lengths as a matter of course. On the other hand, patients generally "accept" a discrepancy if it had already been present preoperatively. A leg length discrepancy that was not present before the operation is the least tolerated outcome, particularly if it exceeds 2 cm. Patients may take legal action if such a difference occurs after a primary procedure. Surprisingly, differences after revision procedures are more likely to be viewed negatively (Table 9.3). Subjective dissatisfaction is greater in the presence of additional limping.

References

1. Abraham WD, Dimon JH (1992) Leg length discrepancy in total hip arthroplasty. Orthop Clin North Am 23: 201–209
2. Cameron HU (1997) Managing length: the too long leg. Orthopedics 20: 791–792
3. Cameron HU, Eren OT, Solomon M, Gollish J: Nerve injury associated with leg lengthening. Can J Surg. In press
4. Edeen J, Sharkey PF, Alexander AH (1995) Clinical significance of leg length inequality after total hip arthroplasty. Am J Orthop 27: 347–351
5. Engelbrecht E, Klüber D, Mahn M (1994) Intraoperative Beinlängenmessung bei totaler Hüftendoprothese. Der Chirurg 65: 1034–1041
6. Green WT, Wyatt GM, Anderson M (1946) Orthoroentgenography as a method of measuring the bones of the lower extremities. J Bone Joint Surg Am 28: 60–65
7. Hoikka V, Paavilainen T, Lindholm TS (1987) Measurement and restoration of equality in length of lower limbs in total hip replacement. Skeletal Radiol 16: 442–446
8. Jasty M, Webster W, Harris W (1996) Management of limb length inequality during total hip replacement. Clin Orthop 333: 165–171
9. Knight WE (1977) Accurate determination of leg lengths during total hip replacement. Clin Orthop 123: 22–28
10. Love BRT, Wright K (1983) Leg length discrepancy after total hip replacement. J Bone Joint Surg Br 65: 103–107
11. McGee HMJ, Scott JHS (1984) A simple method of obtaining equal leg length in total hip arthroplasty. Clin Orthop 194: 269–270
12. Morscher E, Figner G (1977) Measurement of leg length. In: Hungerford DS (ed) Progress in orthopaedic surgery, vol 1. Springer, Berlin Heidelberg New York Tokyo, pp 21–27
13. Nercessian OA, Piccoluga F, Eftekhar NS (1994) Postoperative sciatic and femoral palsy with reference to leg lengthening and medialization/lateralization of the hip joint following total hip arthroplasty. Clin Orthop 304: 165–171
14. Ranawat CHS, Rodriguez JA (1997) Functional leg length inequality following total hip arthroplasty. J Arthroplasty 12: 359–364
15. Turula KB, Freiberg O, Lindholm TS (1986) Length leg inequality after total hip arthroplasty. Clin Orthop 202: 163–168
16. Williamson JA, Reckling FW (1978) Limb length discrepancy and related problems following total hip replacement. Clin Orthop 134: 135–138

CHAPTER 10

Limping

PIA FERRAT

The outcome in terms of limping after a total hip replacement is not always predictable. We analysed a variety of pre-, peri- and postoperative data and correlated the results with limping.

In our patients, obvious limping occurred in 6% of patients after primary total arthroplasties and in 20% of cases after revision procedures. Neither sex nor age had any impact on frequency. Patients without a limp were more satisfied.

In primary operations, the following factors were more likely to be associated with limping: femoral and femoral neck fractures, previous operations, postoperative complications and trochanteric fixation. In the revision patients, second and multiple revisions constituted the main risk for postoperative limping.

As expected, limping was more likely to occur in patients with a shorter walking time, reduced flexion and increased pain. Patients requiring a walking aid or with trochanteric nonunion were also more likely to suffer from a limp.

10.1 Definitions

10.1.1 General

The various types of limping that can occur after a total hip replacement are often difficult to categorise precisely, and full clarification is generally not possible. Unfortunately, the data on limping were not always properly recorded prospectively in our hip documentation. Thus, for example, limping was not recorded on the case report forms preoperatively and could not therefore be compared with the postoperative findings. However, since disabling pain is a crucial factor in the decision to insert an implant, it is probable that many patients suffered a limp to a greater or lesser extent before the operation.

10.1.2 Normal Gait

The normal gait consists of an alternating, rhythmical swinging forward of the leg and foot strike that involves almost all the joints and muscles of the human body. The cycle for each step can be divided into a swing phase (39%) and a stance phase (61%). The stride length and foot strike angle are amenable to simple observation. With every step, the body's centre of gravity plots a wave-shaped profile, each wave being approximately 2.5 cm in height. The centre of gravity is highest in the middle of the stance phase. Observation of the unclothed patient during walking will reveal any deviations from a normal gait in the above parameters.

10.1.3
Limping

Limping can be defined as an asymmetrical gait. It is an extremely fine sign that can disclose even very minor gait problems [4]. While observing a patient's gait, the examiner analyses the harmony and rhythm of the steps, any deviation from temporal and positional symmetry, the combined movement of trunk and extremities and the time at which the deviations occur. The various types of limp are described below:

▪ **Shortening Limp.** This occurs in functional leg shortening and lengthening (see also Chap. 9) and can partly be offset by walking on the ball of the foot on the shorter side or by increased flexion of the knee on the longer side. The common phenomenon of flexion contracture is another type of shortening limping, in which the torso tends to lean forward.

▪ **Protective or Antalgic Limp.** To reduce the pain, the patient shortens the stance phase and does not completely unroll the foot. In a Duchenne limp (inclination of the torso towards the affected side) and a Trendelenburg limp (drooping of the hip on the other side), the body's centre of gravity is shifted closer to the affected hip in order to reduce the load and thus the pain.

▪ **Muscle Weakness Limp.** A muscle weakness limp can arise if the hip joint is dynamically or statically unstable due to an inadequate lever arm of the muscles or weakened abductors. During the stance phase of the affected leg, the hip on the swinging side is not raised (Trendelenburg) and the torso shifts towards the standing leg (Duchenne). This reduces the force required to walk, and thus the force acting on the hip as well, which explains why the type of limping intended to minimise pain also shows positive Duchenne and Trendelenburg signs. Paralysis limping can be classified under muscle weakness limping. Partial or total, flaccid or spastic types of paralysis are responsible for altering the gait picture in a variety of ways.

▪ **Stiff Limp.** Ligament or muscle contractures and ankylosing joints lead to various gait disorders whose common feature is that the swinging forward of the leg is always combined with prior rotation of the whole leg. Hip flexion and adduction contractures produce functional leg shortening during standing and walking, while a hip abduction contracture results in leg lengthening.

10.2
Frequency

10.2.1
Frequency in Our Own Patients

The following data are based on figures recorded prospectively at the 1-year follow-up. Of the 1098 patients receiving a primary implant, 381 women and 487 men were examined in respect of limping, compared with 81 women and 167 men from of a total of 330 patients undergoing revision surgery. The average age at the time of primary and revision surgery was 68 and 71 years, respectively, and ranged, for all patients, from 26 to 90 years.

Postoperative management involved physiotherapy and 6 weeks of partial weight-bearing with underarm crutches. After the operation, the patients continued to attend physiotherapy sessions for gait training and muscle strengthening exercises for 3–4 months.

Overall, limping of a mild, moderate or severe nature was observed in 36% of patients with primary prostheses and 58% of patients after revisions (Table 10.1). For subsequent evaluations, we have divided the patients into just two groups, i.e. patients with an obvious (moderate and severe) limp, and patients with no limp or a slight limp.

▪ **Primary Operations.** The age of the limping patients at operation, i.e. 69 (31–80) years, did not differ significantly from the age of the non-limping patients, i.e. 68 (29–90) years. No sex-related difference in limping was apparent. Limping patients tended to be overweight. The average body mass index (weight divided by the square of the height in metres – BMI) was 26, with a range of 17–36. The normal range for BMI is 18–25.

Patients showed a significantly more pronounced limp if they had received the implant as treatment for

Table 10.1. Frequency of limping after primary implantations and revisions

Limping	(100%)	None	Slight	Moderate	Severe
Primary implantation (n)	868	558 (64%)	258 (30%)	10 (1%)	42 (5%)
Revision (n)	248	104 (42%)	95 (38%)	19 (8%)	30 (12%)

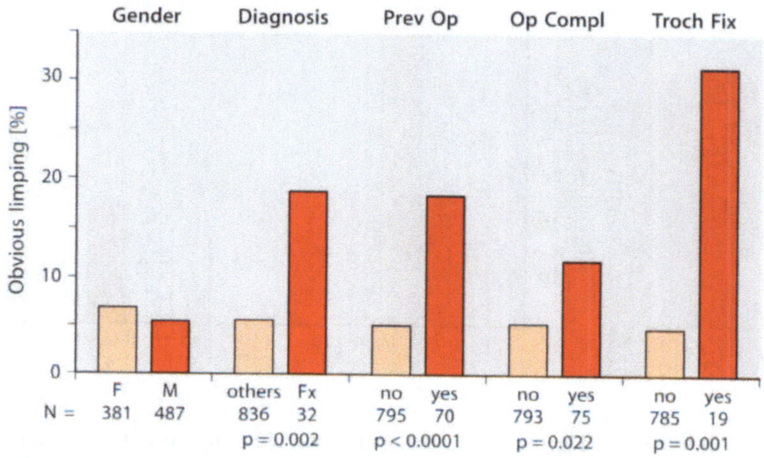

Fig. 10.1. Primary implantations – Initial status: Percentage of limping male and female patients in relation to prostheses implanted because of fractures (*Fx*) and other diagnoses, previous operations (*Prev Op*), operation complications (*Op Compl*) and trochanteric fixations (*Troch Fix*). All factors are significantly associated with obvious limping. *n* Total number of patients, *p* significance level

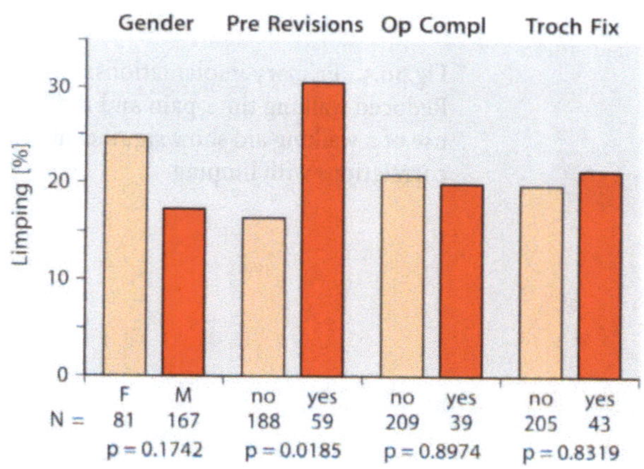

Fig. 10.2. Revision operations – Initial status: Breakdown as for primary operations (see Fig. 10.1). A statistically significant difference for revisions is apparent only for patients with previous revisions

a fracture, had undergone previous surgery in the hip area, if postoperative complications had occurred or if trochanteric fixation had proved necessary (Fig. 10.1). At the 1-year follow-up, limping showed a tendency to occur more frequently in patients with poor flexion of the hip joint, but was significantly more likely to occur in patients with trochanteric nonunion (Fig. 10.3). Obvious limping was also more common in patients with a reduced walking time, while patients with a walking time of over one hour only rarely suffered from a moderate or severe limp. Patients with severe pain or requiring walking aids were also significantly more likely to show obvious limping (Fig. 10.5). We also assessed the ability of the patients with an obvious limp to stand on one leg. Since this depends on various factors (general condition, balance, strength), unsteady standing on one leg cannot readily be attributed to muscle weakness. A third of the patients with an obvious limp were unable to stand on one leg, while almost another third were able to manage this without difficulty. The remainder either showed a positive Duchenne limp or could only stand on one leg for less than 4 s. Ninety-four percent of the non-limping patients and 67% of the obviously limping patients assessed the result of the operation as excellent or good. Overall, 92% of patients expressed satisfaction (Table 10.2).

■ **Revisions.** The average age of the patients with a limp after a revision, i.e. 70 (37–88) years, differed only slightly from that of patients without a limp, i.e. 72 (44–90) years. In contrast with the primary opera-

Table 10.2. Primary implantations: relationship between satisfaction and limping

		Excellent, % (n)	Good, % (n)	Moderate, % (n)	Poor, % (n)
No limping	100 (817)	56 (457)	38 (311)	5 (41)	1 (8)
Obvious limping	100 (52)	21 (11)	46 (24)	21 (11)	12 (6)

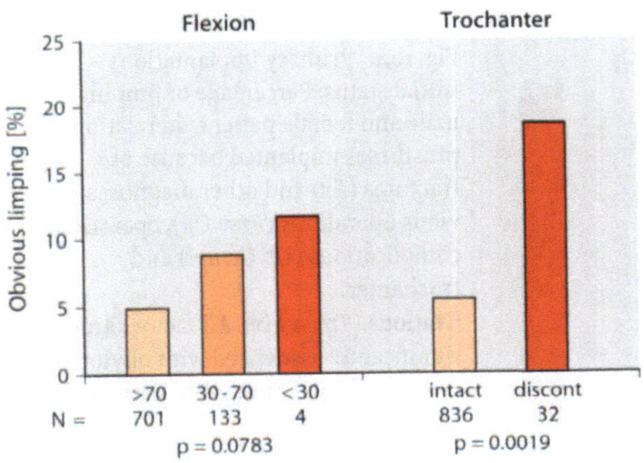

Fig. 10.3. Primary implantations: At the 1-year follow-up we noted a tendency toward a correlation between poor flexion and limping, and a statistically significant correlation between trochanteric nonunion and limping. *n* Total number of patients, *p* significance level

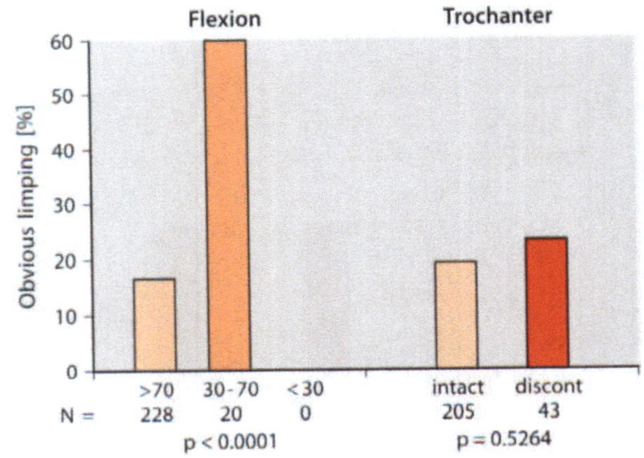

Fig. 10.4. Revision operations: Limping shows a significant correlation with poor flexion, but not with trochanteric nonunion

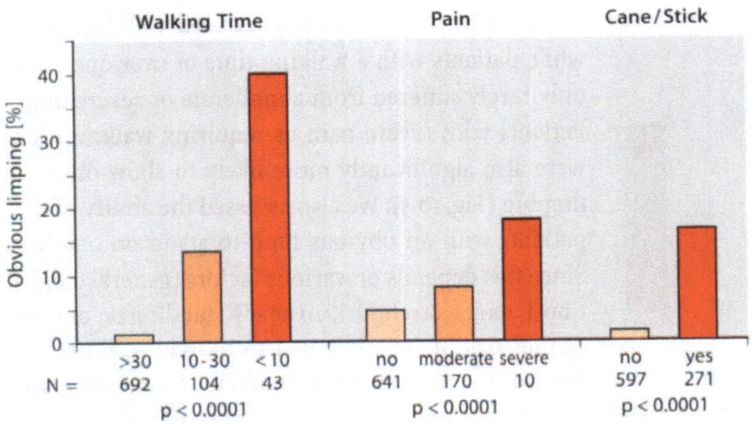

Fig. 10.5. Primary implantations: Reduced walking time, pain and the use of a walking aid show significant correlations with limping

tions, weight and trochanteric fixation did not significantly influence limping, although the existence of previous revisions did have an effect (Fig. 10.2). Also in contrast with the primary procedures, limping was not significantly affected by poor flexion after revisions. Since patients with revisions often have trochanteric problems, patients with trochanteric nonunion were not more likely than the other patients to suffer from a limp (Fig. 10.4). A shortened walking time, pain or the use of walking aids significantly exacerbated a limp (Fig. 10.6). Up to one fifth of the patients with an obvious limp after revision surgery were unable to stand on one leg, while a further quarter encountered no difficulty with this task. By comparison with the primary operations, more patients had problems with standing on one leg for over four seconds. Fewer patients were also able to stand on one leg without restriction. 89% of the non-limping patients and 73% of the obviously limping patients considered the outcome of the operation to be excellent or good. Overall, 85% of the patients assessed the result as excellent or good (Table 10.3).

Table 10.3. Revision operations: relationship between satisfaction and limping

		Excellent, % (n)	Good, % (n)	Moderate, % (n)	Poor, % (n)
No limping	100 (199)	35 (70)	54 (108)	8 (16)	3 (5)
Obvious limping	100 (49)	18 (9)	56 (27)	22 (11)	4 (2)

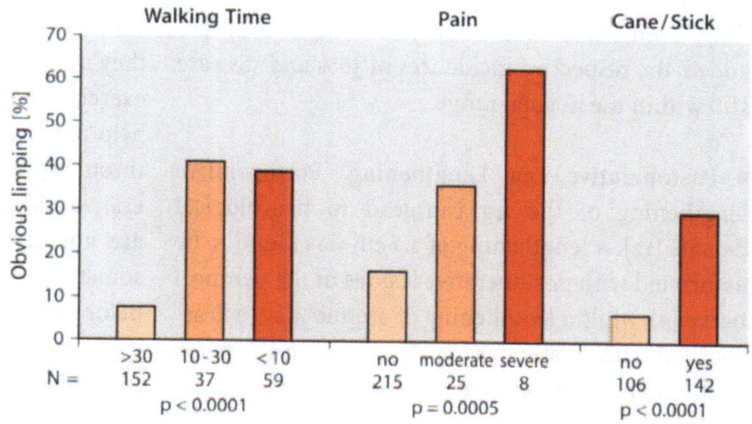

Fig. 10.6. Revision operations: A profile similar to that for primary operations is apparent in respect of reduced walking time, pain and walking aids

10.2.2 Frequency in the Literature

The literature provides figures on the frequency of limping in relation to the surgical approach, risk factors and postoperative leg length discrepancy.

■ **Surgical Approach.** In a study involving 100 patients undergoing primary total hip replacement, the lateral transtrochanteric approach with a Charnley trochanteric osteotomy was compared with the transgluteal approach, modified according to Hardinge [6]. Pain, function and range of motion were compared after 6 months and 1 year; 28% were limping after six months, compared with just 18% after a year. Limping was more common, though not to a statistically significant extent, in the group with the Hardinge approach. No differences were apparent for pain, function or range of motion. Nor was any difference observed in a comparison between a direct lateral approach and a dorsal approach in a total of 50 patients [1]. In another study, the results were investigated in 306 primary and 115 revision procedures employing a lateral approach [11]. Postoperative limping occurred in 18% of cases after primary surgery and in 27% of patients undergoing revision.

■ **Risk Factors and Incidence.** As is apparent in our own patients, postoperative limping is dependent on several factors. Previous surgical procedures [8] and multiple revisions are more likely to result in a poor prognosis for limping. Compared with the revision operations, substantially more patients limped after a primary operation involving a trochanteric fixation or other intraoperative complications. In our population, the incidence of limping was not increased in patients with trochanteric nonunion after a revision operation, but was increased after a primary operation. Reduced postoperative flexion was associated with increased limping after revisions, but only to a very slight extent after primary procedures. Preoperative leg length inequalities greater than 2.7 cm, pre-existing deformities such as hip dysplasia or those resulting from trauma, arthrodesis and established trochanteric nonunion were associated with an increased incidence of limping postoperatively (see also Chap. 9). Overall, 33 patients with an uncemented hip prosthesis were followed up for 4–6 years postoperatively [9]. In a series of uncemented CLS prostheses, limping was observed in just 6% of cases, representing a very favourable result [13]. In a group of 49 uncemented prostheses implanted via a dorsal approach, the number of limping patients fell to 24% after 1 year and 16% after 2 years [2]. The results for 70 uncemented hip implants were compared with those for 66 cemented hip implants after an average of 4.3 years [7]. Limping was present in 26% and 27% of cases respectively. The limping patients complained of pain.

The incidence of limping among our own patients, i.e. 6% after primary operations and 20% after revisions, is within acceptable limits when considering the incidence of patients with a moderate or severe limp. Even when those with just a slight limp are added, the respective incidences of 36% and 58% are still within the normal range.

■ **Postoperative Leg Lengthening.** Postoperative lengthening of the leg can lead to neurological deficits [12]. A lengthening of 2.7 cm was found to be associated with postoperative lesions of the peroneal nerve [5], while a lengthening of around 4.4 cm is associated with sciatic nerve palsy (see also Chap. 11). Both lead to postoperative limping. Paresis is reported to occur primarily as a result of local damage [12] (see Chaps. 10, 11).

10.3 Risk Factors

In the evaluation of our study we sought to determine whether certain factors favour postoperative limping. Ideally, those patients at risk are identified and corresponding preventive measures implemented. The following facts emerged after the implantation of primary prostheses:

- A significantly increased incidence of limping occurred in patients in whom the indication for implantation was a fracture (Fig. 10.1). General health may play an important role here, since this group includes individuals with osteoporotic bone who suffer falls for a variety of causes.
- Patients were also more likely to experience a limp if they had a history of previous operations in the hip area, suffered surgical complications, or underwent trochanteric fixation (Fig. 10.1).

Since limping among patients undergoing a revision operation depended primarily on the number of previous revisions (Fig. 10.2), the severity of the limp correlated with the number of revisions.

10.4 Preventive Measures

A simple and useful measure for reducing the frequency of postoperative limping is preoperative physiotherapy to build up the muscles and teach patients how to walk properly. If patients knew in advance what they could expect after the operation, they might then be able to perform the postoperative exercises properly and more effectively. These can help reactivate muscles that have become atrophied through protective lack of use and facilitate postoperative walking. In practice, however, such exercises are not usually performed. Moreover, patients are sometimes unable to perform the exercises correctly before the operation – often because of pain.

As mentioned above, a strictly observed postoperative physiotherapy plan plays an important role in curbing, or reducing, limping. The anatomical structures must be spared during the operation in order to avoid any postoperative signs of deficit and muscle weakness.

10.5 Treatment

■ **Leg Length Discrepancies.** Depending on the severity, treatment consists of an arch support, heel or sole wedge or, in exceptional cases, an orthosis. The definitive adaptation of the leg lengths should occur only after the extent of the correction required has been clarified by provisional measures, e.g. the wearing of two shoes with differing heights with/without an insole. Guiding factors include a well-balanced spinal column, the disappearance of back pain and the patient's subjective well-being (see also Chap. 9.5).

■ **Muscle Weakness.** The aim of physiotherapy is, firstly, to establish which muscles are affected and, secondly, to develop a targeted training programme that can be continued by the patient and monitored by the physiotherapist. The most important requirement is to instruct the patient concerning the perception of his limp. The main aim of training is to improve the patient's stamina. A successful outcome is only possible if muscles that can be developed through training are present. This is generally the case in postoperative phases, since muscles have often been used incorrectly or insufficiently because of preoperative pain or restricted movement of the hip. Depending on the type of limp, the postoperative physiotherapy generally lasts 3–4 months. A lack of cooperation from the patient and the absence of progress over a prolonged period are reasons for discontinuing treatment.

Generally speaking, patients still showing an obvious limp after one year have a poor prognosis as regards subsequent freedom from limping. In many cases, such patients were already limping badly before the operation because of the aforementioned factors. Other reasons include poor compliance or, more rarely, surgical complications that result in a limp as a result of direct muscle damage.

■ **Nerve Lesions.** Nerve lesions are discussed in Chap. 11.

■ **Management of Pain.** Controlling pain is a key element, and the basic treatment is initiated with NSAIDs, supported if necessary by centrally acting analgesics. Alternative and supplementary methods include physical measures such as high-voltage ultrasound, laser, trigger point treatment, massage or muscle tone reduction by stretching. If necessary, the pain can be alleviated simply by taking the load off the joint.

10.6 Discussion

■ **Importance of Limping for Patients.** Limping is a nuisance for patients, particularly if it is accompanied by pain. According to the observations of our own physiotherapists, patients often fail to notice their gait impairment if it does not cause any pain. The cosmetic aspect is therefore of secondary importance. A constant abnormal posture can lead to disruptive lumbar problems.

■ **Satisfaction.** The question of patient satisfaction is a complex one, since it depends on expectations, preoperative briefing and the objective result. Of 267 patients with a total hip replacement who were monitored for 2–3 years, over 89% were satisfied [10]. The 11% of patients who were dissatisfied complained of persisting pain, leg length discrepancy, a newly occurring limp, dislocations and subsequently required revisions. Patients receiving an uncemented prosthesis were distinctly less satisfied. Our patients assessed the outcome as excellent or good in 92% of cases after primary implantations and in 87% of cases after revisions.

References

1. Barber Th, Roger DJ, Goodman SB, Schurman DJ (1996) Early outcome of total hip arthroplasty using the direct lateral vs. posterior surgical approach. Clin Orthop 19(10): 873–875
2. Barrack RL, Lebar RD (1992) Clinical and radiographic analysis of the uncemented LSF total hip arthroplasty. J Arthroplasty 7: 353–363
3. Cameron HU (1996) Influence of the Crowe rating on the outcome of total hip arthroplasty in congenital hip dysplasia. J Arthroplasty 11: 582–587
4. Debrunner AM (1994) Orthopädie. Orthopädische Chirurgie 3rd ed. Huber Bern pp. 95–103
5. Edwards BN, Tullos HS, Noble PC (1987) Contributory factors and etiology of sciatic nerve palsy in total hip arthroplasty. Clin Orthop 218: 136
6. Horwitz B, Rockowitz N, Goll SR (1993) A prospective randomized comparison of two surgical approaches to total hip arthroplasty. Clin Orthop 291: 154–163
7. Hozack WI, Rothman RH, Booth RE (1993) Cemented versus cementless total hip arthroplasty. Clin Orthop 289: 161–167
8. Hussamy O, Lachiewicz PF (1994) Revision hip arthroplasty with the BIAS (Biologic Ingrowth Anatomic System) femoral component. Three- to six-year results. J Bone Joint Surg Am 76: 1136–1148
9. Lins RE, Barnes BC, Callaghan JJ (1993) Evaluation of uncemented hip arthroplasty in patients with avascular necrosis of the femoral head. Clin Orthop 297: 168–173
10. Mancuso CA, Salvati EA, Johanson NA (1997) Patients' expectations and satisfaction with hip arthroplasty. J Arthroplasty 12: 387–395
11. Moskal JT, Mann JW (1996) A modified direct lateral approach for primary and revision total hip arthroplasty. J Arthroplasty 11: 255–266
12. Nercassian OA, Piccoluga F, Eftekhar NS (1994) Postoperative sciatic and femoral nerve palsy with reference to leg lengthening and medialisation/lateralisation of the hip joint following total hip arthroplasty. Clin Orthop 304: 165–171
13. Robinson RP, Lovell TP, Green TM (1994) Hip arthroplasty using the cementless CLS stem. A 2- to 4-year-experience. J Arthroplasty 9: 177–192

Chapter 11

Neurological Complications

Yves Thomann, Hans Rudolf Stöckli

Any of the following nerves can suffer a lesion in connection with a total hip replacement: femoral nerve, sciatic nerve, superior gluteal nerve and, more rarely, the obturator nerve or the lateral femoral cutaneous nerve. The nerve lesions are generally caused by pressure, overstretching, direct division or overheating.

As regards the severity of the nerve injury, a distinction can be made between neuropraxia, axonotmesis and neurotmesis, although lesions generally involve a mixture of these.

Following a total hip replacement, patients should routinely be examined for neurological deficits. If a neurological complication is detected, we recommend the following procedure: regular clinical examination and, additionally, electrophysiological diagnosis of the paresis after 2 or 3 weeks and again after 3, 6 and 12 months.

In our hospital, the patients were systematically investigated for neurological complications during the period 1988–1996. If a lesion was suspected the affected patient was referred to the neurologist. During this period, 870 primary total hip prostheses were inserted; 296 total implants were partially or completely replaced, or reimplanted after a Girdlestone procedure. The average rate of nerve lesions was 1.9%. The nerves most commonly affected were the femoral (1.3%) and sciatic nerves (0.3%). A nerve lesion occurred in 2.1% of primary operations and 1.4% of revisions.

A neurological complication after a total hip replacement is often very distressful for both patient and surgeon. The recovery phase can last for up to 2 or, in exceptional cases, 3 years, and the uncertainty about the degree of improvement achievable persists for a long time. Detailed information is provided about risk factors and prophylactic measures.

Apart from a few exceptions, treatment is conservative, consisting primarily of physiotherapy and pain management, and occasionally the adaptation of orthoses. A surgical procedure is rare.

Any of the following nerves can suffer a lesion in connection with a total hip replacement: sciatic nerve, femoral nerve, superior gluteal nerve and, more rarely, the obturator nerve or the lateral femoral cutaneous nerve. The associated pareses can severely hinder the affected patients. Depending on the specific nerve that has been damaged, reinnervation can take from 1 year (superior gluteal nerve) to 3 years. The restoration of function is often incomplete. Patients are particularly surprised by a neurological complication if they have not been informed of this possibility during the preoperative briefing. But even with good patient monitoring, coping with the long recovery phase and the uncertainty about the end result can be very distressful for those affected.

Careful examination immediately after the operation, or after the spinal anaesthetic has worn off, will generally reveal the more serious cases of nerve damage immediately. However, the milder forms, or pareses of purely motor nerves, e.g. the superior gluteal nerve, are often detected only during the course of rehabilitation, or may never be recognised at all.

11.1 Definitions

11.1.1 The Injury Mechanisms

The following nerve injury mechanisms can occur in connection with a total hip replacement procedure:

- *Local pressure* on the nerve. This can range from slight irritation, via compression to severe crushing, in the worst case associated with secondary ischaemic damage (vasa nervorum). Occasionally, the injury can also be caused by pressure exerted away from the hip area, e.g. at the level of the spinal column (see also Sect. 11.7.3).
- *Overstretching* of the nerve with functional or structural damage, possibly associated with ischaemic damage.
- *Effect of sharp force* exerted by instruments or screws, with a partial or complete break in continuity.
- *Thermal injury* caused by bone cement.
- *Position-related injury* during or after the operation (e.g. peroneal nerve lesion).
- *Toxic (or mechanical) injury* due to spinal or epidural anaesthesia.
- *Ischaemic injury* as a result of interruption of the arterial circulation, e.g. in connection with a compartment syndrome.

The susceptibility of any nerve to lesions differs depending on the anatomical circumstances. Nerves with little protective epineural or perineural connective tissue, nerves containing a lot of myelin and thick nerve fibres (motor fasciculi), as well as predamaged nerves (polyneuropathy, radicular lesions, etc.) are much more susceptible. An increased risk of injury also applies when nerves are pressed against an abutting surface (bones, joints) or where they run through narrow spaces (tunnels).

11.1.2 Severity of the Nerve Injury

As regards the severity of the nerve injury, a distinction can be made between neuropraxia, axonotmesis and neurotmesis (Fig. 11.1).

- *Neuropraxia*: blocked conduction in a peripheral nerve. The axons and their sheath structures are not disrupted. The resulting functional impairment recovers completely within 2 weeks to 4 months.
- *Axonotmesis*: The axons are disrupted, but the sheath structures, which serve as a guiding splint for regeneration, remain intact. The regeneration occurs under favourable anatomical conditions, and restitution is generally good to satisfactory. Experience indicates that the axons regenerate at a rate of about 1 mm a day. Recovery can take up to 2 years, or even longer in rare cases. It may be complete, but is often only partial.
- *Neurotmesis*: The axons and sheath tissue are completely disrupted. Since the axons no longer have any guiding structures, regeneration cannot be expected to occur. A surgical procedure with microsurgical suturing of the nerves is indicated, although this often results in abnormal nerve sprouting with considerably reduced functionality.
- *Mixed forms*: The clinically observed pareses generally involve mixed forms of this injury pattern.

11.1.3 Severity of Paralysis

The severity of paralysis is subdivided into five grades by the British Medical Research Council:

Paralysis grade	
0	No activity observed in the target muscle
1	Visible/palpable contraction with no motor effect
2	Movements possible with gravity eliminated
3	Movements against gravity possible
3–4	Movements against slight resistance possible
4	Movements against moderate resistance possible
4–5	Movements against strong resistance possible, but to a lesser extent than on the healthy side
5	Full muscle power

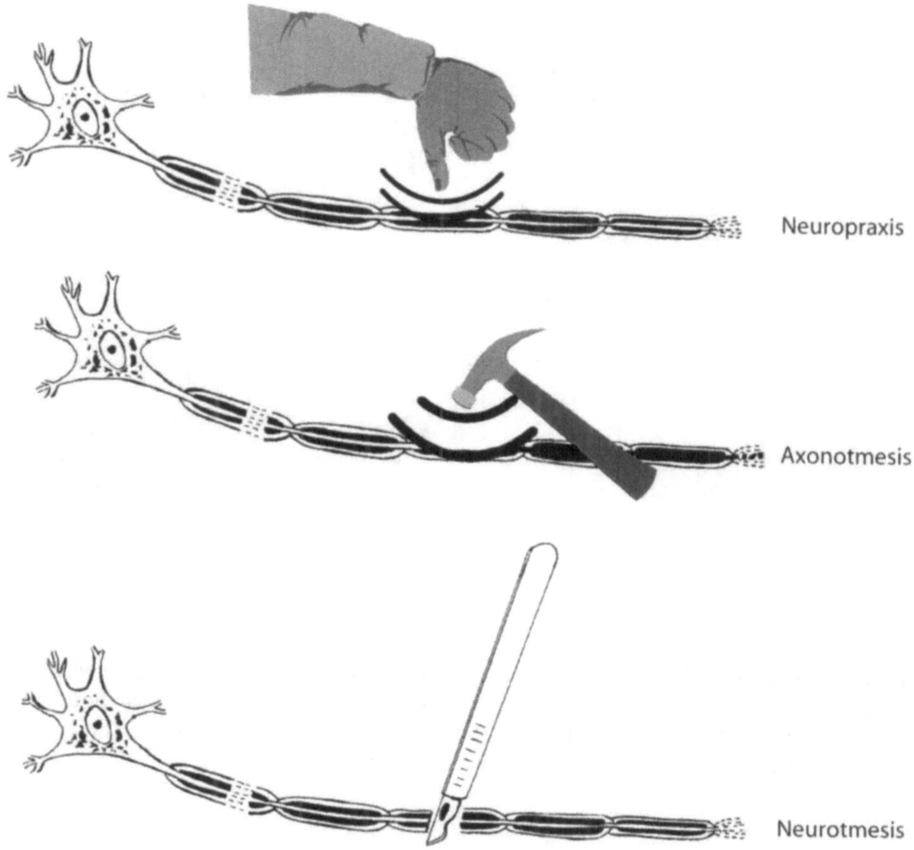

Fig. 11.1. Classification of nerve injuries. In neuropraxia the axons are preserved, while the sheath structures are preserved in axonotmesis. In neurotmesis, the nerve is either cut completely or at least across part of its cross-section

11.1.4 Pain and Nerve Lesions

Although, in many cases, the clinical picture of a nerve lesion is limited to the neurological deficits, occasionally patients can also suffer from severely debilitating pain, including hyperaesthesia and lancinating pains. This pain can sometimes dominate the clinical picture and become a real therapeutic problem (see also Sect. 11.7.2).

11.2 Clinical Pictures and Their Clinical Diagnosis

11.2.1 Sciatic Nerve

An injury to the sciatic nerve is the most serious and most feared nerve lesion that can occur during a total hip replacement procedure (Fig. 11.2, 11.3).

■ **Anatomy.** The sciatic nerve is located roughly in the middle of the line joining the ischial tuberosity and the greater trochanter (Fig. 11.2). It provides motor innervation to the ischiocrural muscles and all the muscles of the lower leg and foot. The sciatic nerve provides sensory innervation to a large part of the skin on the lateral and dorsal aspects of the lower leg and foot. The sciatic nerve consists of two main branches, the common peroneal nerve and the tibial nerve which, even at the proximal end, run next to each other as separate bundles in the main nerve trunk. The common peroneal nerve is located at the level of the infrapiriform foramen, generally lateral to the tibial nerve.

Since it is attached to the fibular head, the peroneal nerve is probably more likely to be overstretched than the tibial nerve. This explains, at least in part, why the peroneal section is always affected in injuries of the sciatic nerve at hip level, while the tibial nerve can even remain uninjured.

If the sciatic nerve fails completely, but the gluteal muscles, extensors and adductors in the thigh remain

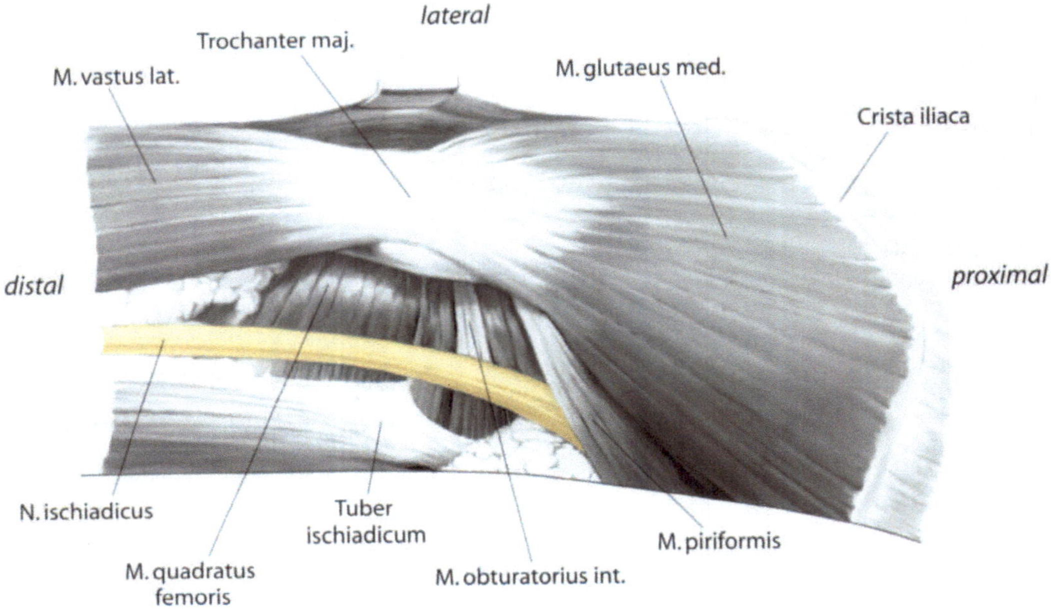

Figs. 11.2. Course of the sciatic nerve. View of the left hip from the back with the patient in a lateral position. The gluteus maximus has been removed. The sciatic nerve appears at the lower edge of the piriform muscle in the infrapiriform foramen, from where it progresses in a lateral-distal direction. Between the femur and the nerve lie the small external rotators and the quadriceps muscle

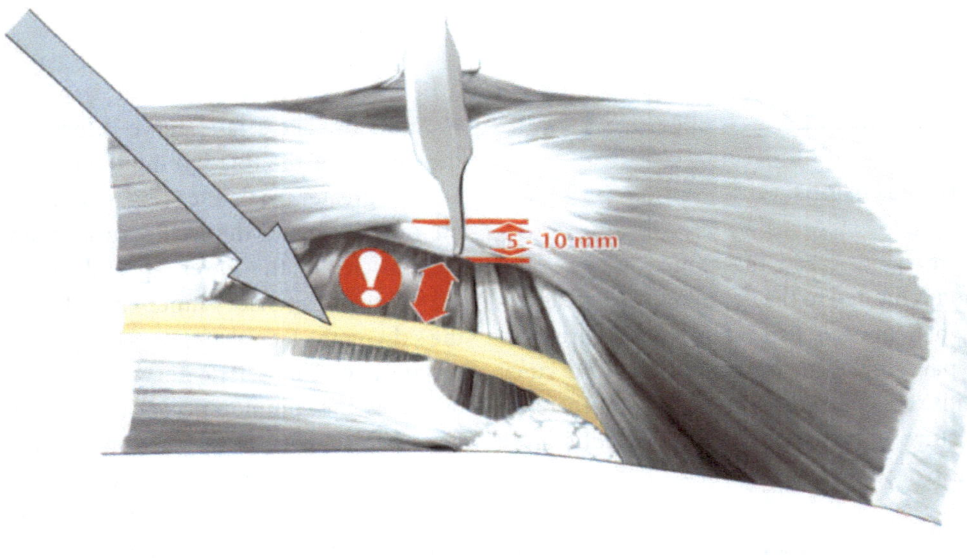

Figs. 11.3. Protective measures for the sciatic nerve: Palpation of the nerve with the finger against the ischial tuberosity. Insertion of the tips of bone levers no more than 5–10 mm beyond the intertrochanteric crest

fully functional, walking is only possible with difficulty because of the lack of innervation to the lower leg and foot muscles. If the common peroneal nerve fails in isolation, a steppage gait is observed as a result of foot drop.

■ **Postoperative Examination.** Examination involves elevation of the foot and toes (peroneal section), lowering of the foot and toes (tibial section), functional checking of the femoral biceps muscle, corresponding inspection of sensation and the Achilles tendon reflex. When the patient is mobile, the motor function can subsequently be checked, ideally by heel and toe walking.

■ **Paresis Prevention Measures**

- Lateral approach (supine position): During the osteotomy of the femoral neck in situ, the saw cut must be protected by blunt bone levers or else the hip must be dislocated prior to the osteotomy.
  If a dorsal bone lever is used to improve the exposure of the greater trochanter, the lever should not project medially beyond the intertrochanteric crest by more than 5–10 mm (Fig. 11.3). If leg lengthening is planned, it is advisable first to loosen the soft tissues dorsal to the greater trochanter by spreading with the scissors, thereby enabling the surgeon to move, or lift off, the sciatic nerve with the index finger in relation to the ischial tuberosity. The tension on the nerve can thus be checked simply during the lengthening procedure.
- Dorsal approach (lateral position): The sciatic nerve can easily be located by dissection of the lower margin of the piriform muscle at the point where it emerges from the infrapiriform foramen (Fig. 11.3).

11.2.2 Femoral Nerve

Injuries to the femoral nerve can be missed if they are not specifically checked. They cause the patient to feel insecure, particularly when walking uphill or downhill or walking up stairs (Figs. 11.4–11.7).

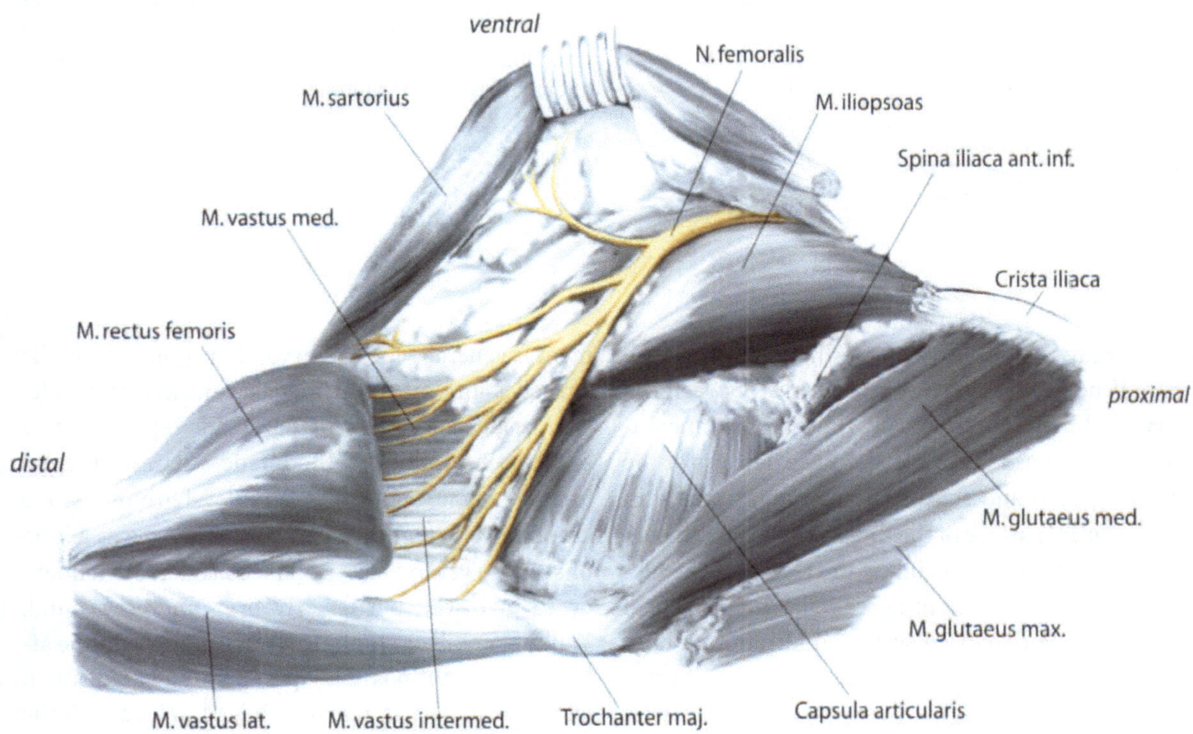

Figs. 11.4. Course of the femoral nerve. Left hip region from the front. The rectus femoris muscle has been detached from the anterior inferior iliac spine and folded back distally. The femoral nerve extends in a fan shape as it advances over the iliopsoas muscle, reaching various sections of the quadriceps and sartorius muscles.

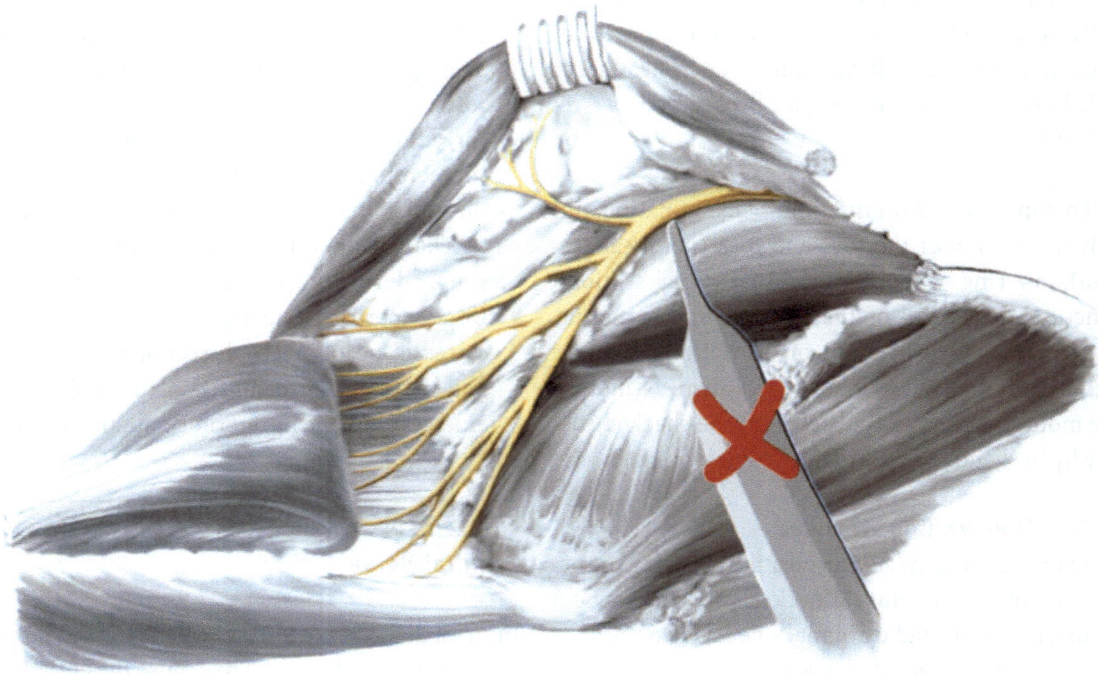

Figs. 11.5. There is a particular risk of injury to the femoral nerve if a bone lever is advanced not directly over the capsule, but through the muscles medially over the acetabular rim

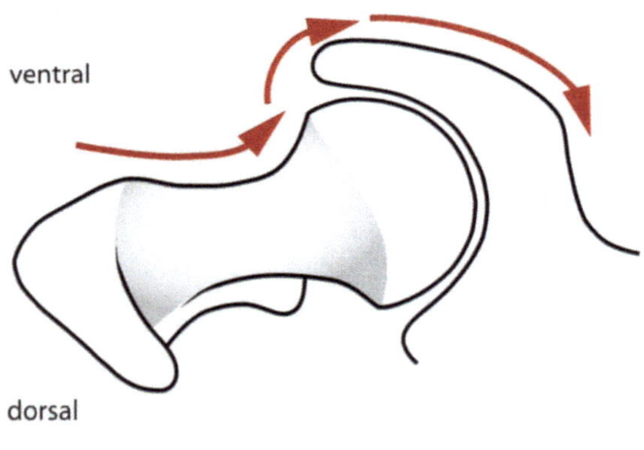

Fig. 11.6. Sagittal section through the hip joint at femoral neck level. The bone lever for adjusting the ventral acetabular rim is advanced directly ventral to the hip joint and the limbus in a medial direction over the acetabular rim. As a result, the femoral nerve is protected from the application of direct force by the iliopsoas muscle

■ **Anatomy.** At the level of the inguinal canal, the femoral nerve is located in the furrow between the psoas and iliac muscles. It provides motor innervation to the iliopsoas muscle and the extensors of the knee (Fig. 11.4) and sensory innervation to the skin on the ventral surface of the thigh and the medial surface of the lower leg, including the region of the medial malleolus (saphenous nerve). The inguinal canal represents a fairly closed system. Infiltration of fluid in this area can cause a dangerous elevation of pressure [25].

■ **Clinical Findings in Pareses.** A lesion of the femoral nerve produced during a total hip replacement is generally located beyond the point where the branches fork off to the iliopsoas muscle. Such a lesion results in paresis of the quadriceps, sartorius and pectineal muscles. In a grade 0 paresis, the patient is only just able to walk on level ground with a slightly overextended knee by using the leg as a kind of stilt. However, there is still a considerable tendency to give way, particularly over uneven ground. Walking uphill or climbing stairs leading with the affected leg is not possible up to paralysis grades 3–4, while the patient is actually obliged to lead with the affected leg while walking downhill. From a grade 4 paresis, while the patient is able to extend the knee against resistance, walking on uneven ground, uphill

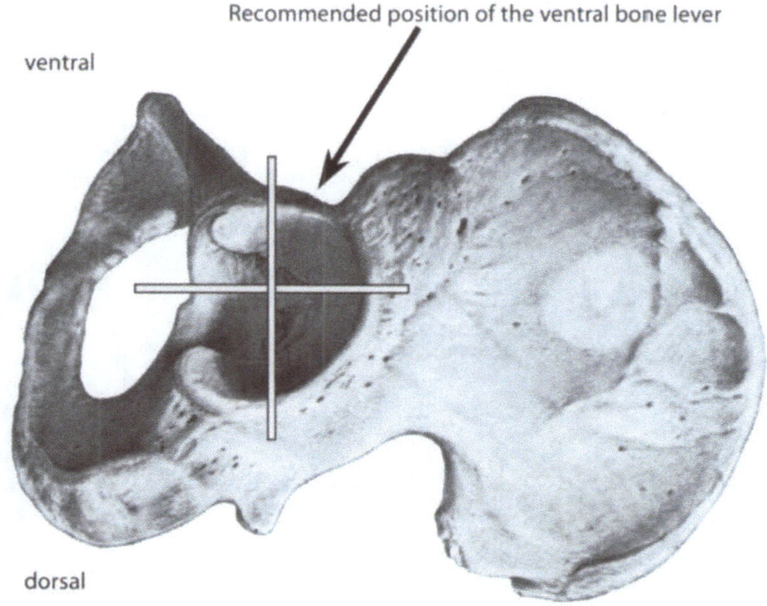

Fig. 11.7. Lateral placement of the ventral bone lever is the safest option (*arrow*), since the femoral nerve runs slightly medially in relation to the acetabulum. This is the safest way to avoid overstretching of the nerve

or downhill is impeded and the patient will often require a stick in such cases. Such low-grade pareses are often only detected after the patient is fully mobilised, i.e. long after the operation.

▪ **Postoperative Examination.** The examiner places his hand below the back of the patient's knee and asks the patient to fully extend the knee. Even if postoperative pain is present, the patient is still able to innervate the quadriceps sufficiently to enable the examiner to observe the raised position of the patella. In the case of mobile patients, step climbing will reveal even fairly minor injuries. Important information can be elicited by examining the patellar tendon reflex or abnormal sensation, which should be checked at the front of the thigh and on the medial side of the lower leg. Sensory abnormalities are not infrequently accompanied by neuralgiform pain.

▪ **Paresis Prevention Measures.** During surgical preparation, tension on the femoral nerve can be reduced somewhat by placing a towel roll beneath the slightly flexed thigh. This roll is left in place throughout the operation (Fig. 3.16).

At the level of the acetabulum, the femoral nerve is located immediately ventral to the iliopsoas muscle. The accidental insertion of a ventral bone lever into this muscle poses a risk of injury (Fig. 11.5). It is particularly difficult to place this lever correctly after repeated operations or in cases of protrusion coxarthrosis. The surgeon must carefully detach the muscles from the hip joint capsule before advancing the bone lever (Fig. 11.6). Since the femoral nerve runs slightly to the medial side in relation to the acetabulum, a lever position towards the lateral side is advisable (Fig. 11.7).

11.2.3 Superior Gluteal Nerve

▪ **Anatomy.** The superior gluteal nerve, a purely motor nerve, exits through the suprapiriform foramen, where the nerve bends sharply around the greater sciatic notch, and then branches out in a fan shape in the layer of connective tissue between the gluteus medius and gluteus minimus muscles (Fig. 11.8). Initially, four to ten small branches fork off to the gluteus medius, after which it branches again one to three times to innervate the gluteus minimus. One of these branches, usually the most cranially located branch, continues in a ventral direction, pierces through the anterior margin of the combined gluteal muscles and, finally, supplies the tensor muscle of the fascia lata. The most caudally located section of the nerve is located 5 cm, on average, proximal to the

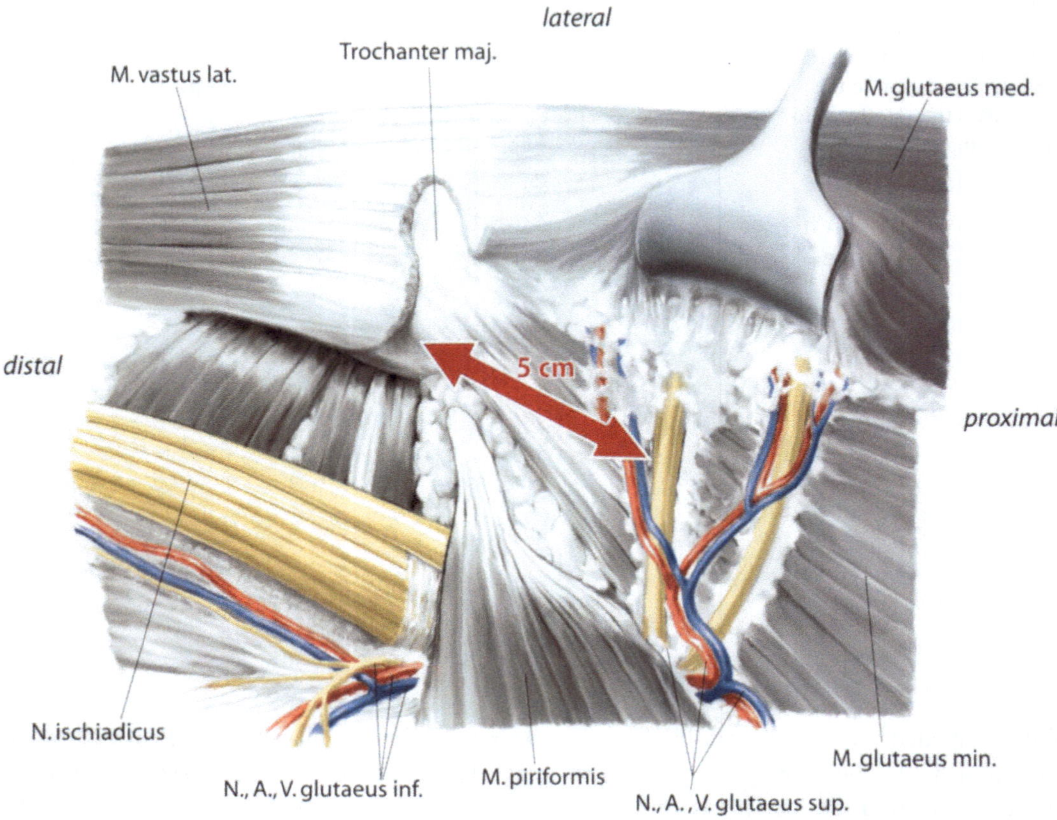

Figs. 11.8. Course of the superior gluteal nerve. View of the left hip from the back with the patient in a lateral position. The gluteus maximus has been folded back in a dorsal-distal direction. The branches of the superior gluteal nerve exit through the suprapiriform foramen. While the superior ramus is exposed to minimal risk, the inferior ramus runs just 5 cm proximal to the tip of the trochanter

most cranial point of the greater trochanter, from where it continues in a ventral and caudal direction (Fig. 11.8).

■ **Clinical Findings in Paresis.** A complete deficit results in weakened abduction in the hip area. The patient walks unsteadily, in severe cases with a Trendelenburg limp.

■ **Postoperative Examination.** Recording the corresponding findings is difficult in the immediate postoperative period. If the postoperative pain has disappeared, the nerve can be tested with the patient in the lateral position by abduction of the leg. Because the patient walks with two sticks during the first few postoperative weeks, a muscle weakness of the abductors is not always apparent and is therefore often overlooked. Once the patient has progressed to full weight-bearing, the diagnosis in obvious cases is made on the basis of the Trendelenburg sign, although other causes should also be borne in mind. Any residual muscle weakness of the abductors is often dismissed and misinterpreted simply as a "weakness that often occurs after a total hip replacement" (inadequate lever arm, etc.). If an abduction weakness persists, we therefore recommend referral to the relevant specialists a few weeks after the operation for neurological and possibly electrophysiological investigation.

■ **Paresis Prevention Measures.** In the Watson-Jones approach, with the patient in a supine position, only the terminal branch to the tensor muscle of the fascia lata is exposed to the risk of division. The main branch may possibly become overstretched by the trochanter lever. In the transgluteal approach, the gluteus medius muscle should not, under any circumstances, be split more than 3–4 cm in the cranial direction, otherwise the inferior ramus may be divided [7, 13] (Fig. 11.8). In very small patients, the extent of the incision will need to be reduced proportionately. Consequently, the incision should not extend more proximally than the distal third of the distance between the greater trochanter and the iliac crest. The surgeon must also be careful to avoid overstretching of the nerve while the soft tissues are retracted cranially to expose the acetabulum or during forced adduction of the thigh during cementation of the stem. In a trochanteric osteotomy, the trochanter generally folds back in a proximal – dorsal direction. This relieves the tension on the nerve and avoids the possibility of damage. In a dorsal approach, the superior gluteal nerve is most likely to suffer damage if the lower border of the gluteus medius muscle is overstretched.

11.2.4 Obturator Nerve

The nerve leaves the psoas muscle at its medial border (Fig. 13.11d), reaches the lesser pelvis via the iliosacral joint and passes along its side wall to the obturator groove. It innervates the adductor muscle group and supplies an area of skin on the medial aspect of the thigh.

Nerve function is tested by simple adduction of the thigh, possibly also by eliciting the adductor reflex. During walking, the predominance of the abductors leads to increased circumduction of the leg. Consequently, this nerve injury is often overlooked initially, and only diagnosed when the patient progresses from partial to full weight-bearing, since the muscle weakness is not apparent during walking with two sticks.

▪ **Paresis Prevention Measures.** One report describes injury to the nerve during drilling of the mediodorsal acetabular wall for screw insertion [10], a possibility also borne out by our own anatomical dissections.

11.2.5 Lateral Femoral Cutaneous Nerve

The nerve leaves the pelvis 2 cm medial and caudal to the anterior superior iliac spine and passes beneath the fascia lata. It is a purely sensory nerve, supplying the anterolateral area of skin on the middle and distal part of the thigh. A nerve injury is most likely to occur during bone harvesting from the anterior iliac crest or during a procedure involving an anterior approach to the hip.

11.3 Neurological Examination

11.3.1 Clinical Examination

A routine examination in respect of possible intraoperative neurological complications is strongly recommended. While major deficits of the sciatic and femoral nerves are easy to diagnose, partial injuries or injuries to the superior gluteal or obturator nerves are often difficult or impossible to detect in the early postoperative phase (see also Sects. 11.2.1–11.2.5).

▪ **Examination in the Immediate Postoperative Period.** During the first few hours, the picture is often obscured by the gradual wearing off of the spinal or epidural anaesthetic. In view of the postoperative pain, muscle power can only be properly assessed in the case of major disorders. The targeted search for sensory abnormalities or reflex asymmetries is more promising during this early phase. However, the absence of sensory abnormalities certainly does not preclude motor deficits, since the motor nerve fibres are often more prone to injury than their sensory counterparts.

▪ **First Few Days After Operation.** Muscle function can only be roughly checked since patients are still generally confined to bed at this stage. Such a cursory examination will enable sciatic or femoral nerve injuries more serious than grade 3–4 to be excluded.

▪ **Mobilisation with Partial Weight-bearing.** Injuries of a serious nature to the sciatic or femoral nerve can be ruled out if the patient's mobilisation, including climbing stairs, proceeds without any problems. It is perfectly possible, however, for definite pareses of the superior gluteal nerve or the obturator nerve to remain completely masked at this stage by the use of two sticks.

▪ **Full Weight-bearing.** If the patient shows a Duchenne-Trendelenburg limp or a disruptive unsteady gait that was not observed prior to operation, then further neurological examination by a specialist is indicated. Even fairly minor impairments can be identified by asking the patient about problems with climbing stairs or toe or heel walking. The prognosis is usually favourable in such cases.

11.3.2 Electrophysiological Diagnosis and Methods

Electrophysiological methods allow a diagnostic distinction to be made between neuropraxia and axonotmesis, i.e. between a simple conduction blockade and structural nerve damage. Unfortunately, no reliable differentiation is possible between axonotmesis and neurotmesis, which is associated with a very poor prognosis.

Electrophysiological Methods

Electroneurography (ENG)

■ **Early Motor Neurography.** Motor neurography recorded approximately 8–12 days after the assumed lesion will show amplitude breakdown of the compound motor action potential.

■ *Neuropraxia.* If, despite obvious paresis or paralysis distal to the injury, a normal amplitude is recorded for the compound motor action potential, then a conduction block is the most likely explanation. The level of the lesion can be located by moving the stimulus until it is just proximal to the lesion.

■ *Axonotmesis or neurotmesis.* A reduction in the amplitude after stimulation both proximal and distal to the lesion. The size of this reduction (compared to the healthy side) is directly proportional to the degree of the nerve fibre deficit or the degree of wallerian degeneration. If all the neurons are degenerated, no potential is evoked.

■ **Early Sensory Neurography**

■ *Neuropraxia.* The distal sensory potentials are preserved and no amplitude breakdown occurs.

■ *Axonotmesis, Neurotmesis.* Axonotmesis leads to a reduction in the sensory action potential. Severe axonotmesis, and of necessity neurotmesis, lead to premature loss of the distal compound sensory action potential.

Electromyography (EMG)

■ *Neuropraxia.* Myography shows a "normal" result, i.e. no denervation potentials or pathological spontaneous activity are observed (fibrillations or positive waves).

■ *Axonotmesis.* Pathological spontaneous activity is observed 15–21 days after the assumed lesion. The severity of the lesion is reflected in the extent of this pathological spontaneous activity, and also in the detection of any voluntary potentials still present. Reinnervation potentials can be expected to appear over the following weeks or months.

■ *Neurotmesis.* At 15–21 days after the lesion, pathological spontaneous activity is seen identical to that observed for axonotmesis, but with no detectable voluntary potentials (although these can also be absent in very severe axonotmesis) and without any subsequent signs of reinnervation.

Other Electrophysiological Methods

Somatosensory evoked potentials (SSEP), motor evoked potentials following transcranial magnetic stimulation (MEP) and other techniques (e.g. F-wave) can be helpful in the search for and objectification of very proximal nerve lesions, but are hardly ever used routinely.

Timetable and Objectives in Electrophysiological Investigations

- In the first few days:
  - ENG for determining the level of a lesion in the event of a strongly suspected sharp nerve injury (neurotmesis)
  - Verification of pre-existing damage caused by old traumatic nerve lesions, root damage, polyneuropathies, etc.
- After 10–12 days: ENG for distinguishing between

neuropraxia and axonotmesis/neurotmesis (amplitude breakdown)
- After 15–21 days:
  - ENG for distinguishing between conduction block and axonotmesis/neurotmesis
  - EMG:
    for distinguishing between conduction block and axonotmesis/neurotmesis
    for the initial quantification of denervation
    for detecting ischaemic or myopathic damage
    for an initial prognostic evaluation
- After 2–3 months and beyond:
  - For a progress assessment
  - For verifying and quantifying signs of reinnervation
  - For detecting secondary deterioration as a result of nerve constriction due to scarring, late haematomas, etc.

Since perioperative nerve damage generally results from pressure or crushing, the first electrophysiological investigation is normally delayed until 3 weeks after the event. The clinical assessment of the situation, however, should be performed as soon as possible.

11.4 Frequency and Course of Neurological Complications

11.4.1 Incidence and Course in Our Patients

No systematic search for neurological complications postoperatively was performed during the first few years of patient documentation. Only from 1988 onward were patients with suspected nerve lesions routinely referred to the neurologist. We shall therefore restrict ourselves to the investigation of the patient population in the period 1988–1996 (Fig. 11.9): 870 primary total prostheses were implanted during this period, while 296 total prostheses were either completely or partially replaced or reimplanted following a Girdlestone procedure.

Of these patients, 1.9% suffered a neurological complication, with annual rates fluctuating between 0 and 3.6%. Neither a significant increase nor decrease has been observed over the years. The commonest lesion involved the femoral nerve (1.3%). The sciatic nerve (0.3%) and the superior gluteal nerve (0.3%) were damaged much less frequently (Table 11.1). Neurological problems were encountered in 2.1% of patients undergoing a primary procedure and 1.4% of patients undergoing a revision.

- *Sciatic nerve:* Three patients suffered a sciatic nerve lesion:
  - One after an intertrochanteric osteotomy
  - One after a total hip replacement as a 4th hip operation
  - One after a primary total hip replacement as a 5th procedure after a hip arthrodesis (Fig. 11.10)

  At the time of diagnosis, all of the lesions were of a serious nature, with grades of paralysis between 0 and 3. The peroneal muscles were affected by the paresis in all cases and the tibial muscles in two cases. Sensory abnormalities were present in all three patients.

  After 1 year, none of the patients showed any sign of recovery. After 2 years, two had completely recovered. In the third case, the condition had improved from complete paralysis of the tibial and

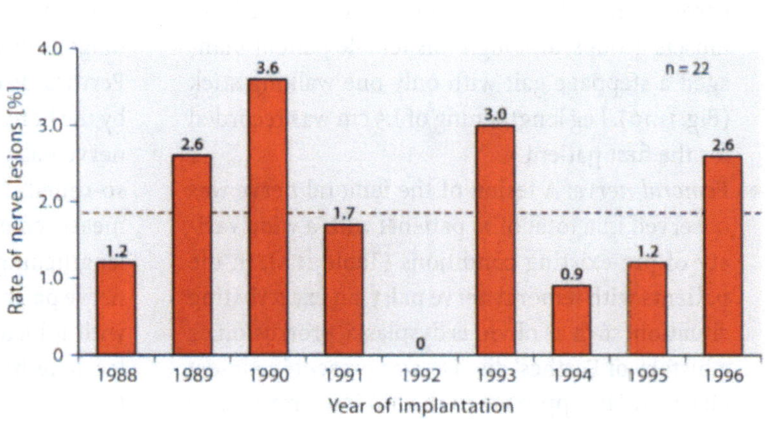

Fig. 11.9. Frequency of neurological complications in our patients after total hip replacement, expressed as percentages in relation to the prostheses implanted/replaced each year

Table 11.1. Nerve lesions 1988–1996

Nerve	Primary THR (n=870)		Revision procedures (n=296)		Total (n=1166)	
	(n)	[%]	(n)	[%]	(n)	[%]
Femoral	12	1.4	3	1	15	1.3
Sciatic	2	0.2	1	0.3	3	0.3
Superior gluteal	4	0.5	0		4	0.3
Obturator	0		0		0	
Lateral femoral cutaneous	0		0		0	
Total	18	2.1	4	1.4	22	1.9

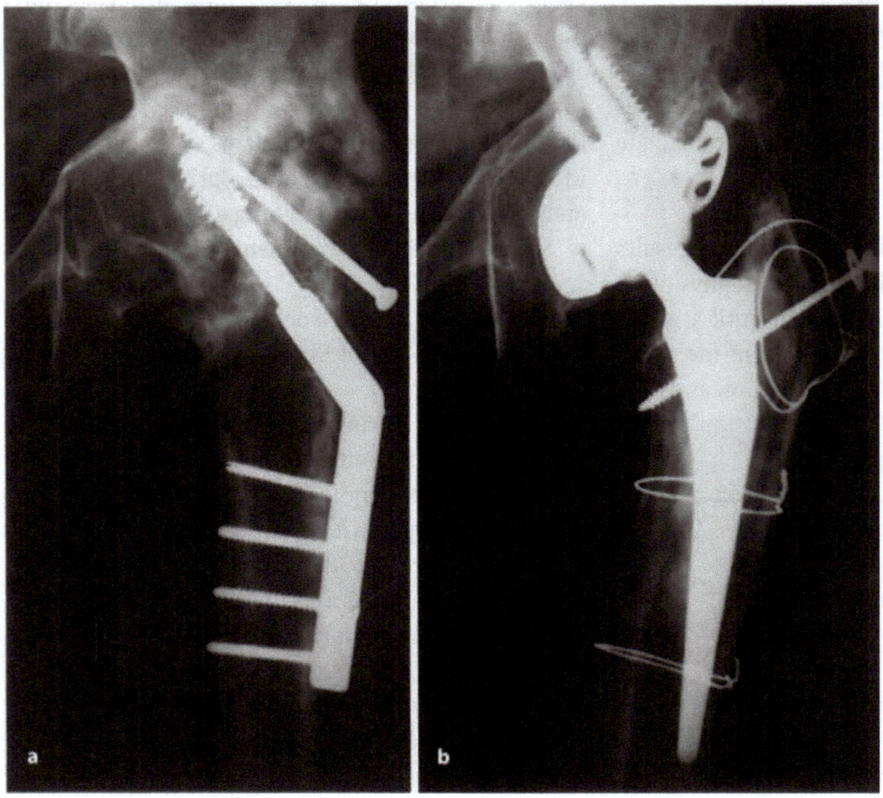

Figs. 11.10a, b. Incomplete recovery from a sciatic nerve palsy 6 years after a total hip replacement. S.H., female, 67 years (O. 3228): **a** Preoperative situation with femoral neck pseudoarthrosis after hip arthrodesis and internal fixation of a fracture. A total prosthesis was inserted during the 5th operation **b** Situation 6 years later. Although the electromyogram recorded 2 years after the lesion showed reinnervation potentials, no further improvement beyond paralysis grade 3–4 occurred up to 3 years postoperatively. Minimal subjective impairment at 6-year follow-up

peroneal muscles to a grade 3 paralysis of both muscle groups, although this female patient managed a steppage gait with only one walking stick (Fig. 11.10). Leg lengthening of 1.5 cm was recorded for the first patient.

- *Femoral nerve*: A lesion of the femoral nerve was observed in a total of 15 patients with a wide variety of pre-existing conditions (Table 11.2). In the patients with femoral nerve palsy, an exacerbating situation, such as obvious dysplasia, protrusion or a history of Perthes' disease, was present in almost all cases. The approach to the hip is aggravated by a protrusion coxarthrosis. Since a substantial bulge is usually present ventrally in patients with Perthes' disease, excessive traction may be exerted by the bone lever on the nerves anteriorly. Femoral nerve palsy was not observed in any patient with so-called "normal coxarthrosis". Radiographic measurements revealed a surgically induced leg lengthening of 26 mm in one patient with femoral nerve palsy. This was the above-mentioned patient with a history of Perthes' disease. No significant leg lengthening was measured in the other patients.

Table 11.2. Type of hip disorder in femoral nerve lesions

Femoral nerve lesions (n=15)	No. of pareses
Dysplastic coxarthrosis	5
Protrusion coxarthrosis	4
History of Perthes' disease	1
Previous intertrochanteric osteotomy	2
Primary coxarthrosis	0
Revision procedures	3

Table 11.3. Recovery trend for femoral nerve lesions (n=15)

Paralysis grades postoperatively	Severe (grade 0–3): 12	Mild (grade 4): 3
Complete recovery after 1 year	3	3
Improved after 1 year	9	
Complete recovery after 2 years	7	
Paralysis grade 4 after 2 years	5	

Course: At the time of diagnosis, a severe lesion, with paralysis grades between 0 and 3, was present in 12 cases. Slight muscle weakness of grade 4 was present in three cases (Table 11.3). Sensory abnormalities were present in all these patients, which suggests that we were only able to identify obvious cases despite systematic controls. One third of all patients showed a residual paralysis with no further improving trend after 2 years.

- *Superior gluteal nerve*: A superior gluteal nerve lesion was documented in a total of four patients, all of whom had undergone primary implantation. In all four cases, the diagnosis was suspected only secondarily on the basis of a Trendelenburg limp when the patients attempted to walk without a stick. A severe grade 2–3 paresis was present in all cases at the time of diagnosis.
  Course: An improving trend was only observed during the first postoperative year, after which the residual pareses remained constant. Only one patient showed a complete recovery, one improved from grade 2 to 3 and one from grade 3 to 4. No improvement occurred in the fourth patient, despite surgical revision. Mild lesions of the superior gluteal nerve, in particular, are probably overlooked since this nerve does not provide sensation to any skin area and any lesions are therefore difficult to diagnose.

11.4.2 Frequency in the Literature

■ **Clinical-Subclinical Nerve Damage.** Rates reported for neurological complications after a total hip replacement range from 0.08% to 2.8% (see Table 11.4). A much higher incidence of nerve damage was reported when changes were documented during or after operation by electrophysiological investigation, even though these were often not clinically detectable (Table 11.5). In 30 consecutively operated patients undergoing electromyographic investigation pre- and postoperatively, a nerve alteration was observed in 21 (70%) cases [27]. In a total of 290 consecutively operated patients, somatosensory evoked potentials of the sciatic nerve were investigated during the operation [21]. The resulting evaluation revealed pathological changes in 31 (11%) of the patients, most of which were of a transient nature.

■ **Risk in Primary and Secondary Procedures.** According to various studies, the risk of nerve damage is higher in revision procedures than in primary operations. In primary total hip replacements, lesions were observed in 0.09% to 1.7% of cases, compared with 0% to 5.6% of cases after revision procedures (Table 11.4). Our own patient population, with fewer lesions after revision operations, represented an exception in this respect (Table. 11.1).

Table 11.4. Literature comparison of nerve lesions after total hip replacement

Author	Study design	Primary THR (%)	Revision (%)	Total (%)
Weber et al. 1976 [27]	retrospective			0.70
Schmalzried et al. 1991 [22]	retrospective	1.30	3.20	1.70
Edwards et al. 1987 [8]	retrospective			1.10
Navarro et al. 1995 [15]	retrospective	0.50	1.10	0.80
Nercessian et al. 1994 [17]	retrospective			0.45
Nercessian et al. 1994 [16]	retrospective	0.9	0	0.08
Rasmussen et al. 1994 [21]	prospective	1.10	5.60	2.80
Rasmussen et al. 1994 [21]	retrospective	1.70	4.40	2.70
Beckenbaugh et al. 1978 [3]	retrospective			1.20
Total		0.90	2.70	0.93

Table 11.5. Literature comparison of nerve lesions in relation to surgical approach

Author	Study design	Nerve lesion in relation to approach (%)	Injured nerve (%)
Weber et al. 1976 [27] *	retrospective	lateral transtrochanteric: 0.7	sciatic: 0.34, femoral: 0.15, sciatic+femoral: 0.15, obturator: 0.05
Weber et al. 1976 [27]	prospective	lateral transtrochanteric: 70	sciatic: 20, femoral: 3, obturator: 27, sciatic+femoral: 3, sciatic+obturator: 17
Weale et al. 1996 [26]	prospective	lateral: 20 posterior: 0	sciatic: 10, femoral: 5, obturator: 10
Schmalzried et al. 1991 [22]	retrospective	lateral transtrochanteric: 1.7	sciatic: 1.3, femoral: 0.16, sciatic+femoral: 0.19
Ramesch et al. 1996 [20] *	prospective	lateral: 23	superior gluteal: 23
Edwards et al. 1987 [8]	retrospective	posterior: 1.14	sciatic: 1.14
Navarro et al. 1995 [15]	retrospective	posterior: 0.5. lateral transtrochanteric: 1.1	sciatic: 0.4, femoral: 0.2, sciatic: 0.9, sciatic+femoral: 0.2
Baker et al. 1989 [1] *	prospective	direct lateral: 34.5 modified lateral: 10.3 posterior:14.3	superior gluteal: 34.5, superior gluteal: 10.3, superior gluteal: 14.3
Black et al. 1991 [5] *	prospective	lateral: 11.8, posterior: 19.3	sciatic:11.8, sciatic: 19.3
Beckenbaugh et al. 1978 [3]	retrospective	lateral transtrochanteric: 1.2	sciatic: 1.2
Kenny et al. 1999 [14]a	prospective	transgluteal: 47 transtrochanteric: 56	superior gluteal

*With prospective electrophysiological examination

■ **Sciatic Nerve.** According to most publications, sciatic nerve lesions were by far the most common type of nerve injury. In retrospectively designed clinical studies, the figures ranged from 0.09% [16] to 2.7% [21]. The corresponding range for prospective studies involving the electrophysiological investigation of all operated patients was between 2.8% [21] and 40% [27]. In our own patients, by contrast, these serious complications were relatively rare.

■ **Femoral Nerve.** Femoral nerve lesions occur less frequently, in both retrospective and prospective studies, with cited incidences ranging from 0 to 0.35% [3, 8, 16, 22, 23]. The percentage of 1.3% observed in our own study seems rather high (Table 11.1). While this high figure may be explained by our concerted efforts to detect these complications in particular, nevertheless the goal of these investigations must be to find measures for reducing the number of lesions (see also Sect. 11.2.2).

■ **Superior Gluteal Nerve, Obturator Nerve.** Reliable figures concerning the frequency of obturator and superior gluteal nerve injuries can probably only be obtained after consistently implemented electrophysiological investigations of all operated patients. The obturator nerve and superior gluteal nerve are rarely mentioned in retrospective studies. Electrophysiological investigations have recorded injury rates of up to 43% [27] and 23% [20], respectively, for the obturator and superior gluteal nerves.

The superior gluteal nerve seems to be exposed to a greater risk of injury with a lateral approach: Pathological readings were recorded in 23% of the patients whose procedures involved a lateral approach, of which over 50% had still not recovered after 9 months [20]. Baker et al. [1] conducted EMG measurements of the superior gluteal nerve in all patients 2 weeks postoperatively after various surgical approaches: After the lateral approach 34.5% of the values were pathological, compared with just 14.3% after a dorsal approach. In a prospective study, Kenny et al. [14] did not observe any difference in the incidence of superior gluteal nerve lesions between the direct lateral and transtrochanteric approaches. Interestingly, they discovered, by means of EMG investigations, that a chronic nerve lesion had been present preoperatively in 48% of the patients. Postoperatively, the EMG for an acutely damaged nerve did not correlate with clinical signs of weakened hip abduction, the Harris hip score or a positive Trendelenburg sign. They therefore viewed the Trendelenburg sign as the product of multifactorial causes, of which damage to the superior gluteal nerve can represent just one factor.

During intraoperative electromyography of the superior gluteal nerve, Siebenrock et al. [24] observed electrical stimulation of the nerve in one of 11 patients in three situations (incision of the superior gluteal muscle, strong retraction during exposure of the pelvis, forced adduction of the femur during cementation of the stem). They therefore considered these three situations to be potentially hazardous in respect of a nerve lesion.

11.5 Risk Factors

Since nerve lesions rarely involve complete severance, i.e. neurotmesis, which is the only lesion that will reliably benefit from surgical revision, the causes of nerve damage are rarely elucidated by findings disclosed at operation. Even if local revisions were to be performed more frequently, local scarring would probably prevent the cause from being detected in many cases. We found only isolated reports in the literature of the cause of the lesion being found during a surgical revision. In other publications, as in our own analyses, one is left with observations of statistical accumulations and probable causes, which in many cases cannot even be considered "very probable".

■ **Approach.** Few publications have compared surgical approaches (Table 11.5). The lateral approach, with or without a trochanteric osteotomy, appears to be more risky than the posterior approach. Only one group of investigators reported a higher incidence of sciatic nerve lesions after a dorsal approach than after a lateral one [5].

■ **Bone Levers.** In several articles, the incorrect placement of bone levers or the overstretching of nerves by excessive traction on the levers during exposure of the hip is mentioned as a cause of nerve lesions [2, 6, 16, 22, 23]. It should be noted, however, that hardly any of the articles offer reliable evidence. Furthermore, it is almost impossible to quantify the traction on a lever. While these reports need to be taken seriously, it is nevertheless the case that wide retraction of the tissues to a substantial depth is required in order to implant an artificial hip. During intraoperative EMG, Siebenrock et al. [24] observed stimulation of the superior gluteal nerve by the acetabular roof lever. This finding also prompted us to pay more attention to the problem of bone levers (see Sect. 11.2). It should be possible to reduce the damage potential markedly by precise placement of the bone levers (Figs. 11.3, 11.5).

■ **Protrusion Coxarthrosis.** The femoral nerve is much more likely to be damaged in cases of protrusion coxarthrosis. Experience has shown that the intraoperative overview is hampered by the deepened acetabulum. In this cramped situation, a bone lever tends to be placed incorrectly at the ventral rim of the acetabulum, thus potentially leading to nerve injury.

■ **Hip Dislocation, Hip Subluxation, Leg Lengthening.** Overstretching of a nerve due to excessive leg lengthening is a commonly described potential cause of muscle paresis or paralysis. However, controversy exists about the precise point from which leg lengthening can be expected to cause neural damage: In their series of 2012 patients, Weber et al. [27] describe just one confirmed case in which a leg lengthening of 3.7 cm resulted in palsy of the sciatic and femoral nerves. Schmalzried et al. [22] postulated that a leg lengthening of 2.5 cm or more was the cause of a neurological deficit in 13 cases out of a total of 3126 operated patients. The sciatic or femoral nerve was involved in five of these patients. There are isolated descriptions in which a leg lengthening of over 2 cm is assumed to be the likely cause of a neuropathology [10, 15].

No precise figures are available on the tolerated extent of lengthening, and the figures vary from one publication to the next. Gill et al. [11], who investigated a large series of 123 patients undergoing a total hip replacement after congenital hip dysplasia, advise against any lengthening in excess of 2 cm, although they fail to provide any actual evidence for this statement. The patient population was therefore extended so that this question could be analysed in greater depth by a second group [9]. In this study, too, no connection was observed with the degree of lengthening obtained. On the other hand, the difficulty of the operation, as recorded on the postoperatively completed case report forms, was described as significantly above average, statistically, in the eight observed cases of paresis. Edwards et al. [8] reported on cases of peroneal nerve lesions after an average leg lengthening of 2.7 cm and the occurrence of sciatic nerve lesions after average leg lengthening of 4 cm.

■ **Haematoma.** The onset of two sciatic nerve lesions due to excessive haematoma formation is described in one article [27]. Two nerve lesions associated with a large haematoma were also observed by Nercessian et al. [17] in a series of 7133 operated patients. Following evacuation of the haematoma, the neurological deficits regressed completely. Schmalzried et al. [22] describe eight cases of nerve lesions in which a large haematoma was postulated as the cause.

■ **Revision Procedures.** Overall, the risk of a nerve injury in revision procedures is much higher compared to primary total hip replacements [5, 15, 21, 22]. Increased scarred adhesions resulting from previous operations make it more difficult to keep nerves out of the way or stretch them freely. In our own patients, the rate of nerve lesions was, surprisingly, higher for primary implantations, at 2.1%, than for the revision implants at just 1.4%.

■ **Other Causes.** The following additional causes are described in the literature:

- Total prosthesis dislocations: two sciatic nerve lesions [27]
- Drill bit/screw: one injury to the obturator nerve (confirmed at operation) [10]
- Bone cement: two femoral nerve lesions [27], two sciatic nerve lesions (confirmed at operation) caused mechanically/by heat [4, 18]
- Overstretching of the nerve during rasping of the femoral shaft/reduction of the total prosthesis [10]

11.6 Preventive Measures

This summary repeats only the most important measures, with cross-references to the corresponding sections in this chapter.

Preoperatively, those patients at increased risk of a nerve lesion will need to be identified. These include patients with pre-existing nerve damage (e.g. radicular or polyneuropathic lesions, see also Sect. 11.7.3), protrusion coxarthritis and who are scheduled for leg lengthening (see Sect. 11.5). Revision operations also generally involve an increased risk.

Measures to be implemented intraoperatively to protect the main individual nerves have already been mentioned in chapter 11.2. The careful use of bone levers is particularly important (Figs. 11.3, 11.5), the selection of patient positions affording the greatest possible slack to the main nerves (Fig. 3.16) and carefully controlled, and not overambitious, leg lengthening (see Sect. 11.5). Particular caution is indicated in the transgluteal approach, which only allows splitting of the gluteus medius over the tip of the trochanter over a length of just 4 cm before running the risk of damage to the superior gluteal nerve (Fig. 11.8).

11.7 Treatment of Nerve Injuries

The spectrum of neurological complications ranges from the obvious, and in some cases severely disabling, paralysis, to transient, mild paresis with no sensory abnormalities. The latter usually remain unrecognised and disappear within a few months during the normal rehabilitation period.

If a neurological complication occurring after the implantation of a hip prosthesis continues to have a negative effect on the outcome beyond the usual rehabilitation period of 3 months, this can be distressful for the patient as well as the operator. The recovery process is often very long and uncertainty can remain about the degree of the expected residual damage. Consequently, when a nerve lesion is diagnosed, the surgeon should talk about the problem and its consequences with the patient, at length and in a sensitive way. The whole postoperative management process, which can be very time consuming, is made much easier by an optimal doctor-patient relationship.

Patients find it difficult to accept the fact that very little can be done to influence the outcome. This is precisely why referral to a neurologist for subsequent joint follow-up can be very useful, since it gives the patient access to an expert who can support him with advice and better explain specific details about neurological healing processes.

11.7.1 Principles of Treatment

The most important principles for targeted follow-up are:

- Careful functional testing of the main nerves in the immediate postoperative period (see Sects. 11.2, 11.3)
- Repeated checks, at regular intervals, for the presence of milder damage to the main nerves, i.e. the sciatic and femoral nerves, and for damage to the superior gluteal nerve and the obturator nerve when the patient is fully weight bearing
- Regular follow-up for any known neurological complications in accordance with Sect. 11.3
- Since a neuropraxia or axonotmesis can generally be assumed to have occurred, conservative treatment, with a few exceptions
- Specialist physiotherapy

11.7.2 Therapeutic Components

■ **Positioning.** During the acute phase, it may be possible to restrict the damage resulting from a sciatic nerve lesion by easing the tension on the nerve, i.e. by extending the hip joint and flexing the knee. The femoral nerve, on the other hand, is slackened by flexing the hip.

■ **Physiotherapy**

- *Management of Damaged Muscles.* This management is based on an assessment of the power of the affected muscles (see Sect. 11.1.3). The assessment should be repeated weekly during the initial stages of treatment, and at increasingly longer intervals thereafter. The gradual restoration of muscle power should be encouraged, without overloading the muscles. Physiotherapy exercises for unaffected compensatory muscles may also be appropriate.

- *Antagonists.* Antagonists should be stretched regularly to avoid contractures.
- *Gait Training.* The aim of gait training is to familiarise the patient with his residual abilities and to help him achieve a steady gait through training exercises. An important part of this tuition is to teach the patient how to recognise and avoid hazardous situations. The main objective in lesions of the femoral nerve is to secure the knee, particularly when walking up- or downhill and when walking on uneven terrain. The main aim in injuries of the sciatic nerve is to enable the patient to cope with foot drop.

Two case studies of injuries resulting from lesions of the femoral nerve:

- Encouraged by the gradual recovery from a lesion of the femoral nerve, the patient became increasingly active. After 1 year, she became unsteady in an unexpected situation, fell and broke her patella.
- Following a change of prosthesis and internal fixation for pre-existing trochanteric nonunion, another patient suffered a femoral nerve palsy. Three months later, she fell and fractured the malleolus on the other side.

Similar accidents are fairly frequent and are directly connected to the nerve palsy. We observed, e.g. a quadriceps tendon tear and a distal radial fracture in patients with a sciatic nerve palsy.

Pain Management. After a nerve lesion, patients can be plagued with severe pain for several months. These neuralgiform symptoms can be alleviated through the use of tri- or tetracyclic antidepressants (e.g. clomipramine, imipramine, fluoxetine), possibly combined with neuroleptics (e.g. haloperidol, levopromazine). The use of carbamazepine, gabapentin, phenytoin or valproate, and possibly also of mexiletene and capsaicin ointment may also be appropriate [12]. All of these preparations, particularly the antiepileptic drugs, should be carefully introduced in gradually increasing doses. Fairly high doses are often required.

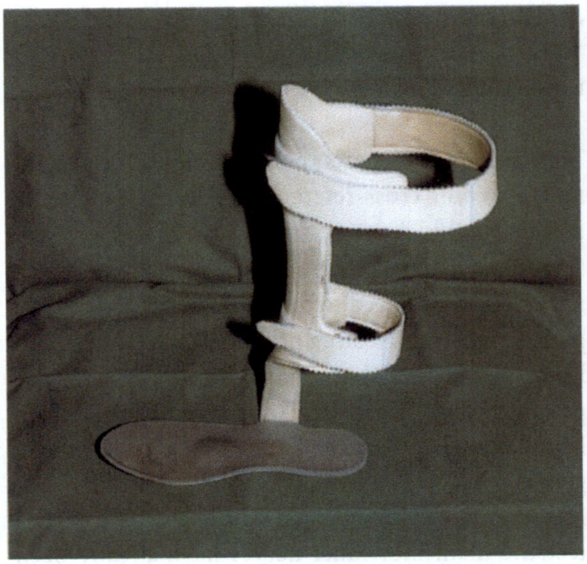

Fig. 11.11. Carbon splint as one way of compensating for weak foot lifting

■ **Orthoses**

- *Foot Drop in Sciatic Nerve Palsy.* The traditional Heidelberg splint and also foot elevators fitted directly to the shoe are often uncomfortable and aesthetically unsatisfactory. Modern carbon splints are much lighter and, because they are fitted on the medial side, much less conspicuous (Fig. 11.11).
- *Knee Stabilisation in Femoral Nerve Palsy.* A knee orthosis is an important provisional aid, particularly during the initial mobilisation phase. Whether a special custom-made device would be appropriate is subsequently decided on the basis of the experience with the individual patient. Important aspects to consider in this decision are the recovery trend for the nerve, the patient's skill and general frailty.

■ **Surgical Measures.** Surgical measures represent the exception.

- Haematoma revision: If a massive haematoma is accompanied by paresis, then revision is indicated (see Sect. 11.5).
- Direct nerve exploration: Surgical revision is indicated if the clinical, neurological and electrophysiological investigations suggest the occurrence of complete or partial nerve severance (neurotmesis). However, this is a rare event. Nercessian

et al. [16] describe a surgical revision for just one patient after the onset of a sciatic nerve lesion in a series of 1284 implanted total prostheses. The revision revealed partial severance of the nerve, and the nerve was sutured by microsurgical techniques [17]. Another case report concerns a revision of the obturator nerve [10]. The damaged part was resected and reconstructed with a free, interposed nerve graft. Two years after this revision, the patient showed an encouraging result, with an improvement in muscle power from an original grade 2 to grade 4. Our own revision of a superior gluteal nerve proved unsuccessful.

- Replacement / palliative surgery: Failure of the superior gluteal nerve is the most likely indication for such a procedure. In one instance, we attempted to alleviate the patient's symptoms by tractopexy, but this produced only temporary success.

■ **Electrostimulation.** The benefits of electrostimulation of the muscles affected by the nerve failure have not been conclusively confirmed and can therefore only be recommended to a limited extent. Electrostimulation has no effect on nerve recovery.

11.7.3 Accompanying Spinal Problems

A previously damaged nerve is more susceptible to further damage (so-called double crush syndrome). Accordingly, any pre-existing clinically mild, or barely detectable, damage means that the nerve is at increased risk of injury. Pritchett et al. [19] report on 21 patients with very pronounced spinal stenosis who suffered neurological deficits following a total hip replacement. None of the patients had complained of weakness in the lower limbs prior to the aforementioned operation. Lumbar decompression was performed for 16 of the 21 patients. Six of these patients recovered completely from their deficits, and a further six experienced at least a partial recovery. No change in the neurological deficits was observed in the remaining four patients undergoing lumbar decompression or in any of the five patients not undergoing a decompression procedure.

References

1. Baker AS, Bitounis VC (1989) Abductor function after total hip replacement. An electromyographic clinical review. J Bone Joint Surg Br 71: 47–50
2. Bauer R, Kerschbaumer S, Poisel S (1986) Operative Zugangswege in Orthopädie und Traumatologie. Georg Thieme, Stuttgart New York, 112–113
3. Beckenbaugh RD, Ilstrup DM (1978) Total hip arthroplasty. A review of three hundred and thirty-three cases with long follow-up. J Bone Joint Surg Am 60: 306–313
4. Birch R et al (1992) Cement burn of the sciatic nerve. J Bone Joint Surg Br 74: 731–733
5. Black DL, Reckling FW, Porter SS (1991) Somatosensory-evoked potential monitored during total hip arthroplasty. Clin Orthop 262: 170–177
6. Bos JC et al (1994) The surgical anatomy of the superior gluteal nerve and anatomical radiologic bases of the direct lateral approach to the hip. Surg Radiol Anat 16: 253–258
7. Comstock C, Imrie S, Goodman SB (1994) A clinical and radiographic study of the "safe area" using the direct lateral approach for total hip arthroplasty. J Arthroplasty 9: 527–531
8. Edwards BN, Tullos HS, Noble PC (1987) Contributory factors and etiology of sciatic nerve palsy in total hip arthroplasty. Clin Orthop 218: 136–141
9. Eggli S, Hankemayer S, Müller ME (1999) Nerve palsy after leg lengthening in total replacement arthroplasty for developmental dysplasia of the hip. J Bone Joint Surg Br 81: 843–845
10. Fricker RM, Troeger H, Pfeiffer KM (1997) Obturator nerve palsy due to fixation of an acetabular reinforcement ring with transacetabular screws. J Bone Joint Surg Am 79: 444–446
11. Gill TJ, Sledge JB, Müller ME (1998) Total hip arthroplasty with use of an acetabular reinforcement ring in patients who have congenital dysplasia of the hip. J Bone Joint Surg Am 80: 969–979
12. Hans G (1998) Recent advances in the therapy of nerve-injury pain. Neurol Clin 16: 951–965
13. Jacobs GH, Buxton RA (1989) The course of the superior gluteal nerve in the lateral approach to the hip. J Bone Joint Surg Am 71: 1239–1243
14. Kenny P, O'Brian CP, Synnott K, Walsh MG (1999) Damage to the superior gluteal nerve after two different approaches to the hip. J Bone Joint Surg Br 81: 979–981
15. Navarro RA et al (1995) Surgical approach and nerve palsy in total hip arthroplasty. J Arthroplasty 10: 1–5
16. Nercessian OA, Piccoluga F, Eftekhar NS (1994) Postoperative sciatic and femoral nerve palsy with reference to leg lengthening and medialization/lateralization of the hip joint following total hip arthroplasty. Clin Orthop 304: 165–171
17. Nercessian OA, Macaulay W, Stinchfield FE (1994) Peripheral neuropathies following total hip arthroplasty. J Arthroplasty 9: 645–651

18. Oleksak M, Edge AJ (1992) Compression of the sciatic nerve by methylmethacrylate cement after total hip replacement. J Bone Joint Surg Br 74: 729–730
19. Pritchett JW (1994) Lumbar decompression to treat foot drop after hip arthroplasty. Clin Orthop 303: 173–177
20. Ramesh M et al (1996) Damage to the superior gluteal nerve after the Hardinge approach to the hip. J Bone Joint Surg Br 78: 903–906
21. Rasmussen ThJ (1994) Efficacy of corticosomatosensory evoked potential monitoring in predicting and/or preventing sciatic nerve palsy during total hip arthroplasty. J Arthroplasty 9: 53–61
22. Schmalzried ThP, Amstutz HC, Dorey FJ (1991) Nerve palsy associated with total hip replacement. J Bone Joint Surg Br 73: 1074–1080
23. Schmalzried ThP, Noordin S, Amstutz HC (1997) Update on nerve palsy associated with total hip replacement. Clin Orthop 344: 188–206
24. Siebenrock KA, Rösler KM, Gonzalez E, Ganz R (2000) Intraoperative electromyography of the superior gluteal nerve during lateral approach to the hip for arthroplasty. J Arthroplasty 15: 867—870
25. Slater N, Singh R, Senasinghe N, Gore R, Goroszenink T, James D (2000) Pressure monitoring of the femoral nerve during total hip replacement: an explanation for iatrogenic palsy. J R Coll Surg Edinb 45: 231 – 233
26. Weale AE et al. (1996) Nerve injury after posterior and direct lateral approaches for hip replacement. J Bone Joint Surg Br 78: 899–902
27. Weber ER, Daube JR, Coventry MB (1976) Peripheral neuropathies associated with total hip arthroplasty. J Bone Joint Surg Am 58: 66–69

Chapter 12

Periarticular Ossification

Joachim Vaeckenstedt

Periarticular ossification, or ossification near the trochanter, after a total hip replacement occurs more frequently in men and affects about one third of patients. The aetiology is not fully understood. The extent of ossification only correlates partially with observed movement restrictions. Since the frequency and severity in our patient population were not sufficiently influenced by the prophylactic administration of ibuprofen to men, this drug was subsequently discontinued. The literature on non-steroidal anti-inflammatory drugs is critically reviewed.

While numerous risk factors are known to favour the onset of ossification, only a few have been conclusively confirmed. The latest studies suggest that radiotherapy in the immediate preoperative period is the most reliable, and also the least expensive, form of prophylaxis.

The surgical technique for removing obstructive ossification is described.

12.1 Introduction

Periarticular ossification (PO) occurs with varying frequency and severity after total hip replacements and involves the formation of genuine bone in the periarticular soft tissues, which can be differentiated radiologically from calcification. Countless articles in the literature have been written on this subject, most of which are concerned with drug-based prophylaxis.

The pathogenesis of periarticular ossification is not fully understood. Some authors have postulated that mesenchymal cells differentiate into osteoblasts, which then form non-mineralised bone matrix (osteoid) [7, 8]. Another possible explanation is that particles of living bone enter the muscles surrounding the hip during reaming of the acetabulum or rasping of the femoral shaft and thus form an initial focus for bone formation. Recent analysis contradicts this view (see Sect. 12.8).

As the number of total hip replacements increases worldwide, many publications dealing with the prophylaxis of PO have appeared in recent years. We make a distinction between drug-based and radiological (radiotherapy) prophylaxis, and have only resorted to the latter method in exceptional cases (Fig. 12.1). We have, however, investigated our own patients prospectively in order to assess the value of ibuprofen in the prophylaxis of ossification.

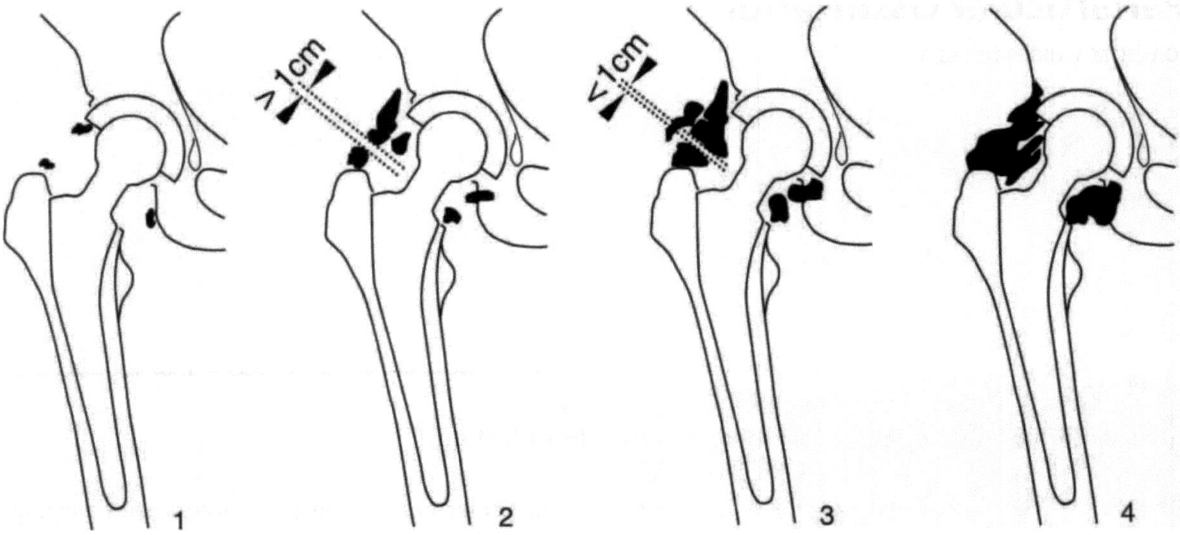

Fig. 12.1. Classification of ossification according to Brooker [5]: class 1: Islands of bone formation within the periarticular soft tissues; class 2: Bone spurs from the iliac bone and/or greater trochanter; class 3: As for class 2, but the bone spurs are closer together; class 4: "Ankylosis". We believe that this term is misleading, however, since several islands of bone can simulate bridging and be associated with considerable range of motion

12.2 Definitions

■ **Periarticular ossification** is extraosseous ossification near the joint that forms in the muscles and in the area of tendinous and other connective tissues. Histologically, it is indistinguishable from orthotopic bone. Tendinitis calcarea, pseudogout and neoplastic bone formation are not classified as ossification [7].

■ **Trochanteric ossification** is directly related to the greater trochanter and should be mentioned in conjunction with periarticular ossification to the extent that it spreads in the direction of the joint. A definite cause worth noting at this point is the lifting off of bone lamellae during a transgluteal approach.

12.3 Classification

No clinical classification exists. The Brooker classification [5], based solely on radiological criteria, has become established internationally. In this classification, the postoperative radiograph must be compared with a preoperative image in order to avoid pre-existing islands of bone from being classified incorrectly as heterotopic ossification. In his original paper, Brooker distinguishes between four classes (Fig. 12.1).

No statement or prognosis can be made about the clinical course of ossification with this classification, nor does the extent of radiologically visible ossification correlate in individual cases with the restriction of movement [1] (Fig. 12.2). A radiological class IV "ankylosis", for example, often involves an overprojection of different islands of bone which can simulate bridging and which still allow an acceptable range of motion. A definite diagnosis of ankylosing ossification is only possible by means of radiographic documentation in two projections and the analysis of hip mobility. The more accurate CT scan is prone to interference from the implants.

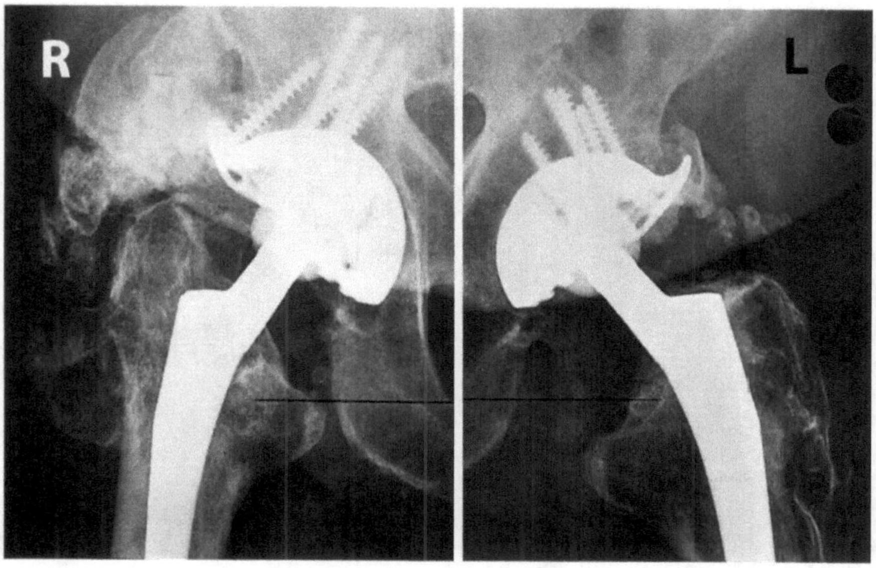

Fig. 12.2. Periarticular ossification, class 3 according to Brooker *right*, class 2 *left*. W.E., male, 58 years (O. 649). Situation 5.5 years after the primary operation. Flexion: 105° on the right, 100° on the left

12.4 Aetiology

In the differentiation of mesenchymal cells into osteoblasts already mentioned in the introduction [6], two types of precursor cells that can differentiate into osteoblasts after tissue trauma are described [8]:

- Inducible osteogenic progenitor cells: bone precursor cells that migrate and circulate and are capable of differentiation. Various differentiation factors can be involved (e.g. BMP: bone morphogenic protein).
- Determined osteogenic progenitor cells: local cells from the bone marrow that can differentiate into osteoblasts. These cells are thought to be responsible for the new bone formation that occurs in autologous cancellous bone grafts.

12.5 Clinical and Radiological Presentation

The radiological picture of periarticular ossification does not allow any direct conclusions to be drawn about the clinical status of the patient. During the first 3–6 months after a total hip replacement, a patient will occasionally complain of interfering and irritating non-specific symptoms during the formation of ossification. The patient then notices a gradual decline in range of motion (Fig. 12.3). Radiographs initially show ill-defined condensation structures resembling tufts of wool. After 3–6 months, these shadows become denser and more mineralised with sharper contours (Fig. 12.3).

Even with substantial ossification, a patient's range of motion can still be perfectly respectable (Fig. 12.2). Only rarely does the patient's range of motion become severely restricted, though this can then develop into ankylosis (Fig. 12.4). Surgical removal remains the exception, indicated only in cases of severely restricted mobility, particularly in flexion, or if severe local irritation is present.

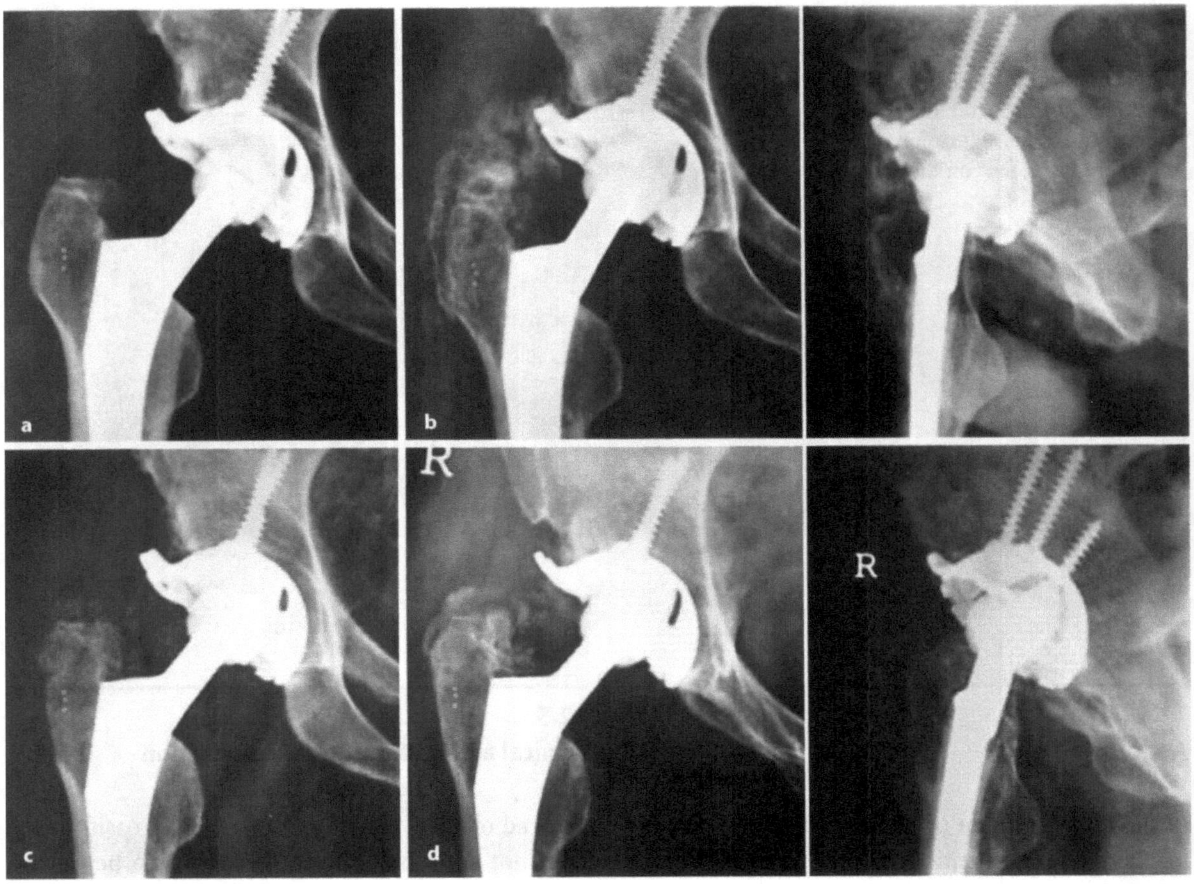

Figs. 12.3a–d. Removal of ossification 2.5 months after primary THR with prior radiotherapy. B.H., male, 58 years (O. 13172)

a Flexion/extension of 90–5–0° before implantation of a total prosthesis. On discharge, the range of motion was 100–0–0°

b After 2.5 months the range of motion dropped to 40–5–0° in the presence of massive ossification

c Situation after preoperative radiotherapy and removal of ossification

d Four months later, range of motion of 100–0–0°, occasional fatigue pain

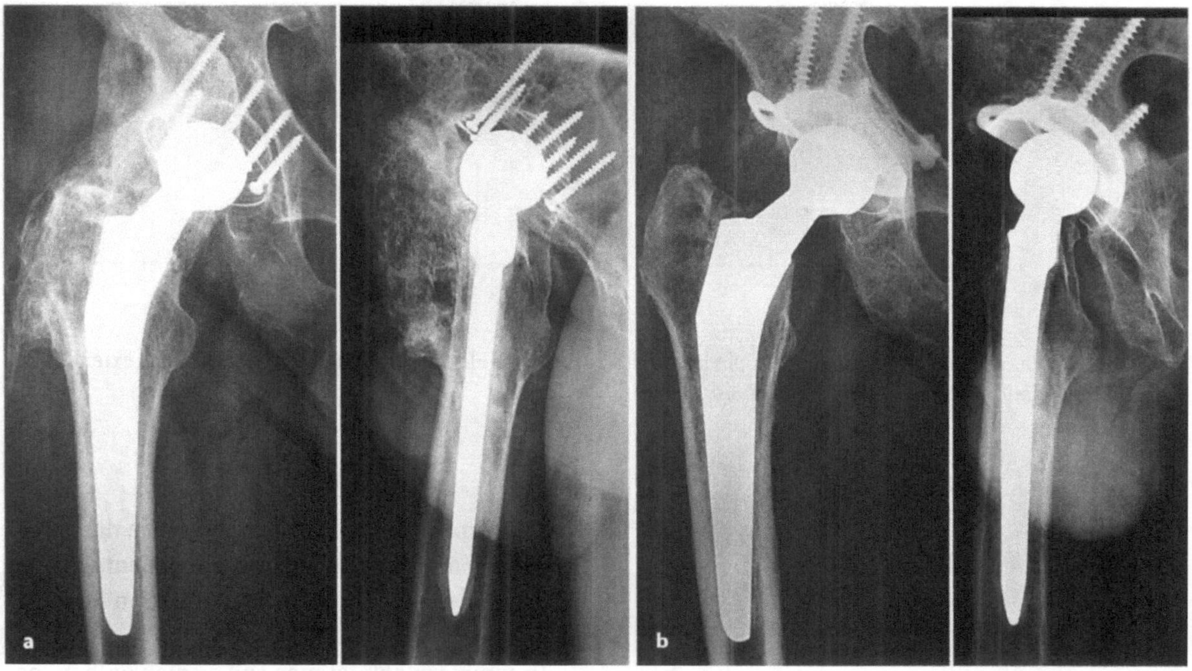

Figs. 12.4a,b. Removal of complete bone bridge after radiotherapy. M.G., male, 47 years (O. 16862)
a Hip almost completely stiffened and painful, with minimal pseudoarthrosis ventral to the cup
b Situation 2 years after removal of ossification after irradiation with 700 rads. Occasional slight pain. Flexion/extension 110-0-0, internal/external rotation 15-0-40

12.6 Frequency

12.6.1 Frequency in Our Own Patients

Material and Methods

The degree of ossification and flexion after 1 year was determined prospectively in 528 primary total hip replacements with an SL cup and a straight stem. The ossification was classified as mild, moderate or severe, on the basis of classes I-III used in the Brooker classification [5] (Fig. 12.1). In this context, the follow-up forms for hip implants developed by M.E. Müller (IDES) were evaluated.

Ibuprofen was administered from the 1st to the 18th postoperative days at a dosage of 400 mg (3 1), starting with one sugar-coated tablet on the evening before the operation and a further two tablets on the day of operation.

Ossification prophylaxis was not administered during the period 1989–1991, but was administered to all men during the period 1993–1995. The women were not treated during these periods and served as comparator groups, enabling us to determine whether the two periods represented comparable populations. The average ages of the women and men were 69.5 (40–89) years and 67 (41–85) years, respectively. A total of 145 untreated men were compared with 156 treated men. The comparator group consisted of 227 women.

Results

Of the 227 women in the two groups, 24% showed ossification, subdivided into 15% with mild, 3% with moderate and 6% with severe ossification.

Of the 145 men without ibuprofen, 35.5% showed ossification, subdivided into 23% with mild, 3% with moderate and 9.5% with severe ossification (Fig. 12.5).

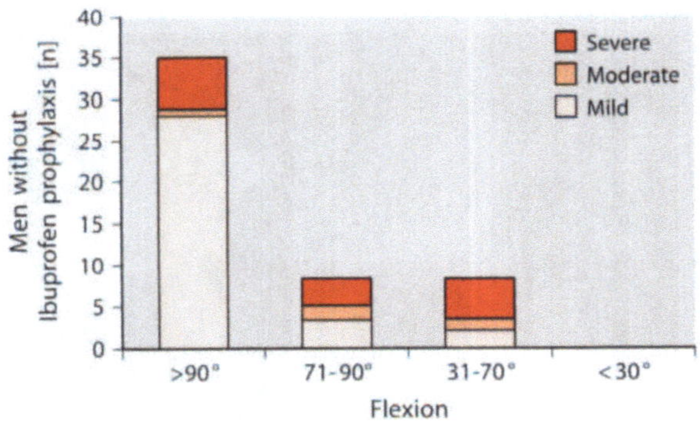

Fig. 12.5. Flexion in men not receiving prophylaxis with ibuprofen in relation to the extent of ossification

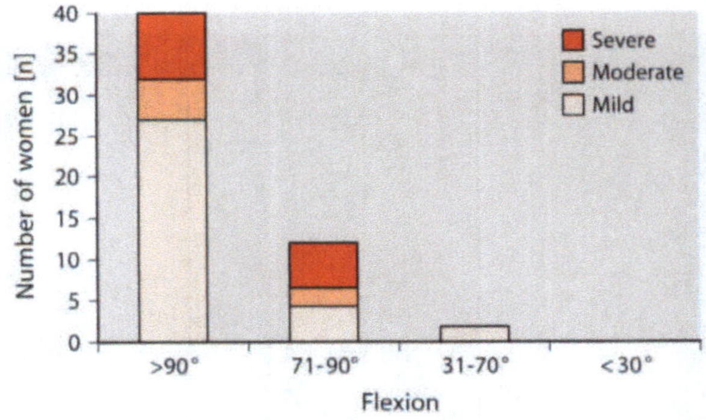

Fig. 12.7. Flexion in women in relation to the extent of ossification

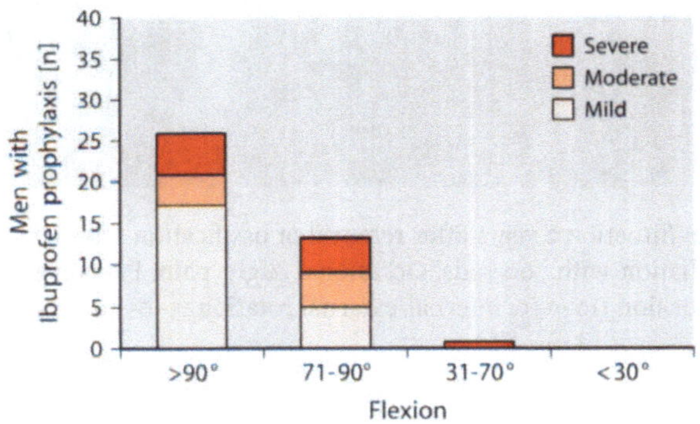

Fig. 12.6. Flexion in men receiving prophylaxis with ibuprofen in relation to the extent of ossification

Of the 156 men with ibuprofen, 23% still showed ossification, subdivided into 14% with mild, 5% with moderate and 4% with severe ossification (Fig. 12.6).

This reduction in ossification was not statistically significant ($p<0.6$). No ankylosis was observed during the period under review. The ossification was classified according to the evaluation employed in the aforementioned follow-up form for hip implants developed by M.E. Müller. On this form, mild ossification corresponds to Brooker class 1, moderate to class 2, while severe ossification is covered by Brooker classes 3 and 4.

As regards flexion, 40 (74%) of the women with ossification showed flexion of >90°, irrespective of the degree of ossification (Fig. 12.7).

Of the men not taking ibuprofen, 16 (31%) showed a reduction in flexion, and were equally divided between the two restricted flexion groups. Fairly advanced ossification (severe) was evenly distributed across all three groups (Fig. 12.5).

Of the men taking ibuprofen, 13 were in the 71–90° flexion group (28%), while just one patient with severe ossification was restricted to a flexion of 31–70° (Fig. 12.6).

In summary, 90% of men and women without ossification were able to achieve flexion of >90°. The extent of flexion in men with ossification was slightly improved by ibuprofen (13% more with flexion of >90°, but just one more with flexion of >70°). This improvement was not statistically significant ($p<1.2$). Absence of osteointegration of the SL cup due to ibuprofen administration was not observed, and seam formation around the SL cup was present in seven men with ibuprofen and seven without.

12.6.2 Frequency in the Literature

While the frequencies cited in the literature are subject to considerable fluctuation, approximately one patient in three can be expected to show ossification after a total hip replacement [2, 5]. Over 80,000 total hip prostheses are implanted each year in the Federal Republic of Germany, which means that the annual incidence of periarticular ossification involves some 25,000 patients [2].

The frequency of impairment is contentious. Ahrengart [1], for example, showed that, among 145 patients undergoing total hip replacement, those with Brooker class 3 and 4 ossification showed higher muscle power in flexion, with no flexion deficit, 2 years postoperatively compared to patients with mild or no ossification. The distribution pattern for ossification and percentage grading matches that of large-scale studies: 29% of men with ossification, 11% of which are severe cases [16].

12.7 Risk Factors

Predisposing factors cited in the literature include various skeletal disorders (e.g. dysostosis) and serious trauma and disorders affecting the brain or spinal cord with comatose states and paresis of the extremities [1,3,5,7]. Known risk factors are listed below:

- Pre-existing periarticular ossification (ipsi- or contralateral)
- Ankylosing spondylitis
- Male gender, massive osteophytes of the hip
- Revision of a total hip replacement or repeated previous hip operations
- Diffuse idiopathic hyperostosis (Forestier's disease)
- Post-traumatic arthritis

12.8 Preventive Measures

12.8.1 Overview of Possible Measures

The available prophylactic measures can be subdivided according to the time of implementation:

Intraoperative measures:
- Atraumatic surgical technique
- Meticulous haemostasis
- Excision of devitalised tissue
- Extraction of small bone particles
- Prevention of infections

Perioperative measures:
- Drugs (e.g. indomethacin, ibuprofen)
- Pre- and postoperative irradiation of the hip (10 Gy in fractionated doses or 8 Gy as a single dose)

12.8.2 Literature on Prophylactic Measures

Intraoperative Measures

▪ **General Rules of Conduct.** Measures during the operation are difficult to quantify and are therefore frequently mentioned but rarely investigated, apart from the irrigation process.

▪ **Irrigation.** A randomised investigation of intraoperative irrigation has recently been published [22]. One group of patients was irrigated in a straightforward manner with 500 ml Ringer's solution, while the other group was irrigated by "jet lavage" with 3 l Ringer's fluid. No appreciable difference was observed between the two groups. The conclusion, i.e. that bone particles remaining in the soft tissues rarely cause serious ossification, is surprising but should not be dismissed out of hand.

Perioperative Measures

▪ **Nonsteroidal Anti-inflammatory Drugs.** In our own investigations, the group of men taking ibuprofen did not differ significantly from the group without ibuprofen, either in respect of the ossification itself or the degree of possible flexion.

Numerous variants concerning the type and duration of administration of nonsteroidal anti-inflammatory drugs have been tried [7, 12, 15]. Their biochemical mode of action involves the inhibition of cyclooxygenase and a consequent reduction in arachidonic acid derivatives (prostaglandins). However, the precise connection with a reduction in ossification has not yet been proven biochemically.

In a major review of the literature, Eulert [7] points to differing levels of success in relation to drug-based prophylaxis of heterotopic ossification. In his own prospective study, 685 patients were randomly allocated to four different drug regimens: Indomethacin prophylaxis for 7 and 14 days (2 × 50 mg) and administration of diclofenac (2 × 75 mg) did not show any significant differences in respect of the development of ossification. The outcome was significantly worse for patients receiving aspirin 3 × 750 mg for 14 days. The article does not state whether any differences were observed in the range of motion, but simply evaluates the results according to Brooker's radiological classification. The study by Amstutz [3] is an example of a structured statistical evaluation. In this investigation, an at-risk population received indomethacin for 10 days postoperatively. After 1 year, he reported statistically significant differences in the incidence of serious ossification after primary and second procedures. While indomethacin is the drug for which significant differences are most consistently reported in the literature [3, 7, 12, 13, 15, 16, 18, 19], it is often inappropriate in practice because of its pronounced gastrointestinal side effects [16].

Ibuprofen is associated with fewer gastrointestinal problems compared to indomethacin and does not appear to have an adverse effect on the osteointegration of the acetabular component [6, 9, 12]. Studies have shown that the administration of naproxen and ibuprofen for four weeks does not affect the frequency of aseptic loosening over the following 5 years. Our own investigations, which are not based on an at-risk population, have, however, not shown any significant differences in respect of ossification or degree of flexion.

■ **Perioperative Radiotherapy.** Postoperative radiotherapy, either as fractionated or single doses, should be administered, or initiated, within the first 5 postoperative days [2, 4]. According to other analyses, the effectiveness of postoperative irradiation diminishes after 72 h [21]. The objective is to prevent the transformation of pluripotential mesenchymal cells into osteoblasts at an early stage of differentiation. This radiotherapy is administered mainly to patients who have already had areas of ossification removed surgically or with ossification on the contralateral side.

More recent studies have confirmed that the radiotherapy can also be administered up to 4 h preoperatively. In three prospectively randomised studies, the preoperative administration of a single dose of 7 Gy did not show any significant differences in respect of the onset of ossification according to Brooker compared with postoperative radiotherapy [10, 11, 20]. Irradiation even 16–20 h preoperatively should be effective [14], although to a lesser extent compared with administration 4–8 h preoperatively [21]. Preoperative irradiation therefore should take place on the day of operation. In two of these studies, the Harris hip score was used as a clinical parameter for checking function [11, 20]. Preoperative administration is much simpler for the care team and the patient. Our own experience over 1 year is positive, although the corresponding investigations are not yet concluded.

Because of the side effects of radiation, it is not advisable to administer such radiotherapy routinely to younger patients or those wishing to have children [2].

12.9 Management of Ossification

12.9.1 Procedure in Our Hospital

The following basic principles apply:

- Surgical removal of periarticular ossification that is clearly demarcated on radiographs is not generally performed within the first 6–9 months following the primary operation.
- The surgical procedure:
  - Place the patient in the supine or lateral position depending on the location of the main ossification site.
  - Do not remove the periosteum from the ossification, but carefully and gradually expose the ossification with the scalpel or scissors, leaving a fine layer of tissue. Carefully lift off the muscles from the areas of ossification. While it is advisable to chisel off as large fragments as possible when removing the ossified areas, it is often necessary to remove the ossification in stages in order to spare adjacent nerves or intervening muscle strands.
  - After removing all ossification sites, irrigate liberally and perform meticulous haemostasis.
  - Ensure good drainage by inserting thick drains, leave these in place for 3–4 days and possibly remove them in stages.
  - If necessary, use a Cellsaver during the operation.
  - Maximise blood recovery postoperatively.
  - Radiotherapy on the 1st postoperative day, or possibly preoperatively, with a single dose of 600 rads (Fig. 12.7).
  - Physiotherapy: the aim is to achieve full extension in the 1st week, concentrating on flexion and rotation in the 2nd week.

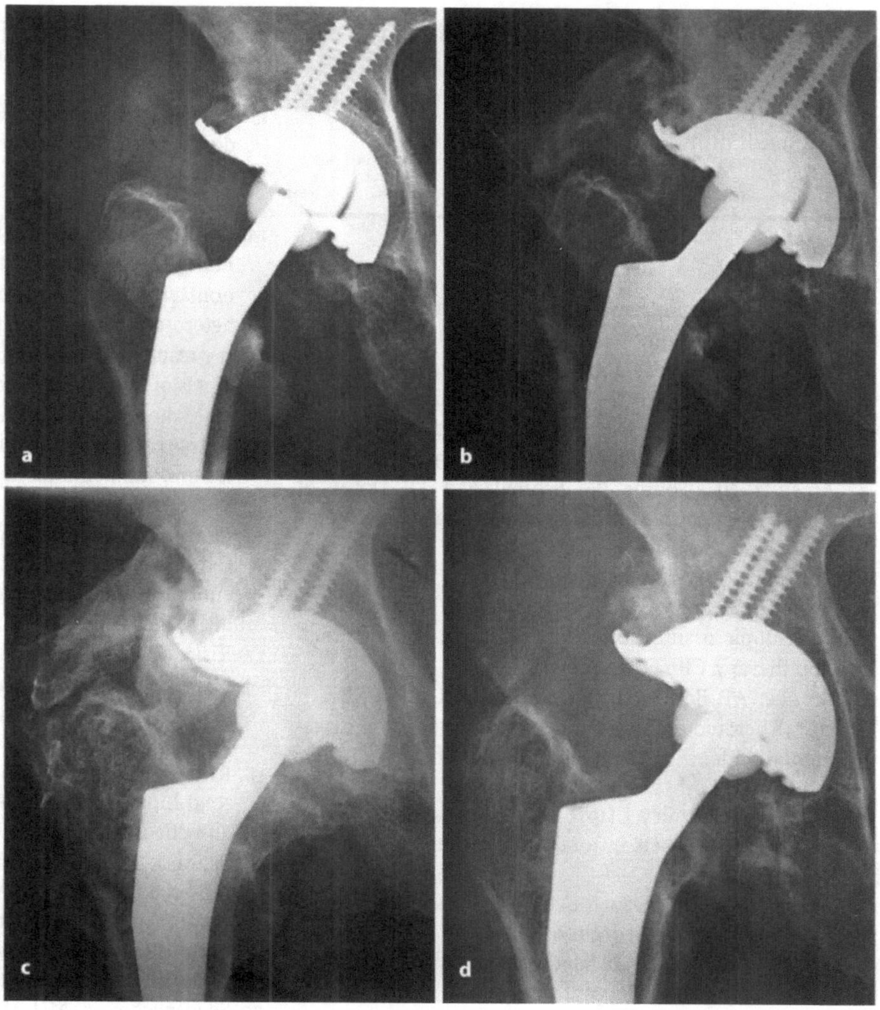

Fig. 12.8a–d. Moderate functional improvement after removal of ossification with subsequent radiotherapy. L.F., male, 70 years (O. 1364)
a Situation after the primary operation
b Ill-defined ossification after 4 months, flexion/extension 70–25–0°
c 5 years postoperatively, flexion/extension 50–20–0
d Six months after removal of ossification with subsequent radiotherapy, flexion/extension 70–20–0°

The results after surgical removal, combined with prior or subsequent radiotherapy, have ranged from satisfactory to very good. A substantial reduction in ossification is achieved in most cases. Occasionally, an impressive improvement in mobility is also achieved (Figs. 12.3, 12.4). In other cases, the initial mobility is only moderate, despite successful removal of the ossified areas (Fig. 12.8).

12.9.2 Literature on the Management of Ossification

There are no detailed descriptions of the surgical procedure for the removal of periarticular ossification in the hip area. In 1979, Riska [17] reported on just six patients undergoing surgical removal of extra-articular ossification after a total hip replacement. A free fat graft was successfully performed in these cases after excision of the ossification.

12.10 Conclusions

In view of the results of our investigations, we have abandoned the prophylactic use of ibuprofen. We administer radiotherapy in the immediate preoperative period to patients with functionally disabling ossification and those who have undergone ossification removal after a total hip replacement on the other side. Patients with a pronounced tendency toward ossification, e.g. those with ankylosing spondylitis, or those scheduled for ossification removal also receive radiotherapy beforehand (single dose of 600 rads).

The surgical removal of ossification involves only a very small number of patients.

References

1. Ahrengart L, Lindgren U (1989) Functional significance of heterotopic bone formation after total hip arthroplasty. J Arthroplasty 4: 125–131
2. Alberti W, Krahl H, Quack G, Löer F, Pohl M (1995) Strahlentherapie nach endoprothetischem Hüftgelenksersatz. Dtsch Ärztebl 92: A1236–1243
3. Amstutz HC, Fouble VA, Schmalzried TP, Dorey FJ (1997) Short-course indomethacin prevents heterotopic ossification in a high-risk population following hip arthroplasty. J Arthroplasty 12: 126–131
4. Ayers DC, Pellegrini VD, Evarts CM (1991) Prevention of heterotopic ossification in high-risk patients of radiation therapy. Clin Orthop 263: 87–93
5. Brooker AF, Bowerman JW, Robinson RA, Riley LH Jr (1973) Ectopic ossification following total hip replacement. Incidence and a method of classification. J Bone Joint Surg [Am] 55: 1629–1632
6. DeLee JG, Charnley J (1976) Radiological demarcation of cemented sockets in total hip replacement. Clin Orthop 121: 20–32
7. Eulert J, Knelles D, Barthel T (1997) Heterotope Ossifikationen. Unfallchirurg 100: 667–674
8. Friedenstein AJ (1995) Marrow stromal fibroblasts. Calcified Tissue Int 56: Suppl 1: 17
9. Gebuhr P, Skovgaard K, Sperling K (1997) Naproxen given to prevent heterotopic ossification does not increase prosthetic loosening. Orthopaedics 5: 21–23
10. Gregoritch SJ, Chada M, Pelligrini VD, Rubin P, Kantorowitz DA (1994) Randomized trial comparing preoperative versus postoperative irradiation for prevention of ossification following prosthetic total hip replacement: Preliminary results. Int J Radiat Oncol Biol Phys 30: 55–62
11. Kantorowitz DA, Muff NS (1998) Preoperative vs. postoperative radiation prophylaxis of heterotopic ossification: a rural community hospital experience. Int J Radiat Oncol Biol Phys 40: 171–176
12. Keller JC, Trancik TM, Young FAS, Mary E (1989) Effects of indomethacin on bony ingrowth. J Orthop Res 7: 28–34
13. Kjaersgaard-Andersen P, Nafai A, Teichert G (1993) Indomethacin for prevention of heterotopic ossification. A randomized controlled study in 41 hip arthroplasties. Acta Orthop Scand 64: 639–642
14. Kölbl O, Knelles O, Barthel T, Raunecker F, Flentje M, Eulert J (1998) Preoperative irradiation versus the use of nonsteroid anti-inflammatory drugs for prevention of heterotopic ossification following total hip replacement: the results of a randomized trial. Int J Radiation Oncology Biol Phys 42: 390–401
15. McMahon JS, Waddell JP, Morton J (1991) Effect of short course indomethacin on heterotopic bone formation after uncemented total hip arthroplasty. J Arthroplasty 6: 259–264
16. Metzenroth H, Publig W, Knahr K, Zandl C, Kuchner G, Carda C (1991) Ossifikationsprophylaxe nach Hüfttotalendoprothesen mit Indomethacin und ihr Einfluss auf die Magenschleimhaut. Z Orthop 129: 178–182
17. Riska EB, Michelsson JE (1979) Treatment of para-articular ossification after total hip replacement by excision and use of free fat transplants. Acta Orthop Scand 50: 751–754
18. Ritter MA, Vaughan RB (1983) Ectopic ossification after total hip arthroplasty. Predisposing factors, frequency, and effect on results. Science 220: 680–686
19. Schmidt SA.,Kjaersgaard-Andersen P, Pedersen N, Kristensen SS, Pedersen P, Nielsen JB (1988) The use of indomethacin to prevent the formation of heterotopic bone after total hip replacement: a randomized, double-blind clinical trial. J Bone Joint Surg [Am] 70: 834–838
20. Seegenschmiedt MH, Martus P, Goldmann AR, Wölfel R, Keilholz L, Sauer R (1994) Preoperative versus postoperative radiotherapy for prevention of heterotopic ossification (HO): first results of a randomized trial in high-risk patients. Int J Radiat Oncol Biol Phys 30: 63–73
21. Seegenschmiedt MH, Makoski H, Micke O (2001) Radiation prophylaxis for heterotopic ossification about the hip joint – a multicenter study. Int J Radiat Oncol Biol Phys 51: 756–765
22. Sneath RJS, Bindi FD, Davies J, Parnell EJ (2001) The effect of pulsed irrigation on the incidence of heterotopic ossification after total hip arthroplasty. J Arthroplasty 16: 547–551

CHAPTER 13

Vascular Injuries

PETER E. OCHSNER, BERNHARD NACHBUR

While vascular injuries during total hip replacements can be potentially life threatening, in most cases they pose at least a serious threat to the affected leg. Intraoperative injuries include open or concealed massive bleeding, which can lead to shock. Perioperative vascular thrombotic occlusions are easily overlooked because of their insidious nature. Postoperatively, pseudoaneurysms and arterioarterial emboli can result in an ischaemic syndrome in the affected leg. The most serious consequences for the affected leg are generally apparent by the end of the procedure at the latest. Since the aforementioned later occurring consequences are not acutely life-threatening, time is available for more precise diagnostic measures to be implemented.

The point at which a threat is present depends on the nature and mechanism of the underlying vascular injury. The vessels most commonly injured are the external iliac and common femoral arteries and their branches and accompanying veins in the hip area. The injuries are caused primarily by the use of pointed bone levers in the acetabular roof and by acetabular implants or cement fragments protruding into the lesser pelvis. Screw cups and their self-tapping threads, screws, chisels, and even guide wires, can also cause vascular injuries.

In numerical terms, life-threatening vascular injuries are relatively rare, with an incidence of around 0.2%. As a preventive measure, bone levers should be placed ventral to the acetabulum under visual control or with finger protection. Penetration of cement into the lesser pelvis should be avoided at all costs, and any excess cement carefully removed. Screws should be inserted in the direction of the iliosacral joint. Particular caution is indicated with the acetabular reinforcement ring and the antiprotrusio cage. In the event of a massive haemorrhage during operation, all means should be used to staunch the bleeding locally and immediately locate and clamp off the external iliac artery by means of a lower anterior retroperitoneal lumbotomy. The arterial reconstruction should then be left to the vascular surgeon.

13.1 Introduction, Definitions

Although vascular injuries arising in connection with total hip replacements are rare, they are particularly dangerous since they can lead to amputation or even to the death of the patient. A subsequent vascular reconstruction can result in almost intractable neurogenic pain of the de-efferent type (Fig. 13.5). An overall view of the problem can be obtained by a review of the literature or a perusal of liability reports. In addition to a number of summary publications incorporating a literature review [3, 6, 7, 13, 14, 16, 18], there are also numerous case descriptions, just a selection of which is mentioned here.

Injuries can be subdivided according to the

- Time of clinical manifestation
- Type of vascular injury
- Cause of the injury
- Affected artery/vein

13.1.1 Time of Clinical Manifestation

The prognosis for serious vascular injuries depends on the rapidity of detection – ideally immediately after their occurrence – and the implementation of appropriate emergency measures. In the case of haemorrhages developing at a later stage, there is usually time to make an in-depth diagnosis or consult a vascular surgeon.

■ **Intraoperative Massive Bleeding.** Manifest massive haemorrhaging into the surgical field. This is impossible to overlook and is usually amenable to plugging, during which the external iliac artery can be located via a separate approach (anterior retroperitoneal lumbotomy, see also Sect. 13.5.1) and clamped off within minutes to staunch the bleeding.

In the fairly rare cases of concealed or occult massive bleeding, the blood flows into the lesser pelvis. This event manifests itself by a drop in blood pressure and circulatory collapse and is very dangerous because it is liable to be misinterpreted and underestimated initially. The cause can, however, rapidly be elucidated by ultrasonography (see also Sect. 13.3.2, Case 5).

■ **(Immediate) Postoperative Manifestation of an Ischaemic Syndrome.** A growing, massive haematoma, circulatory collapse, peripheral ischaemia or a combination of these symptoms may become apparent during postoperative monitoring. If these signs are obvious, there is an acute risk to the very survival or vitality of the limb on the same side. If a fairly major haemorrhage only comes to light after several hours as a result of increasing tachycardia, drop in blood pressure and dwindling Doppler signal, there is generally still sufficient time for more specific investigations (e.g. contrast angiogram, MRI with gadolinium, CT scan).

■ **Threatening Ischaemic Syndrome Without Bleeding.** Particularly insidious, and also hazardous in terms of liability, are dissections resulting from the intimal fracture of arteriosclerotic plaques, which can lead to complete or subtotal thrombotic occlusion and a total or subtotal ischaemic syndrome, for example if the femoral bifurcation is affected.

These thrombotic occlusions of arteries at a strategically important site are insidious because no external or internal bleeding has disturbed the routinely satisfactory progress of the hip replacement and consequently no suspicions are aroused because the blood pressure readings remain unchanged. With careful investigation, however, the ischaemic syndrome can be detected as early as the end of the operation. Symptoms reported by the patient (pain in the lower leg) are nevertheless often underestimated as a normal consequence of the operation, suppressed with fairly large doses of opiates, then possibly misinterpreted as thrombophlebitis and finally, and too late, corrected by vascular surgery. If the leg can be preserved, as is often the case, the patient may be left with lifelong, severely disabling, neurogenic pain of the de-efferent type which, in functional respects, can have much worse consequences than a below-knee amputation with a prosthesis.

In this situation however, and almost without exception, patients will prefer to keep a painful and unusable foot with no feeling rather than undergo a below-knee amputation that may be much more advantageous in terms of function and social and physical rehabilitation.

■ **Delayed Manifestation.** In the case of delayed manifestation, conspicuous, or even alarming, signs of poor perfusion or a tumour with a flow sound, can occur unexpectedly a few days or even weeks later. A causal connection with the hip operation is usually obvious.

■ **Late Manifestation.** Circulatory disorder that often occurs only after several years, e.g. in connection with the migration of a loosened cup. Since the corresponding problems tend to develop in the form of a protracted crescendo, relevant investigations can be planned in good time.

13.1.2 Type of Vascular Injury

A wide variety of vascular injuries can be involved [13].

■ **Arterial Injuries.** These include direct, full-thickness wall injuries usually caused by pointed objects, injuries to the intima usually caused by blunt force, thromboses caused by intimal dissection or heat generated by the polymerisation of bone cement, a false aneurysm, an arteriovenous fistula and arterioarterial emboli (emboli that break away from a thrombus in the hip area and cause an occlusion distally).

A particularly impressive phenomenon is the sudden onset of arterial bleeding during extraction of a subsided acetabular component, usually as a result of the slitting open of the external iliac artery by an adjacent sharp fragment of cement.

■ **Vein Injuries.** Vein injuries are rarely so dangerous as to require revision. However, while they are generally more amenable to plugging, they can still behave like untameable animals and pose their own special risks. It has even been known for pelvic veins to become wound up in a rotating Kirschner wire. Haemostasis in such vein injuries is much more difficult than in arterial injuries, and a functional pelvic vein block, with the clinical consequences of a so-called post-thrombotic syndrome, is one possible outcome [13].

13.1.3 Causes of Injury

■ **Instrument.** The primary culprits are bone levers, drill bits and self-tapping threads for screw cups, while curettes, chisels, Kirschner wires, etc. can also be involved.

■ **Implants.** Particularly important in this context are bone cement, screws and screw cups, and possibly a whole migrating acetabular component in protrusion with adherent bone cement. Bone cement can cause mechanical and thermal damage to major arteries.

■ **Intraoperative Manipulation.** Overstretching of the vessels by dislocation and reduction manoeuvres can prove particularly harmful when severely arteriosclerotic vessels with pre-existing damage are compromised. A particularly hazardous procedure is the removal of acetabular implants and sharp cement fragments that have penetrated into the lesser pelvis during the first operation. Any excess cement must therefore be removed with meticulous care (see Sect. 13.1.2) if it cannot be left in place.

13.1.4 Affected Arteries/Veins

The external iliac artery, followed by the common femoral artery are generally agreed to be the most frequently injured vessels. Much less frequently affected are the deep femoral, superficial femoral and lat./med. circumflex femoral arteries and their accompanying veins. Injuries to the branches of the internal iliac or obturator arteries represent the exception [3, 7, 13, 18]. The bifurcation of the common femoral artery can be located at differing heights [22], which explains why, for example, different vessels can be injured by the insertion of a bone lever tip ventrally to the acetabulum (Fig. 13.1).

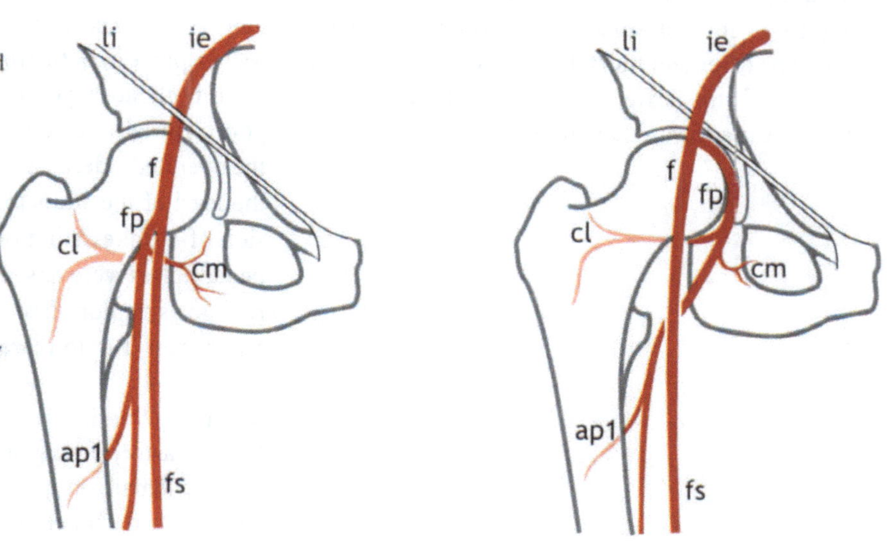

Fig. 13.1. The arterial blood supply in the hip area (*left*) and one of its numerous variants (*right*) [21]. *li* Inguinal ligament, *ie* External iliac artery, *f* Common femoral artery, *fp* Deep femoral artery, *cl* Lateral circumflex artery, *cm* Medial circumflex artery, *fs* Superficial femoral artery, *ap1* Superior perforating artery

13.2 Frequency

13.2.1 Frequency in Our Own Patients

Three serious arterial haemorrhages occurred overall in our patient population: one during a primary implantation and two during revision procedures. Only one matched the description of a typical incident that would be classed as a high-risk situation (see also Sect. 13.3.1).

13.2.2 Frequency in the Literature

■ **Frequency of Vascular Injuries.** Figures are cited only by Nachbur et al. [13, 14]. The authors observed a frequency of 0.25% among 8000 procedures. When the subject was reviewed 10 years later, the figure was slightly lower among patients treated under the auspices of the M.E. Müller Foundation, although the percentage of revision operations had increased. Vascular complications are much more likely to occur during revision procedures.

■ **Mortality Risk, Amputation Risk.** Several review studies provide corresponding figures. In the series of 25 cases investigated by Nachbur et al. [13], no patient died of this complication. In two literature reviews, the mortality among 36 and 68 recorded cases was 14% [3] and 7% [18], respectively. The corresponding risk of amputation was 4%, 8% and 19%, respectively. The divergent mortality statistics may be a reflection of the extent of cooperation between orthopaedic and vascular surgeons.

13.3 Known Causes of Vascular Injuries

13.3.1 Our Own Cases

■ **Case 1.** Injury of the arteriosclerotically altered external iliac/common femoral arteries with a bone lever.

G.A., female, 80 years (O. 1680). Because of the poor view into the acetabulum, the usual bone lever placed ventral to the acetabular roof was supplemented by the additional insertion of a pointed lever ventrally and as medially as possible on the anterior acetabular roof. A bleed soon occurred when tension was applied. Since no cause was found during the search for a source with a repeatedly moved Langenbeck retractor, the operation was continued. A pronounced drop in blood pressure occurred over the next quarter of an hour. Assuming that an intrapelvic haemorrhage had occurred, the surgeon plugged the wound. The vascular surgeon was notified, the abdominal wall covered with fresh drapes and an anterior lower lumbotomy performed (Fig. 13.12). Moderate bleeding only was present above the inguinal ligament, but massive bleeding was found to have occurred distal to this point. The haemorrhaging area was compressed pending the arrival of the vascular surgeon. A 6-cm section of severely arteriosclerotic artery was resected just proximal to the bifurcation of the common femoral artery and replaced by an 8 mm diameter Goretex graft of corresponding length. The resected section showed a tear approximately 2 cm long. At a check-up 7 years later, the femoral pulse was palpable in both groins, though weakened equally on both sides, possibly owing to the pre-existing poor arterial circulation in this elderly patient. On the operated side, an arterial flow sound was heard at the level of the adductor canal, probably an expression of a pre-existing obliterating arteriopathy. The pedal pulses were absent on both sides. The patient remains symptom free in respect of her hip and arteries even after 10 years.

■ **Case 2.** Arterial bleeding from a branch of the deep femoral artery during an iatrogenic shaft perforation.

S.E., female, 81 years (O. 12036), fractured steel curved-stem Müller prosthesis. Although the tip of the prosthesis stem could be grasped and knocked out after proximal drilling, the shaft was perforated and split during the removal of cement residues, whereupon a branch of the deep femoral artery began to bleed profusely. With the leg in flexion, it seemed to be possible to stop the bleeding with a ligature. Postoperatively, following the insertion of a Wagner revision stem, massive bleeding occurred, requiring surgical revision of a haematoma. Although an early infection necessitated revision and irrigation-suction drainage, a complete recovery was the eventual outcome. Today, this type of postoperative bleeding would probably be amenable to embolisation (see also Sect. 13.4.3).

■ **Case 3.** Intraoperatively noted bleeding from the superior gluteal artery: C.M., male, 36 years (O. 15924). History of two previous revision operations due to infection and a huge, fist-sized acetabular defect, with particularly extensive destruction of the posterior pelvic wall. Although the surgeon was able to remove the acetabular implant at operation, with the patient in the lateral position, a massive bleed from the main branch of the superior gluteal artery occurred at the posterior rim of the cavity during curettage of the acetabular bed. The operator managed to grasp the vessel, but was only able to ligate it after careful chiselling away of adjacent bone sections. There were no other problems postoperatively.

13.3.2 Supplied Case Studies with Fatal Outcome

■ **Case 4.** The following extremely instructive case study forming the subject of an expert report was supplied by Dr. A. Siegel, Endoklinik Hamburg.

At the age of 68, a female patient with pronounced dysplastic coxarthrosis years after a Schanz osteotomy complained of severe pain (Fig. 13.2a). An uncemented prosthesis was inserted (Fig. 13.2b). Five years later, the patient was advised to undergo a cup revision as treatment for mild pain and incipient cup loosening (Fig. 13.2c).

The operation report for the acetabular revision describes the removal of a very thick neocapsule surrounding the joint. A bone lever was carefully inserted (ventrally?), and the knee was flexed at an angle of 35° to safeguard the neurovascular bundle. The acetabular bed was then reamed out to a size-64 reamer. Massive bleeding occurred while the cup was being screwed in place. Central venous pressure dropped to −3 cm on the water column and a blood loss of 4 l was reported.

Over the next hour the operator tried to stop the bleeding, initially by plugging with an abdominal pad and subsequent cauterisation, and then with suture ligatures. A period of temporary recovery was followed by another drop in blood pressure. Although the bleeding was eventually stopped with the aid of numerous vascular clamps, the blood loss increased to approximately 6.5 l by the end of this hour, and the patient went into circulatory arrest. Cardiac activity was resumed by resuscitation. Half an hour later, a summoned vascular surgeon performed an anterior lower lumbotomy as a second access route. Locally, the external iliac vein and artery had been caught by the threads of the screw cup and screwed in between the cup and the bone. The vein defect of approximately 6 cm was bridged by an endogenous vein, while the gap in the artery was bridged by an approximately 3-cm Dacron graft. Twenty-three units of blood, with additional plasma, were administered from the start of bleeding until the end of the operation.

Despite all these measures, the patient's pupils were described as wide and fixed after a good 3 hours. Until her death 2 days later, the patient suffered major blood losses as a result of a severe clotting disorder and the circulation was never properly stabilised. The autopsy merely revealed cardiac findings appropriate to the patient's age.

■ *Comments.* This case illustrates how screw cups, particularly in revisions, can injure the ventral rim of the acetabulum. Protection of this site by bone levers is important and allows the implant to be screwed in under visual control. Although the operator was able to staunch the massive bleeding via the hip incision after 1 hour by clamping the major vessels, the resulting circulatory collapse led to irreversible brain damage. This incident underlines the importance of the following recommendation to perform an anterior lower lumbotomy immediately as a second access route in cases of massive bleeding of uncertain origin (see also Sect. 13.5.1, Case 1, Fig. 13.12).

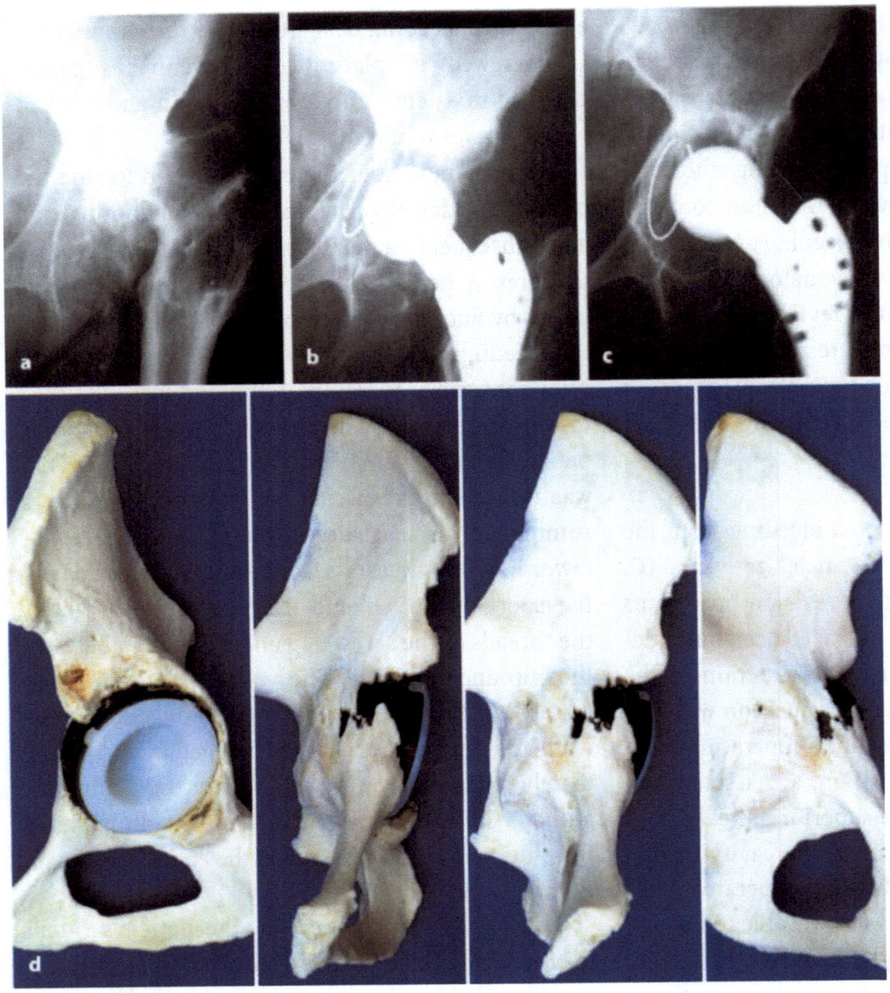

Figs. 13.2a–d. Tearing of the external iliac artery and vein during insertion of a Zweymüller screw cup, with fatal outcome

a Pronounced dysplastic coxarthrosis 24 years after a Schanz osteotomy with high subluxation

b Before reaming and implantation of a 54-mm-diameter Endler polyethylene screw cup, the acetabular bed was driven into the lesser pelvis with a tamp in order to move the acetabulum to a more central position

c Five years later, the cup is moderately loosened. The bone contours are clearly protruding into the lesser pelvis and appear to be widened towards the cranial end

d Macerated preparation of the operated pelvic half with a 64-mm-diameter Zweymüller screw cup. The screw cup fits precisely in the custom-tapped threads. Ventrocranially and immediately lateral to the ant. inf. iliac spine, the cup has split the acetabulum and its threads project 1–3 mm beyond the outer contours of the bone into the soft tissues

■ **Case 5.** The following important case is based on personal communication.

In a stand-alone orthopaedic hospital, an acetabular revision was performed on a 57-year-old female patient in good general health. The acetabulum was prepared using three bone levers, one of which was placed ventral to the acetabular roof. The loosened cup was removed, whereupon the anaesthetist announced that the patient had gone into hypovolaemic shock. The operator was unable to locate any source of bleeding in the surgical field, including the anterior acetabular rim. No perforation through the bony wall into the lesser pelvis had occurred. The surgeon decided to conclude the operation, and the anaesthetist managed to stabilise the circulation only with great difficulty.

Twenty minutes after extubation, the patient complained of abdominal pain and again went into shock. An ultrasound scan revealed the presence of a haemoperitoneum.

The patient was urgently transferred to the central hospital, where her abdomen was explored via a median laparotomy. Exploration of the inguinal area revealed two small tears at the junction of the external iliac artery and vein with the common femoral artery and vein. These were repaired, resulting in primary stabilisation of the circulation. The ventral bone lever over the acetabular roof was considered to be the only possible explanation for the injury.

Shortly thereafter, the patient suffered another circulatory collapse. A catheter inserted to treat the shock caused a mediastinal haematoma as a result of injury to the brachiocephalic trunk and the adjacent vein. The catheter placement in the neck had been aggravated by a previous operation for a malignant thyroid tumour. Even an emergency sternotomy was unable to prevent the patient's death.

■ *Comments.* The following conclusions can be drawn from this case:

- Even if there is no obvious bleeding into the surgical field, a vascular injury during the operation can still be responsible for the sudden onset of hypovolaemic shock.
- Concealed massive bleeds can be triggered not just by screws, drill bits or Kirschner wires perforating through the bony wall into the lesser pelvis, but also by bone levers at the anterior acetabular rim.
- If the situation is life threatening, active investigation via an anterior lower lumbotomy (see also Sect. 13.5.1) is indicated.
- If an orthopaedic department is not incorporated in a central hospital, the emergency procedure in the event of vascular injuries must be established and a vascular surgeon must be contactable.

13.3.3 Case Studies from the Literature

The following scenarios were chosen partly because of their relative frequency and partly because of their particularly hazardous nature.

During or immediately after operation (massive bleeding, shock, ischaemia):

- A bone lever ventral to the acetabulum can injure the external iliac artery or the common femoral artery or their branches immediately after the bifurcation [7, 13, 21]. In the attempt to suture the presumed source of bleeding, one author reports that the common femoral artery had to be ligated several times. A femoral nerve lesion was found at revision as well [3].
- The removal of loosened acetabular implants during revision procedures, particularly if protrusion or large intrapelvic cement fragments are present, can lead to bleeding and thromboses [13, 14, 17, 18]. Injury to any intrapelvic vessels is possible (Fig. 13.3).
- Massive bleeding [4] or thrombosis [11] can occur during reaming of the acetabulum [12], tapping for

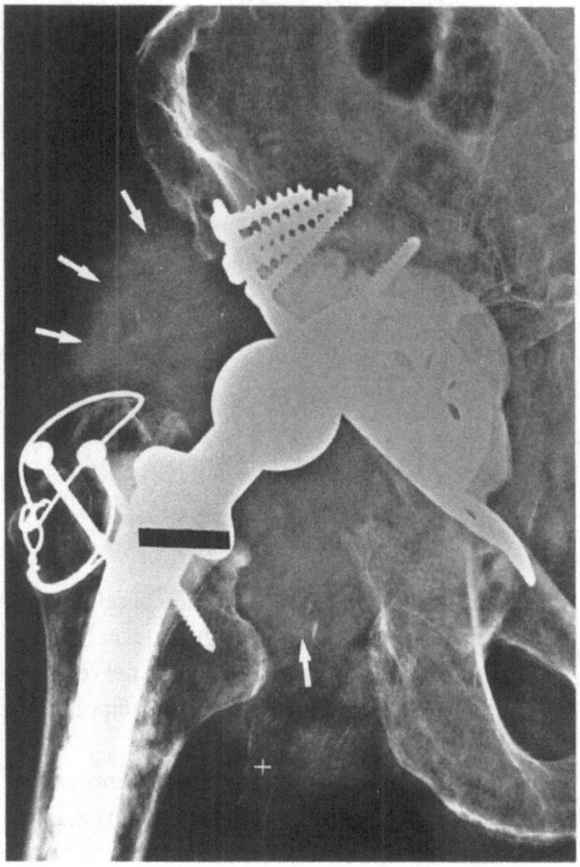

Fig. 13.3. Central breakthrough of an antiprotrusio cage into the lesser pelvis years after its implantation together with prosthesis dislocation. Spherical soft tissue shadow (*arrows*) originating from a massive haematoma. During removal of this implant, the posterior wall of the external iliac artery was slit open by the sharp cement edges

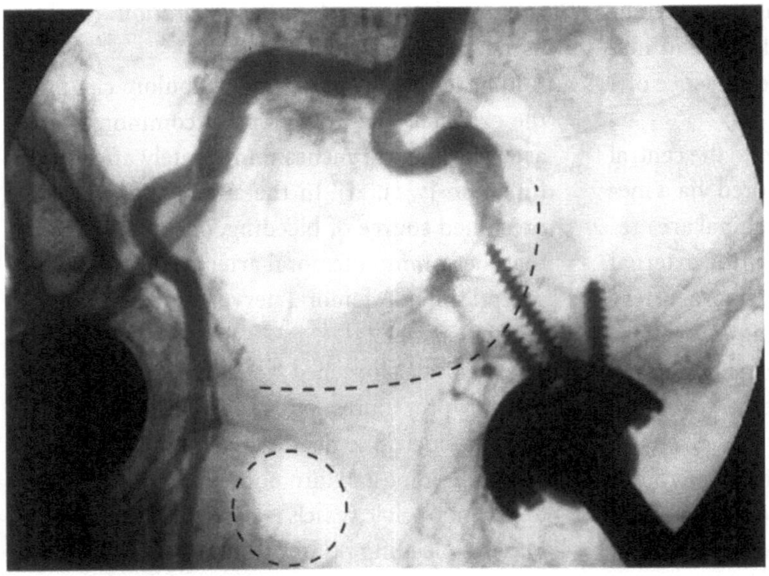

Fig. 13.4. Intimal dissection of the common femoral artery during screw fixation of an uncemented cup. *Dotted line*: Terminal line of pelvis. Ascending thrombotic occlusion up to the bifurcation of the common iliac artery. The resulting ischaemia was observed straightaway and fully corrected by immediate endarterectomy and thrombectomy

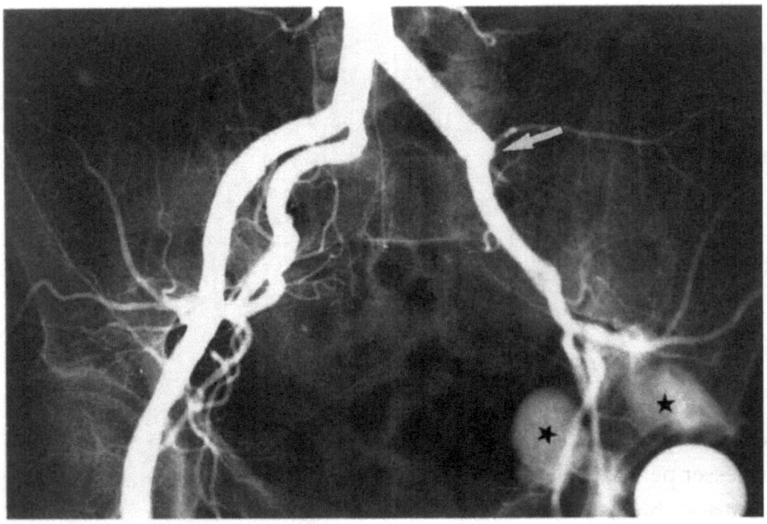

Fig. 13.5. Thrombotic occlusion of the external iliac artery, ascending up to the bifurcation of the common iliac artery (→), probably as a result of heat of polymerisation liberated by cement that had penetrated into the lesser pelvis through a bone defect (*asterisk*). Clinically, the patient suffered severe and constant pain, particularly in the toes, from the moment she awoke from the anaesthetic. This was interpreted in the hospital as normal pain associated with the operation. During the first follow-up appointment after discharge from the hospital, the internist noted absent leg pulses. The emergency surgical recanalisation resulted in a normal malleolar arterial occlusion pressure. As a consequence of the ischaemic damage, however, the patient continued to suffer from almost intractable neuralgia, probably as part of a persistent de-efferent neuropathy

conical screw cups or the insertion of self-tapping conical screw cups. Not just the external iliac artery and vein, but also the femoral nerve can simultaneously be injured by a self-tapping cup [11].

- Screw fixation of acetabular components can occasionally lead to vessel injuries (Fig. 13.4). Here, too, the external iliac artery and its branches are affected in particular [7, 9, 8, 10]. Even a thread-tipped Kirschner wire protruding into the lesser pelvis has caused a fatal haemorrhage in a patient undergoing DHS implantation as a result of injury to the external iliac vein [19].

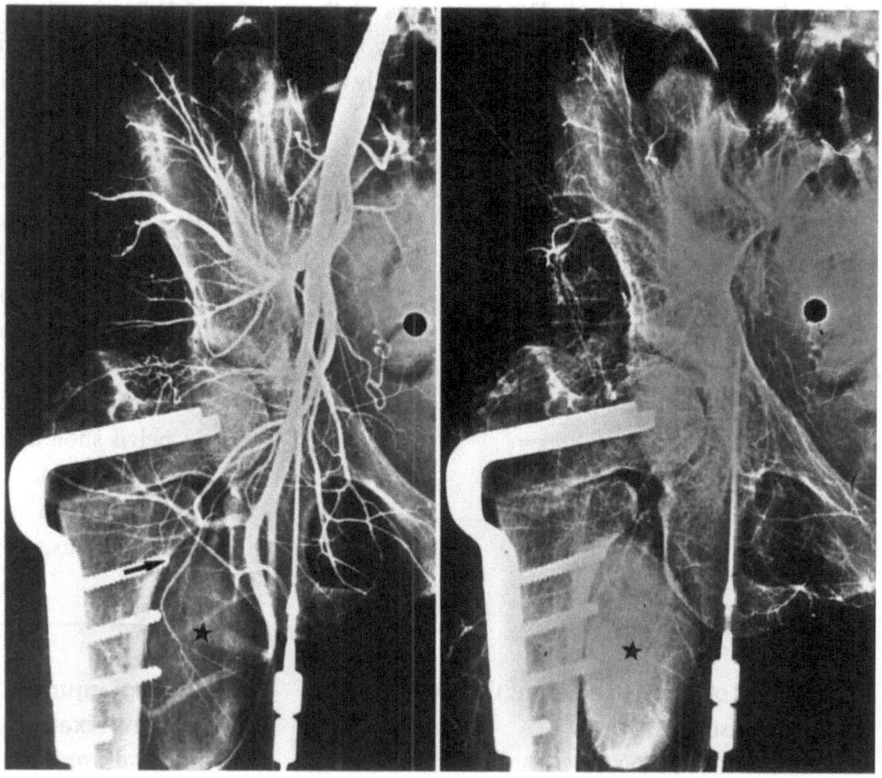

Fig. 13.6. Arteriographic presentation of a false aneurysm (*asterisk*), probably caused by the predrilling for the topmost screw (→) in connection with an intertrochanteric osteotomy. The treatment consisted of ligation of the descending branch of the lateral circumflex artery

First few days/weeks (ischaemia, massive haematoma):

- Acetabular implants and cement fragments protruding into the lesser pelvis, screws (Fig. 13.4) and the tips of bone levers can cause circulatory impairment by the exertion of local pressure on arteries and veins, mechanical or heat-induced (Fig. 13.5) intimal damage [7, 13, 17], or a false aneurysm (Fig. 13.6) [13].
- Vigorous leg manipulations, e.g. during dislocation/reduction of the hip, are thought to be a cause of intimal tears and arterial and venous thromboses [18, 20], particularly if advanced arteriosclerosis is present (Fig. 13.7).
- The removal of a gentamicin cement chain ended in tearing of the femoral vein, which necessitated subsequent disarticulation [5], partly also because of an existing hip infection.

After several months/years (ischaemia):

- The increasing protrusion of loosened acetabular components can lead to compression of a major artery with interruption of the blood flow [1, 17]
- Arterioarterial emboli arising from intravascular thromboses and resulting in peripheral occlusion

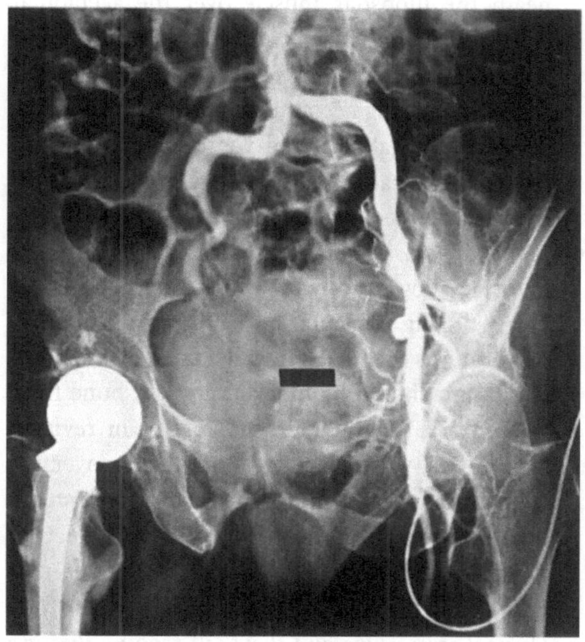

Fig. 13.7. Thrombotic occlusion of the external iliac and common femoral arteries, probably caused by overstretching of a vessel with pre-existing degenerative damage during manipulations associated with the total hip replacement. This resulted in an intimal tear with apposition thrombosis

have been described [15]. The symptoms of the acute arterial occlusion, which is surgically rectified, generally appear first. The source is only discovered secondarily.

13.4 Preventive Measures

The probability of a vascular injury, and thus the risk of a fatality or amputation associated with the onset of this complication, can be reduced through targeted measures.

13.4.1 Measures to Reduce the Frequency of Injury

The primary objective is to avoid the most common causes (see also Sect. 13.3.3).

- *Bone levers*: Bone levers should be advanced ventrally only under visual control or control with a finger covering the tip, and as laterocranially as possible directly over edge of the bone and beneath the iliopsoas muscle over the acetabular rim. These precautions are similar to those designed to protect the femoral nerve (Figs. 11.5–11.7). During acetabular revisions involving a destroyed acetabular roof ventrally, the use of a soft tissue retractor (e.g. a Langenbeck retractor) is recommended for elevation of the soft tissues.
- *Cementation*: Under no circumstances must cement be allowed to reach the inside of the lesser pelvis during cementation (Fig. 13.5). Accidental perforations of the pelvic wall during primary implantation should be blocked up with bone from the femoral head. Our own practice in revision procedures, which has proved effective over the years, is to never remove any medial periosteum after removal of the cup and to seal any defects of the acetabular floor with thin disks of bone prepared from frozen allogeneic femoral heads.
- *Conical screw cups and their self-tapping threads*: Since the ventral acetabular contouring immediately adjacent to the ant. inf. iliac spine can be destroyed during insertion of the self-tapping thread or screw cup (Fig. 13.2d), the placement of a bone lever at this point so as to allow the procedure to be performed under visual control is urgently recommended. To avoid overstretching of the femoral nerve in the supine patient, a roll should be placed under the thigh to flex the leg slightly (Fig. 3.16). If the aforementioned part of the acetabulum is already destroyed, the use of a different type of cup is recommended.
- *Removal of loosened acetabular components with pronounced protrusion and intrapelvic cement fragments*: It is safer to perform this operation in a hospital with a vascular surgery department. The removal of isolated cement fragments from the lesser pelvis should be restricted to cases of clinical need (Fig. 13.3), e.g. with concurrent infection. The use of pointed or sharp instruments is intrinsically dangerous.

13.4.2 Prevention of Injuries During Screw Fixation of Acetabular Implants

A common feature of the SL cups, acetabular reinforcement rings and antiprotrusio cages used by ourselves is that the holes used for anchorage are oriented mainly in the direction of load-bearing bone stock (Fig. 3.1). The screw holes are usually drilled in a cranial direction with medial and dorsal deviations of 20° in each case (Fig. 3.2). We strongly recommend drilling in stages (Fig. 3.21).

Using the aforementioned three types of implant, Heiner Reichlin and Mathias Klein conducted an unpublished cadaver trial with the objective of ascertaining which vessels and nerves are potentially exposed to injury. Two representative sizes of each implant were inserted according to the recommendations in Chap. 3. Screws were inserted into two holes on the cranial flange of the acetabular reinforcement ring and into all screw holes on the inside of the implants such that, where technically feasible, the screws projected beyond the cortical bone on the other side.

- **Uncemented SL Cup** (Fig. 13.8): During correct implantation of the size 52 SL 1 cups (Figs. 2.6, 3.1c), no vessels or nerves were endangered, while the psoas muscle, at most, was placed at risk. If the cup is implanted too steeply, screw perforation medi-

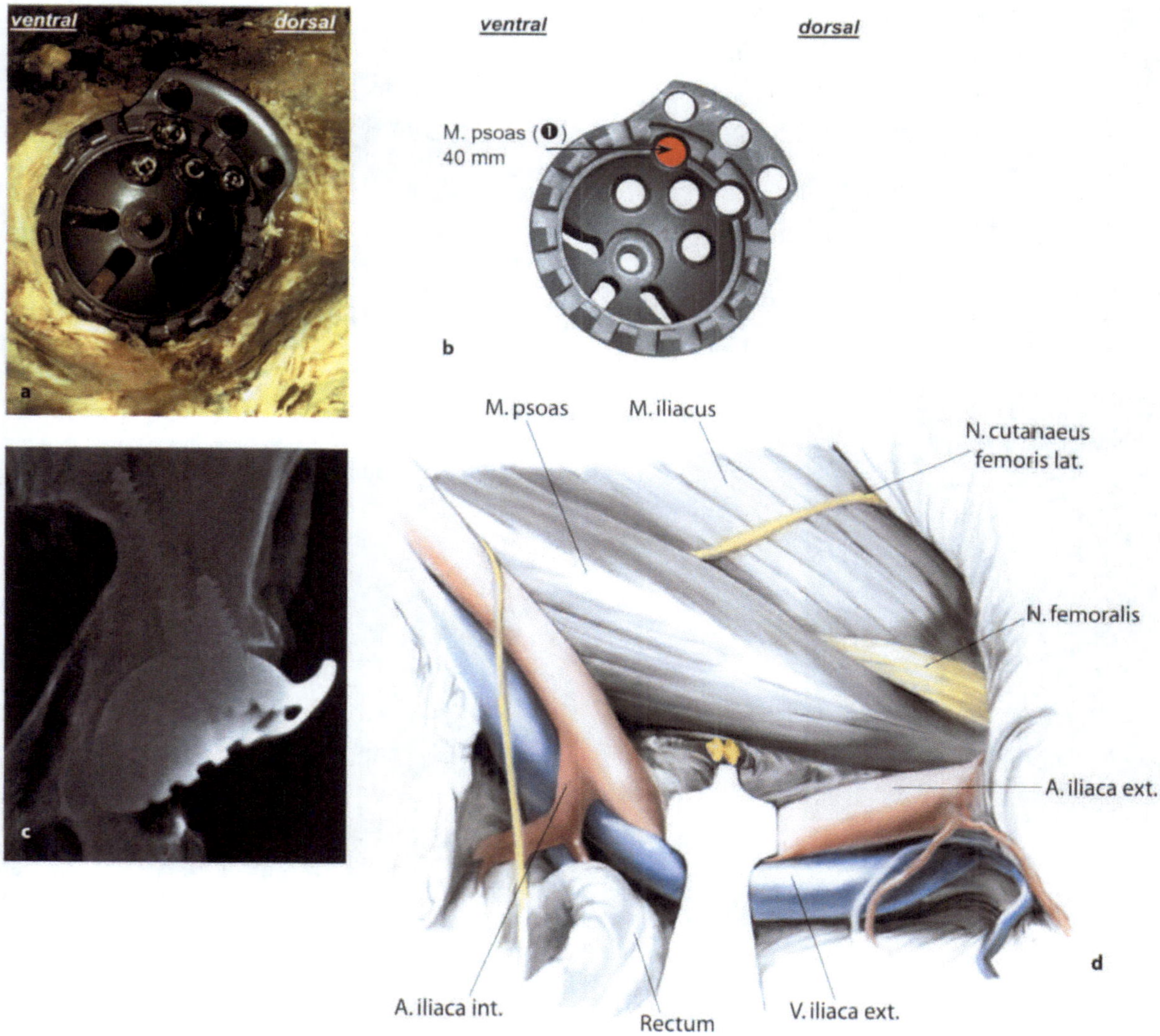

Figs. 13.8a–d. SL titanium shell 1 (52 mm Ø; see also Fig. 2.3). The numbers in the individual figures denote the same screws in each case

a SL cup inserted in the left hip

b Diagram: dangerous screw. Distance in mm from the bone to the mentioned anatomical structure

c ap radiograph: where possible, the screws were deliberately oriented in the medial direction. One of the overlapping long screws corresponds to screw 1

d Inside the lesser pelvis, cranial to the acetabulum and looking onto the external iliac artery and its companion vein: the ventral of the two lateral screws perforates the psoas muscle after 40 mm

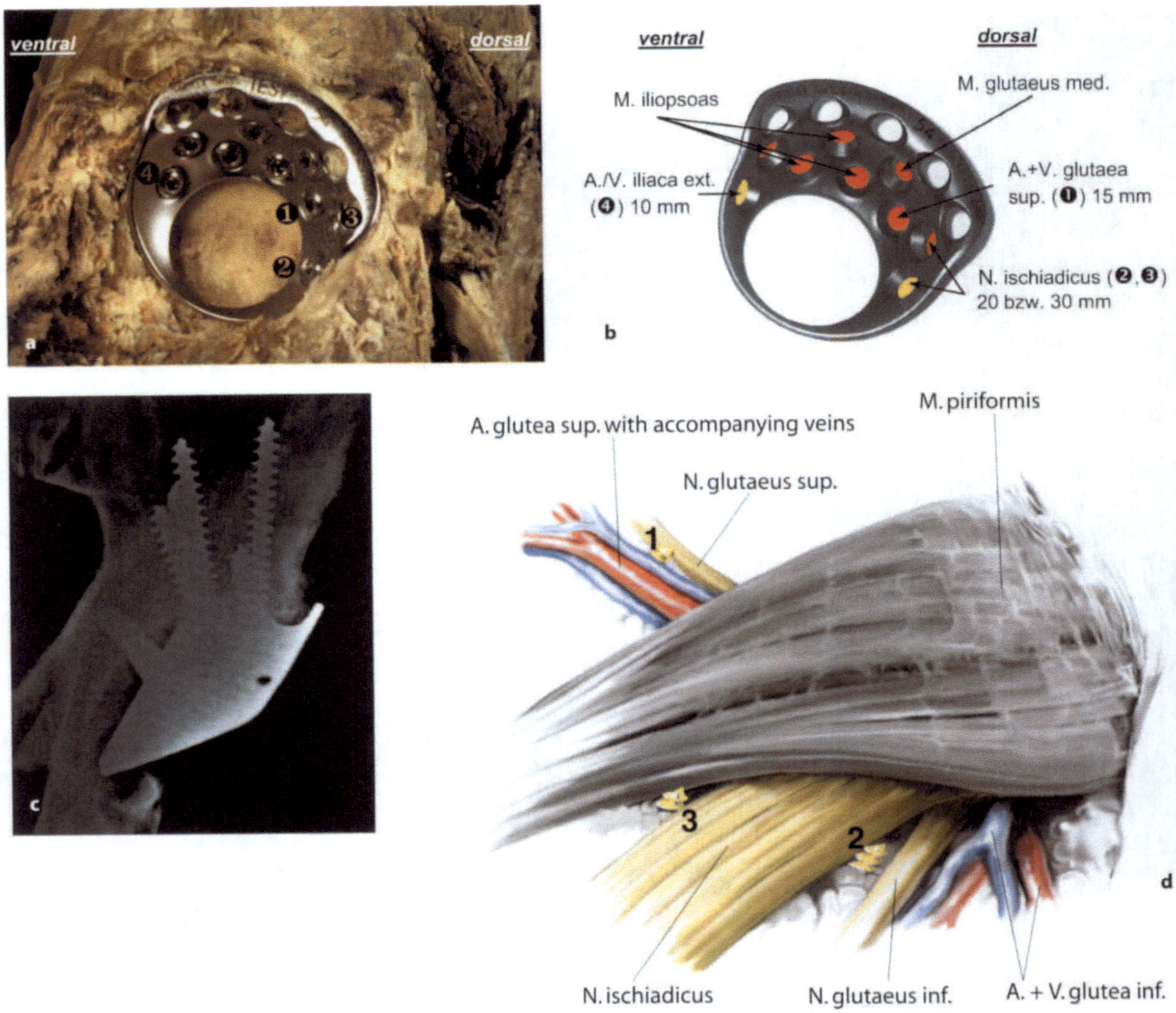

Figs. 13.9a–d. Acetabular reinforcement ring (old) according to M.E. Müller, size 54 (Ø 58 mm; see also Fig. 13.9). The numbers in the individual figures denote the same screws in each case

a Acetabular reinforcement ring inserted in the left hip

b Diagram: screws in the medial ventral and medial dorsal positions are particularly dangerous. The yellow-coloured holes have been omitted in the latest version

c ap radiograph. All screws perforated the corresponding muscles

d Interior view of the lesser pelvis, dorsal section: possibility of injury to the superior gluteal artery and vein (*1*) and the sciatic nerve (*2, 3*), which surfaces below the piriform muscle

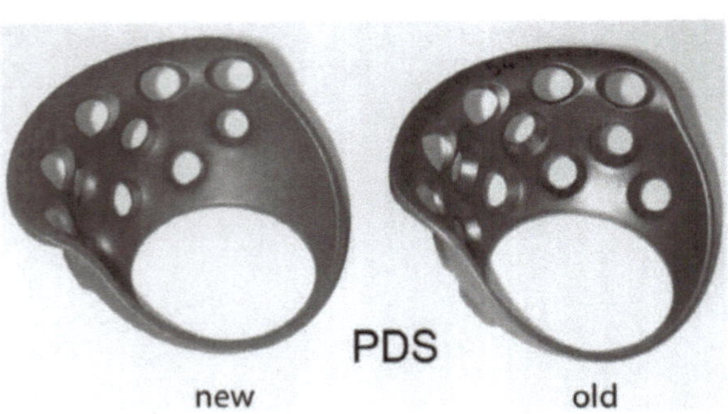

Fig. 13.10. Acetabular reinforcement ring according to M.E. Müller in its current (*left*) and old versions. In the new model, the most ventrally and dorsally positioned screw holes were omitted in order to minimise the threat to the external iliac artery and vein and the sciatic nerve. At the same time, the outer surface of the titanium implant was more coarsely textured

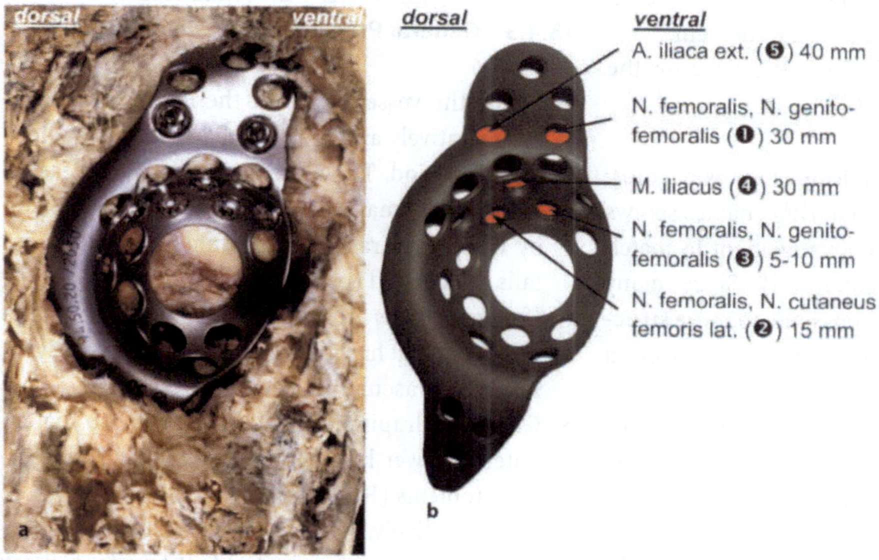

Fig. 13.11a-d. Antiprotrusio cage according to Burch-Schneider, size 50 (Ø 54 mm; see also Fig. 3.10). The numbers in the individual figures denote the same screws in each case
a Antiprotrusio cage inserted in the right hip. The flange points in the cranial – ventral direction
b Diagram: many screws can reach sensitive structures.

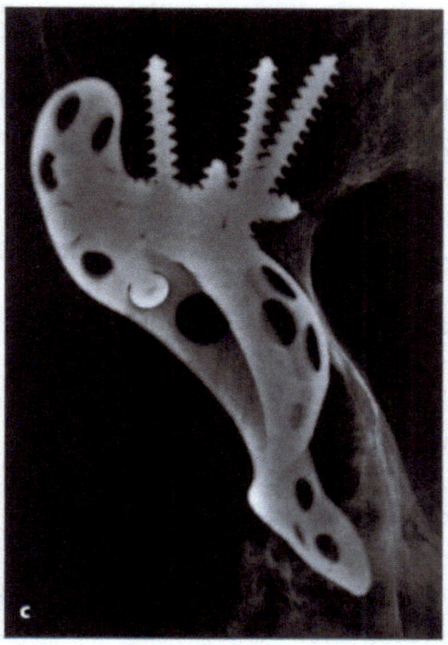

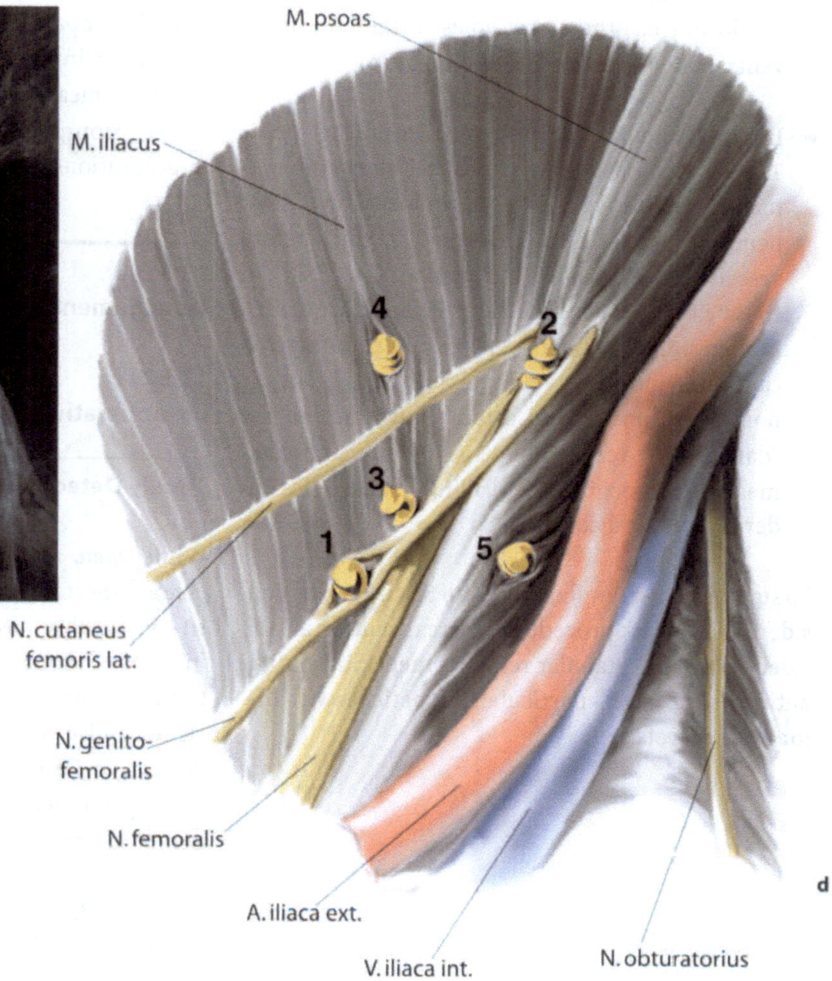

c a.p. radiograph
d Interior view of the lesser pelvis. All numbered screws, if relatively overlength, will be in the immediate vicinity of sensitive structures. Screw 1 perforates the genitofemoral nerve. Screw 2 is directly next to the lateral femoral cutaneous nerve

ally is a possibility. Ventral screws might then jeopardize the external iliac artery and vein.
The layout of the screw holes is the same for the new SL 2 cup (Fig. 2.6).

- **Acetabular Reinforcement Ring** (Figs. 13.9, 13.10): The acetabular reinforcement ring enables screws to be fixed in the optimal arrangement to match the pre-existing bone conditions. Since many more screw directions are possible, so more structures are potentially at risk. Screws placed in an excessively ventral or dorsal position, in particular, will reach the external iliac artery after just 10–15 mm and the sciatic nerve after 20–30 mm. Consequently, drilling in stages is especially important with this implant.
  As a precautionary measure on the implant side, we do not use the screw holes in the outermost ventral and dorsal positions (Fig. 13.10).

- **Burch-Schneider Antiprotrusio Cage** (Fig. 13.11): The same applies as for the acetabular reinforcement ring, although in this case most screws must penetrate a muscle layer roughly 1 cm thick before vessels and nerves are threatened. The risk can thus be reduced appreciably if the holes are drilled in stages. Since patients requiring an antiprotrusio cage often have a very difficult bone situation, it is not always possible to avoid using some of the "dangerous" screw holes. As a precautionary measure, we recommend drilling critical holes under radiological control.

To sum up: the screw fixation of an SL cup can be considered a low-risk procedure, whereas caution is indicated with the acetabular reinforcement ring and the antiprotrusio cage – particularly in patients with major bone defects.

13.4.3 General Precautionary Measures

- Check the vessel status of the lower extremities preoperatively and then in the immediate postoperative period. The easiest method is to measure (and record) malleolar arterial occlusion pressure by Doppler ultrasound. Examiner-dependent details of palpated (pedal) pulses is unreliable.
- If obvious risks are present (e.g. a loosened, dislocated cup that has migrated into the lesser pelvis), notify the vascular surgeon in advance.
- Generous draping of the surgical field, so that an anterior lower lumbotomy can be initiated without problems (Fig. 13.12).
- Postoperatively, starting directly after the procedure and continuing for the first few days, check and compare the vessel status, even if no discernible injury is present. The pre- and postoperatively measured, and recorded, malleolar arterial occlusion pressure is the best protection against accusations from outside (see above).

13.5 Management of Vascular Injuries

13.5.1 Intraoperative Massive Bleeding

Timely Detection

While *open, massive haemorrhage* is unmistakable (see also Sect. 13.3.2), the possibility of *concealed massive intrapelvic bleeding* should be considered, even in cases of moderate or slight bleeding, if the anaesthetist reports a sudden drop in blood pressure and a rising pulse rate (see also Sect. 13.3.1, Case 1; Sect. 13.3.2, Case 5).

Surgeons generally tend to underestimate the urgency of the situation intraoperatively if no open massive haemorrhage is present. Ultrasonography is the only additional investigation capable of providing further useful information immediately.

Intraoperative Emergency Procedure: Lower, Anterior Lumbotomy

Basic principles:

1. Controlling the bleeding is accorded *top priority!*
2. Accidental arterial bleeds are most reliably controlled by arterial clamping at the *next higher stage.*
3. Since it is not usually sufficient just to clamp off the arterial afflux, the injured arterial segment should also be clamped off completely so as to control the arterial reflux.
4. To this end, the surgeon should not shrink from creating sufficiently wide access to the pelvic arteries so as to facilitate the subsequent arterial reconstruction.
5. The most reliable way of rapidly controlling open or occult bleeding is an *anterior lower lumbotomy* (see below).

Rapid and targeted termination of both open and occult massive bleeding via the hip access takes too long, and a definitive solution is not possible via this route (see also Sect. 13.3.2, Case 4).

Sequence of immediate measures:

1. Local plugging with pads and application of fist pressure to the groin. The effectiveness of this measure is checked.
2. The vascular surgeon is notified.
3. Additional supplies of blood and fresh frozen plasma obtained. If not already in operation, a blood recovery system is set up.
4. The patient is repositioned on his back and the draping is extended (Fig. 13.12).
5. Anterior lower lumbotomy (Fig. 13.12) by the orthopaedic surgeon, with exposure of the external iliac artery and vein and clamping of same with vascular clamps (see box below).
6. If the bleeding is staunched by this procedure, and depending on the experience of the orthopaedic surgeon in each case, the surgeon performs a preparatory search for the vessel distally and stops the reflux. If the bleeding is not staunched, a branch of the internal iliac artery or the artery itself, or a branch of the external – possibly internal – iliac vein may be affected, which requires energetic plugging of the actual bleeding source(s). Compression is applied proximally and medially in the lesser pelvis.
7. Definitive exposure and bridging of the defects by the vascular surgeon. Vein grafts are used primarily, though synthetic implants may also be used. Ligation of the trunk vessels should be avoided, since many of these patients already suffer from pronounced arteriosclerosis and potentially preexisting peripheral arterial occlusive disease.

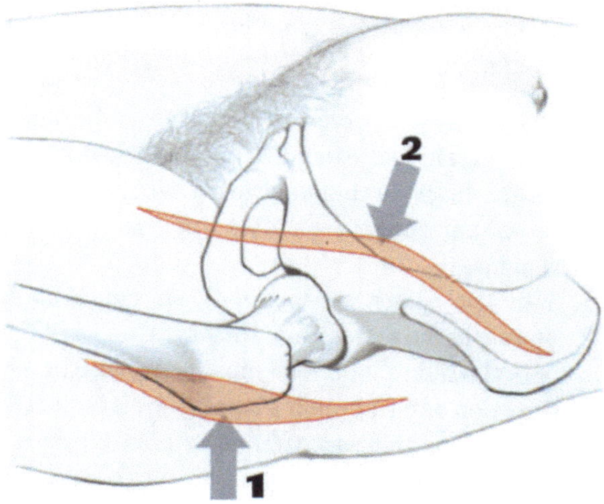

Fig. 13.12. Anterior lower lumbotomy as a second access route (2) for the emergency correction of vascular injuries noted during operation. The lumbotomy is totally separate from the lateral (or dorsal) access route for the total hip replacement (*1*). The incision follows the inguinal fovea at a distance of approximately two finger widths and then curves away distally around the saphenous hiatus

Procedure for anterior lower lumbotomy (see also Fig. 13.12):

1. Make a slightly curved skin incision in the lateral hypogastrium extending to about two finger widths from the inguinal fovea (approximately 10–12 cm long, depending on the patient's weight).
2. Split the aponeurosis of the external oblique muscle in the direction of the fibres.
   Split the internal oblique muscle, likewise in the direction of the fibres. If a better view is required, divide this muscle transversely by thermocautery (caution: entry into the abdominal cavity with possible concealed bowel injury). The muscle fibres should therefore only be divided down to the fascia of the transverse muscle. Carefully open the fascia, insert two fingers and cut open separately with scissors to the extent required.
3. Enter the retroperitoneum by pushing back the unopened peritoneal sac by hand or using a swab on a stick. Take care to preserve the ureter, which crosses over the common iliac artery proximally in the area of the bifurcation with the internal iliac artery, and the spermatic cord structures.
4. The source of the bleeding can now be located and the subsequent procedure adapted accordingly. If no vein injury is present, the pelvic veins do not need to be dissected, a procedure that is rather more delicate than the corresponding dissection of the more robust artery.
5. Immediately clamp off the bleeding vessel proximally using an atraumatic clamp, and then clamp off the segment distal to the vessel lesion to prevent reflux. Vein injuries require a combination of plugging and targeted suture ligatures. Anatomical reconstruction can be very time consuming.
6. If vascular reconstruction extending beyond the joint proves necessary, the lymph nodes below the inguinal ligament, together with the lymphatic vessels, are pushed as a complete package away from the trunk vessels, from the lateral to the medial direction, thus allowing detailed dissection of the femoral artery and vein.

13.5.2 Detection of Postoperative Bleeding or Ischaemia

■ **Danger Signals.** Signs of bleeding include a rapidly growing haematoma, circulatory collapse or a cold or dysaesthetic lower leg or foot. Severe pain, which is often underestimated and suppressed with opiates, may be an indication of ischaemia alone without local bleeding in intimal injuries or an aneurysm.

■ **Investigation.** The first priority is to ascertain the pulse status. If no pedal pulses are present, the malleolar arterial occlusion pressure is measured by Doppler ultrasonography. Members of the orthopaedic team themselves should know how to manage this investigation technique and interpret the results. Ultrasonography can also provide valuable information rapidly.

If the malleolar arterial occlusion pressure is below the critical level of 40–50 mmHg, the site of a suspected occlusion will then need to be determined. In critical situations in the immediate postoperative period, the urgently consulted vascular surgeon will be responsible for deciding what kind of additional investigations can still be performed in time before any surgical correction without definitively jeopardising the leg.

The most important diagnostic tool is the contrast angiogram. In bleeds outside the trunk vessels, this technique can also be used for embolisation (see also Sect. 4.3, Fig. 4.2). Colour-coded ultrasound takes longer and is less suitable for documentation purposes. In patients with pre-existing renal impairment, the MRI scan with contrast visualisation may be the method of choice.

■ **Case Report.** K.A., male, 54 years (O.26565). Two days after a total hip replacement in another hospital, this patient underwent revision of a haematoma, which secondarily proved to be infected. Antibiotic therapy was initiated. Over the course of the next 4 weeks, two further revisions were implemented for recurrent haematomas. Two days after the last revision, the patient became so unstable, with a falling blood pressure and haemoglobin despite fluid and blood replacement, that he had to be transferred to the high-dependency unit. Arteriography revealed a profusely bleeding injury of the ascending branch of the lateral circumflex femoral artery, which was selectively embolised using two 4-mm coils. The circulation subsequently remained stable. Ten days later, by which time the patient's general condition had stabilised, an encapsulated haematoma was evacuated.

References

1. Al-Salman M, Taylor DC, Beauchamp CP, Duncan CP (1992) Prevention of vascular injuries in revision total hip replacements (comment). Can J Surg 35: 261–264
2. Bergqvist D, Carlsson AS, Ericsson BF (1983) Vascular complications after total hip arthroplasty. Acta Orthop Scand 54: 157–163
3. Bindewald H, Ruf W, Heger W (1987) Die Verletzung der Iliacal- und Femoralgefäße – eine lebensbedrohliche Notfallsituation in der Hüftprothesenchirurgie. Chirurg 58: 732–737
4. Bullrich A, Miltner E (1989) Tödliche Blutung bei TEP-Reimplantation. Kasuistik und rechtliche Gesichtspunkte. Unfallchirurg 92: 187–190
5. Fiddian NJ, Sudlow RA, Browett JP (1984) Ruptured femoral vein: a complication of the use of gentamicin beads in an infected excision arthroplasty of the hip. J Bone Joint Surg [Br] 66: 493–494
6. Freischlag JA, Sise M, Quinones-Baldrich WJ, Hye RJ, Sedwitz MM (1989) Vascular complications associated with orthopaedic procedures. Surg Gynecol Obstet 169: 147–152
7. Fruhwirth J, Koch G, Ivanic GM, Seibert FJ, Tesch NP (1997) Gefäßläsionen in der Hüftgelenkchirurgie. Unfallchirurg 100: 119–123
8. Hwand SK (1994) Vascular injury during total hip arthroplasty: the anatomy of the acetabulum. Int Orthop 18: 29–31
9. Keating EM, Ritter MA, Faris PM (1990) Structures at risk from medially placed acetabular screws. J Bone Joint Surg Am 72: 509–511
10. Kirkpatrick JA, Callaghan JJ, Vandemark RM, Goldner RD (1990) The relationship of intrapelvic vasculature to the acetabulum: implications in screw-fixation of acetabular components. Clin Orthop 258: 183–190
11. Krenzien J, Gussmann A (1998) Arterielle Gefäßverletzungen bei Hüftprothesenimplantation. Zentralbl Chir 123: 1292–1296
12. Mallory TH (1972) Rupture of the common iliac vein from reaming the acetabulum during total hip endoprosthesis: a case report. J Bone Joint Am Surg 54: 276
13. Nachbur B, Meyer RP, Baumgartner J (1989) Vaskuläre Komplikationen in der Hüftgelenkchirurgie. Orthopäde 18: 552–558
14. Nachbur B, Meyer RP, Verkkala K, Zürcher R (1979) The mechanisms of severe arterial injury in surgery of the hip joint. Clin Orthop 141: 122–133
15. Neal J, Wachtel TL, Garza OT, Edwards WS (1979) Late arterial embolization complicating total hip replacement: a case report. J Bone Joint Surg Am 61: 429–430
16. Reiley MA, Bond D, Branick jr, Wilson EH (1984) Vascular complications following total hip arthroplasty. A review of literature and a report of two cases. Clin Orthop 186: 23–28
17. Schätzer A, Heilberger P, Möllers M, Stedtfeld H-W, Raithel D (1997) Arterielle Gefäßläsionen nach totalem Hüftgelenkersatz. Unfallchirurg 100: 531–535
18. Shoenfeld NA, Stuchin SA, Pearl R, Haveson S (1990) The management of vascular injuries associated with total hip arthroplasty. J Vasc Surg 11: 549—555
19. Siegel A, Schulz F, Püschel K (2001) Tödliche Beckenvenenverletzung durch Führungsdraht bei Anwendung der dynamischen Hüftschraube (DHS). Unfallchirurg 104: 182–186
20. Stamatakis JD, Kakkar VV, Sagar S, Lawrence D, Nairn, D, Bentley PG (1977) Femoral vein thrombosis and total hip replacement. Br Med J 2: 223–225
21. Todd BD, Bintcliffe IW (1990) Injury to the external iliac artery during hip arthroplasty for old central dislocation. J Arthroplasty (Suppl) 5: S53–S55
22. Töndury G (1981) Angewandte und topographische Anatomie, 5th edn. Thieme, Stuttgart

Chapter 14

Pain

Peter E. Ochsner

Pain after a total hip replacement means that the treatment has failed. Exclusion of the usual suspects – haematoma, infection, loosening, trochanteric nonunions, formation of ossification – is often followed by a time-consuming search for the actual cause. Detailed history-taking, regular standardised check radiographs, hip aspiration and arthrography, ultrasound scans, neurological examination, test infiltrations and, if applicable, a pain analysis can prove helpful, as can an MRI scan occasionally.

Rare causes of groin pain include mechanical irritation of the anterior acetabular rim and impingement problems. Trochanteric pain can be caused by snapping or poor muscle healing. Thigh pain may originate from poor healing of an uncemented prosthesis, a stem fracture or cement leakage from the femoral shaft. Other possible causes to be considered include pain resulting from a nerve injury or ischaemia and polymyalgia rheumatica. Scar pain also occurs occasionally. From the standpoint of differential diagnosis, it is particularly important to take the back into account. In some cases, the pain cannot be controlled, or can only be partially controlled.

A total hip replacement is performed primarily to alleviate pain. Consequently, residual pain in the operated hip is often rightly viewed by the patient as indicative of failure. The patient is particularly unhappy if the pain interferes with the use of the hip immediately, or shortly, after the operation. The surgeon should initially think of the more common causes, particularly a haematoma, early infection, developing ossification, etc. If there are no indications of such complications, targeted physiotherapy followed by a further check-up after 1–3 months is worth considering. Not infrequently this can actually cause the pain to disappear or at least be alleviated to a significant extent. If no improvement occurs, however, further investigation is needed, and this can prove very time-consuming in some cases. Generally, however, the effort pays off in the end. The patient feels that he is being taken seriously and, if given a credible explanation, does not lose his willingness to recover. If pain remains, the patient feels that the doctor ought also to take an active part in the search for an explanation. In so doing, the doctor gains the patient's trust and there is no suspicion that the doctor may be concealing a cause of which he is perfectly aware. If the patient suspects that active commitment on the doctor's part is lacking, he may soon feel inclined to change his doctor.

14.1 Exploratory Options – Investigations

▪ **History.** History-taking is the most important tool in the search for the cause of pain and serves to record the development, time, intensity and localisation of the symptoms. If the patient's history is too complex, asking the patient to complete a pain diary over a certain period has proved to be a useful measure.

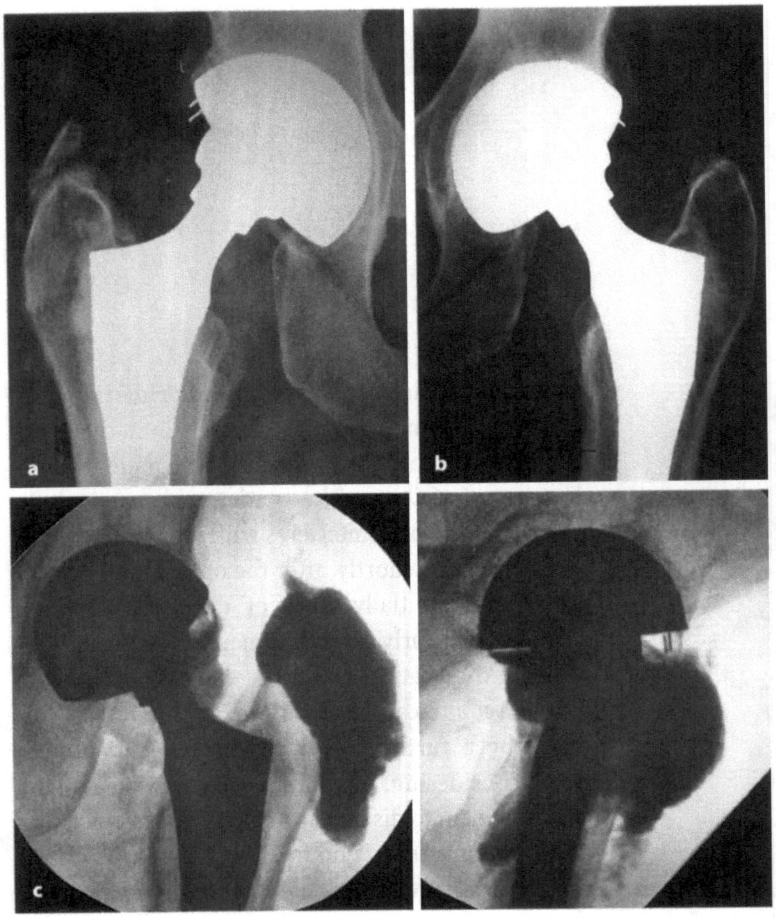

Fig. 14.1a–c. Pain due to cup loosening (*right*), bald patch on the trochanter (*left*). M.M., female, 58 years (O. 13795). Case 3
a Groin pain with a right-sided PCA acetabular component with seam. No improvement in the situation following a cup change (acetabular reinforcement ring, cemented polyethylene cup)
b Left-sided hip pain and Trendelenburg limp, cup with seam craniolaterally
c Arthrography with irrigation with contrast medium all around the greater trochanter confirms the failed integration of the pelvitrochanteric muscles. The patient did not wish the situation to be rectified on the left side because of the failure on the right

▪ **Standard Radiographs.** The basis for any follow-up observation of a patient suffering from pain is repeated and standardised radiographic investigation (see also Sect. 3.4.1). Comparison with the postoperative picture allows the surgeon to rule out obvious causes. If the pain is intractable and several standardised radiographs are already available, then a migration measurement may prove worthwhile (EBRA, see also Sect. 3.3.1) for detecting any loosening that is not immediately visible. Another useful measure is to check the implant position, particularly the anteversion of the cup and torsion of the stem, since this can provide evidence of possible impingement (see also Chap. 6).

▪ **Functional Examination Under the Image Intensifier.** Suspected phenomena such as subluxations and impingement can occasionally be verified by this technique.

▪ **Hip Aspiration and Arthrography.** These investigations are primarily designed to rule out an infection (see also Sects. 5.2.3 and 5.2.5, Fig. 5.7), but can also reveal surprising findings, for example failed healing of the hip abductors (Fig. 14.1).

▪ **Ultrasound.** Ultrasonography is preferred over the other imaging techniques for investigating soft tissue structures in the immediate vicinity of the implants. An ultrasound scan can detect a bursa at the ventral acetabular rim arising from mechanical irritation between the projecting implant and the tendon of the iliopsoas muscle. However, it is also worth looking for surprise findings such as a trochanteric bursa or other soft tissue changes. The significance of such findings is not always clear from the outset.

▪ **Scintigraphy.** A bone scan will almost invariably show hyperactivity in the first year after implantation. The regression profile for such hyperactivity varies considerably from one individual to the next, and its value is often overestimated.

■ **Neurological Examination.** If pain does not respond to treatment for a prolonged period after a total hip replacement, then additional neurological examination can be useful, particularly if limping is also present. The possibility of neurogenic pain should also be borne in mind.

■ **Magnetic Resonance Imaging (MRI).** Despite the presence of a prosthesis, an MRI scan is still capable of, for instance, providing information about the condition of the hip abductors. Muscle deficits, incorrect insertions, etc. can also be diagnosed, as can abscesses and other soft tissue swellings cranial to the implants.

■ **Test Infiltration.** While a test infiltration with a local anaesthetic can help locate the pain, it will not necessarily shed light on its cause. Combination with a contrast medium and examination under the image intensifier can provide further clarification (Fig. 14.1).

■ **Pain Analysis.** When all the possible somatic causes have been investigated, there should be no excessive delay in referring the patient to a pain specialist for investigation, since the chances of recovery diminish with increasing delay.

14.2 Pain Associated with Common Organic Complications

The most common causes of pain after surgery are a haematoma (Chap. 4), an early or delayed infection (Chap. 5), trochanteric nonunion (Chap. 8) or developing periarticular ossification (Chap. 12). If the patient complains of pain during the months following surgery, the above-mentioned more common causes first need to be ruled out. If the pain occurs only years after the operation, then the most likely cause to consider is a loosened prosthesis.

The absence of any obvious signs to explain the pain does not mean that the situation is necessarily without danger. Since pain requiring treatment is rare, the treating doctor, but particularly the operator, is inclined to play down the pain and not believe the patient sufficiently. The operator, especially, would do well to bear other possible causes in mind.

14.3 Foreign Body Sensation

While many patients who feel well are not even aware of the presence of their artificial hip, others are very conscious of something being "different" in the hip, but are unable to provide a more precise description of the difference. Patients with hard bearing couples in particular, e.g. metal-metal or ceramic-ceramic, may notice a more or less obvious click when resuming an activity after a period of relaxation. The phenomenon is thought to be caused by abrupt complete joint closure resulting from the resumption of muscle activity in a (still) lax joint capsule. Thus, for example, one patient with a metal-metal joint regularly noticed a squeaking noise, which so irritated him that he carried a tape recorder in his trouser pocket to record the sound and then play it back to the doctor at his next appointment. Since the patient was also concurrently suffering from pain caused by a cemented titanium stem, the surgeon decided to replace the stem and insert a polyethylene-ceramic pairing at the same time. This measure eliminated all the symptoms. Apart from this particular case, none of our other patients felt particularly handicapped by a foreign body sensation.

14.4 Rare Pain Phenomena

Despite the presence of a well-functioning total hip prosthesis, a not inconsiderable number of patients can suffer from pain which, in some cases, can be experienced subjectively as very pronounced. They repeatedly make appointments to see the surgeon who, despite checking all the traditional causes, finds nothing. The following case studies from our own records are used as examples to indicate possible causes. The selection of cases also demonstrates that freedom from pain cannot always be achieved in every instance. The cases are subdivided according to the main location of the pain.

14.4.1 Groin Pain

■ **Mechanical Irritation of the Iliopsoas Muscle by the Acetabular Component.** During a primary im-

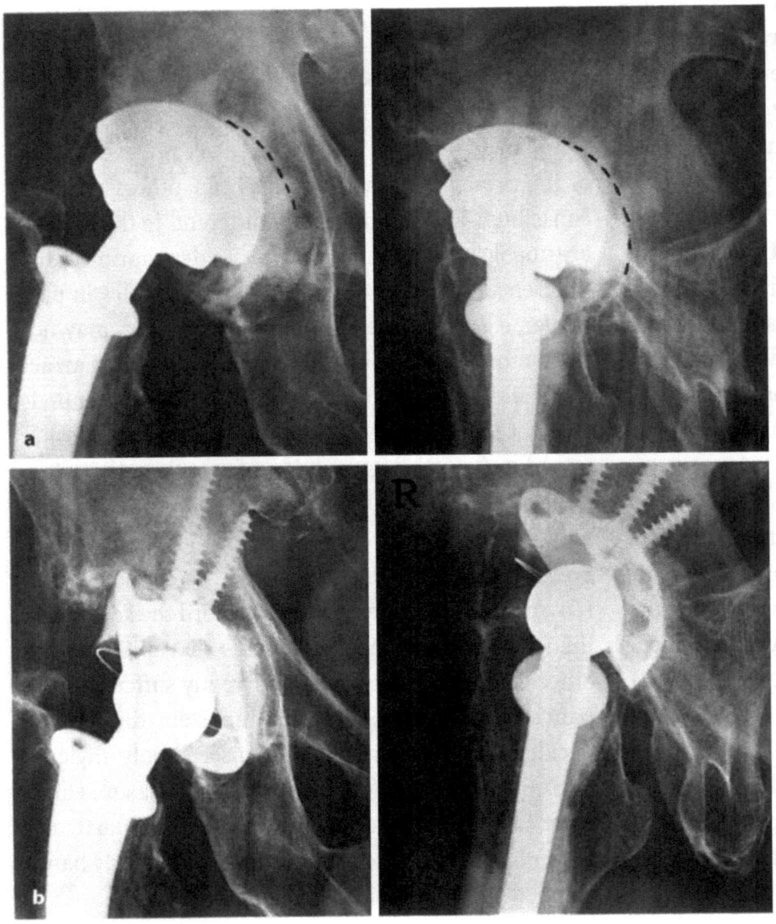

Fig. 14.2a,b. Groin pain with incorrect ventrolateral positioning of the acetabular implant. R.F., male, 75 years (O. 2295), Case 1

a Pronounced ventrolateral protrusion of the acetabular component with substantial gap dorsally and distally in relation to the bony acetabular base (*dotted line*). Since the implantation, increasing, painful snapping during hip movement, particularly during rotation of the extended leg. In addition, the patient was suffering from weight-bearing-related adduction and groin pain

b After the cup was changed, the patient remained permanently free of symptoms. Check radiograph after 5 years

Fig. 14.3a–h. Groin/thigh pain – impingement – dislocation. I.E., female (O. 7). Case 2. Patient also suffering from tendovaginitis, carpal tunnel syndrome, varus gonarthrosis, osteoarthritis of the upper ankle

a Pain in the groin, radiating into the thigh, walking distance 300–400 m

b Four months after a total hip replacement with a metal-metal joint and cemented stem, the patient is free of symptoms, apart from a rapidly recovering femoral nerve palsy. The "faux profil" radiograph shows retrotorsion

c Following further episodes of thigh pain, stem subsidence of 9 mm was observed after 4.5 years. The stem was replaced by a Virtec stem. Accidental leg lengthening of 1 cm. Bacillus subtilis was found in one of three samples. After a period of laborious rehabilitation with tensing of the thigh and buttocks muscles, the patient eventually became symptom-free once more

d Following a further recurrence of thigh pain, a seam is apparent proximally around the cement, which was thought to be the cause of the pain

e The slightly loosened stem was replaced with an SL revision prosthesis. The metal pairing was replaced at the same time. Following the revision, the patient complained of severe pain in the groin and subluxation phenomena, particularly during flexion

f Dorsal dislocation 1 year after the revision

g Revision with cementation of a polyethylene cup with distinct anteversion – recognisable by the wire ring – into the secured SL cup. Following temporary exacerbation of a previous femoral nerve palsy, the patient is now largely symptom-free

h Subsequent analysis of the metal pairing removed 4 years ago revealed distinct impingement with drag marks on the metal cup rim and a ventral notch on the neck (*arrows*)

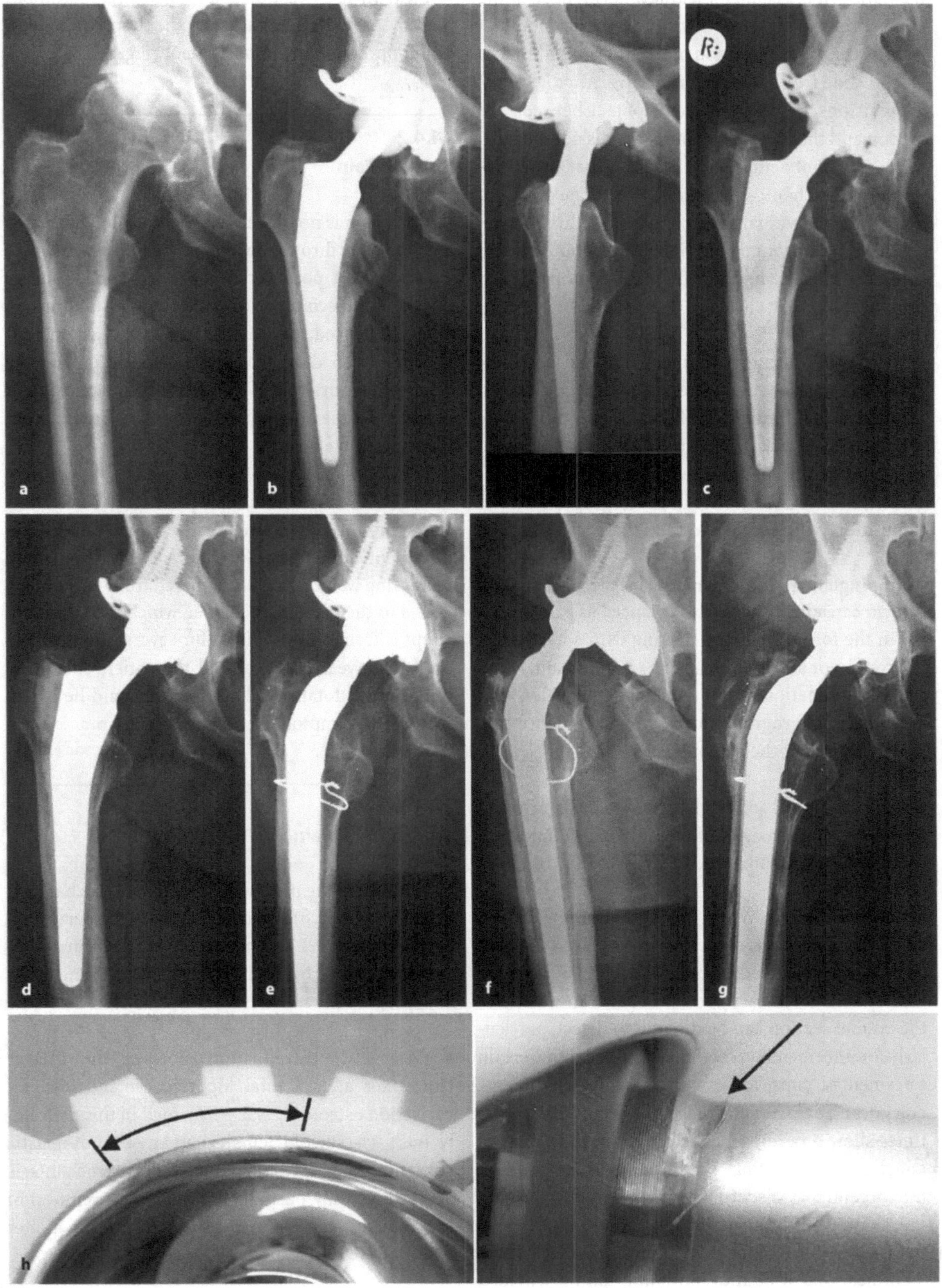
R:
a
b
c
d
e
f
g
h

plantation, it is assumed that the anterior edge of the cup is protected by the bony rim of the acetabulum. In this scenario, the tendon of the iliopsoas muscle is able to slide freely in its usual groove. After acetabular revisions, however, a direct contact between the tendon and the acetabular component is not unusual. While it cannot definitely be assumed that any corresponding mechanical irritation will actually lead to groin pain, individual cases confirm that this is a possibility. An ultrasound scan (bursa formation) and local infiltration (temporary freedom from pain) can provide important clues.

■ *Case 1.* Replacement of a cup that had been implanted in an excessively lateral and ventral position resulted in the elimination of regular snapping in the groin area (Fig. 14.2). We investigate cases of groin pain and groin snapping with "faux-profil" radiographs, ultrasound scans, hip arthrography and test infiltrations with local anaesthetics.

■ **Impingement.** Impingement (see also Chap. 6) on its own can sometimes be experienced as pain, possibly in the form of painful clicking with a hard bearing couple, or as vague, unspecified groin pain. Functional examination under the image intensifier, with or without arthrography, can provide evidence of a possible cause of the symptoms.

■ *Case 2.* Inguinal and thigh pain were misinterpreted for a long time as signs of loosening, until impingement symptoms manifested themselves (Fig. 14.3).

■ **Cup Loosening.** While this is the most common cause of groin pain, even very pronounced cases of cup loosening with advanced destruction of the bone stock do not necessarily result in pain. Loosening in the cranial section can be difficult to detect, particularly for uncemented acetabular components. Certain uncemented cups, for example, the Harris-Galante cup [3], and occasionally the Sulmesh cup, may sometimes show a radiographic seam as an indication of failed osteointegration. During a revision, however, the surgeon may discover very firm fibrous interlocking. Consequently, a cup change did not always lead to disappearance of the troublesome pain.

Indications of painful loosening can be provided by arthrography with the concurrent administration of long-acting local anaesthetics.

■ *Case 3.* The correction of a loosened cup accompanied by presumed irritation of the iliopsoas tendon did not produce any improvement (Fig. 14.1).

14.4.2 Buttock Pain

Buttock pain is not infrequently associated with protrusion coxarthrosis. But it can also be observed in isolation as a postoperative phenomenon, causing the patient discomfort when sitting or standing up and experienced, for example, as a stabbing pain. Buttock pain can disappear spontaneously during the course of the first year. The differential diagnosis will need to take the possibility of symptoms arising from the spine into account.

■ *Case 4.* A 47-year-old male patient (N.W., O. 4323) was symptom free 6 weeks after implantation of an uncemented prosthesis (SLS cup, CLS stem) but, with increasing weight-bearing, suffered from severe pain dorsal to the greater trochanter, which forced him to adopt a Trendelenburg limp for several months. Not until the 1-year check-up did the patient feel fairly well. He was totally well after 2 years, and he is still completely symptom free after 9 years.

14.4.3 Trochanteric Pain

In addition to the previously mentioned trochanteric problems (Chap. 9) associated with trochanteric fractures, osteotomies and nonunions, patients are occasionally plagued by trochanteric pain associated with snapping. Four cases are described below:

■ *Case 5.* Increased protrusion of the greater trochanter after a total hip replacement. Bilateral varisation osteotomy was performed in this delicately built 47-year-old female patient with dysplastic coxarthrosis. This resulted in pain in the trochanteric area, which only partially subsided after removal of the angled blade plate and the insertion, at a later date, of a CDH prosthesis.

■ *Case 6.* In a female patient with severe cerebral damage caused by a shooting injury, a total prosthe-

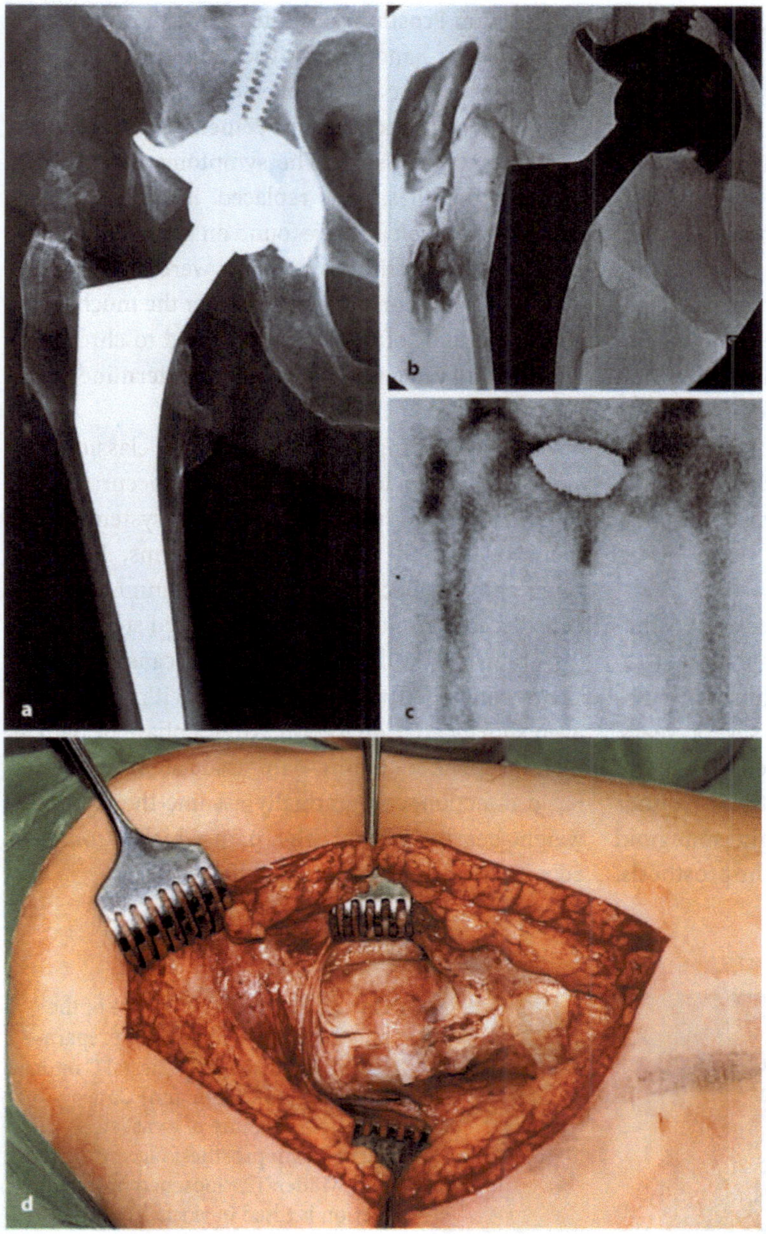

Fig. 14.4a–d. Pain with "trochanteric bald patch". W.R., female, 70 years (O. 12814). Case 7
a Following a total hip replacement, the patient was left with trochanteric pain and a Trendelenburg limp
b Investigation with localised contrast medium revealed an extensive trochanteric bursa. The pain disappeared temporarily after infiltration
c A bone scan revealed accumulation primarily in the area of the greater trochanter. Infiltration in this area alleviated the symptoms
d Extensive bald patches were found on the trochanter at operation. Almost the whole of the pelvitrochanteric muscles had lost contact with the greater trochanter. Careful transosseous anchorage of the muscles. Significant improvement 3 months after operation

sis was inserted because of femoral head necrosis. This was followed by the onset of superior gluteal nerve paralysis. An insufficient gluteus medius muscle and a very prominent greater trochanter led to trochanteric pain and snapping. The pain was alleviated somewhat by tractopexy.

■ *Case 7.* Bald patch on the trochanter: Failed insertion of the trochanteric muscles. Tractopexy improved the situation (Fig. 14.4).

Residual adduction contracture after a total hip replacement for coxarthrosis following an acetabular fracture. No improvement after tractopexy (see case 13).

Intractable trochanteric pain can also remain after repeated attempts at correction. The symptoms persisted in one female patient, for example, both after stabilisation of trochanteric nonunion and after additional tractopexy. Troublesome trochanteric pain is a problem that needs to be taken seriously and one that often stubbornly persists in patients.

14.4.4 Thigh Pain

■ **Diffuse Pain Without Loosening.** Thigh pain in patients with uncemented stems is not always an indication of failed integration. In our hospital, for example, the implantation of 36 uncemented SL prostheses according to M.E. Müller with attached collars (Fig. 2.9a) led to seven cases of persistent thigh pain. Detectable signs of loosening necessitated a revision in just two patients. No loosening occurred in the other cases. Today, more than 10 years after implantation, all of these implants are firmly anchored and the patients are either largely or completely free of symptoms.

■ *Case 8.* After receiving an uncemented SL prosthesis according to M.E. Müller, this female patient reported pain radiating into the thigh, which only subsided, without fully disappearing, after several years. The prosthesis remained firmly anchored over an observation period of 10 years. However, the surrounding cortical bone became increasingly spongioid along the full length of its contact with the prosthesis.

■ **Titanium Prostheses.** An increased loosening rate [2] on the one hand, and diffuse, sometimes nagging, thigh pain with no detectable loosening on the other, have been observed after the cemented implantation of titanium prostheses. The symptoms disappeared after the prosthesis was replaced. In other patients *traces of corrosion* [5] were found on the femoral component. Whether these symptoms were directly connected with the corrosion, or whether the much lower elastic modulus of titanium, compared to chromium and steel, played a role is not easy to determine.

■ **Stem Loosening.** Thigh pain is the classical key symptom in stem loosening, but rarely occurs during the first 10 years in proven cemented systems. With the introduction of uncemented stems, however, thigh pain has become much more commonplace. A considerable proportion of uncemented stems fail to integrate or show delayed integration, causing the patients concerned to be confronted with thigh pain even shortly after operation. After a phase of pain at rest, the pain, including pain associated with a delayed infection, can gradually assume the nature of weight-bearing-related thigh pain, which is connected with the onset of prosthesis loosening.

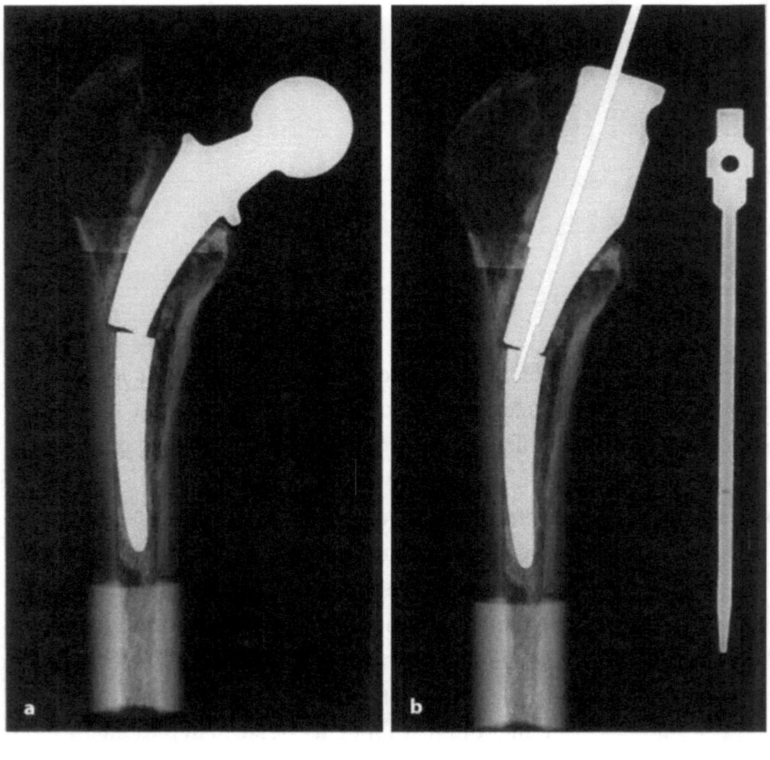

Fig. 14.5a,b. Fatigue fracture of the prosthesis stem. Macerated preparation (Path. Institute of Liestal Cantonal Hospital, Prof. Wegmann) Case 9
a Fatigue fracture of a cast steel curved stem prosthesis according to M.E. Müller. The loosened proximal section is tilted in varus. The distal portion is firmly anchored in cement
b A centering component modelled on the proximal part of the prosthesis is tapped onto the distal tip. A hardened steel bit is used to drill a hole centrally into the distal section.
A tapering threaded rod (on the right of the picture) is screwed into this hole and connected to an extraction mallet for subsequent removal of the distal portion

■ **Fracture of the Stem.** Stem fracture primarily affects patients whose implant has already remained in situ for a few, or even many, years. If the stem gradually loosens from the proximal end while the tip of the stem remains securely cemented, this can produce fatigue loading in the transitional area (Fig. 14.5). Most first-generation prostheses were cast and were not adequately tested in respect of fatigue resistance. As a result, fatigue fractures occurred in isolated cases. Although this was not usually experienced as a fracture incident by the patient, it generally provoked immediately obvious pain.

■ *Case 9.* Example of a prosthesis fracture, noted by the pathologist (Fig. 14.5).

■ **Fracture of a Ceramic Component.** The patient generally experiences the fracture of a ceramic component as a loud crack. The fracture can be triggered by material irregularities of the head, cone damage and inappropriate loading of the ceramic cup as a result of excessive inclination.

■ **Cement Leakage from the Stem.** As prophylaxis against a fat embolus, we create a 3.2-mm diameter ventilation hole approximately 2 cm distal to the cement plug to enable the pressure to be equalised (see also Chap. 3). If the hole is placed slightly too proximally, a certain amount of cement leakage may occur during stem cementation. Generally this small bulge does not cause any symptoms, even if we explain its existence to the patient, although pain is occasionally reported.

■ *Case 10.* A female patient suffered from thigh pain in connection with a cemented titanium prosthesis (see also Sects. 14.3, 14.4). During replacement of the prosthesis we performed a shaft biopsy in order to gain a better insight into the problem. Unfortunately, cement escaped through the small hole and caused the patient pain (Fig. 14.6). The symptoms were significantly alleviated following removal of this cement. The patient consulted a lawyer because of this problem, though the latter declined to take legal action.

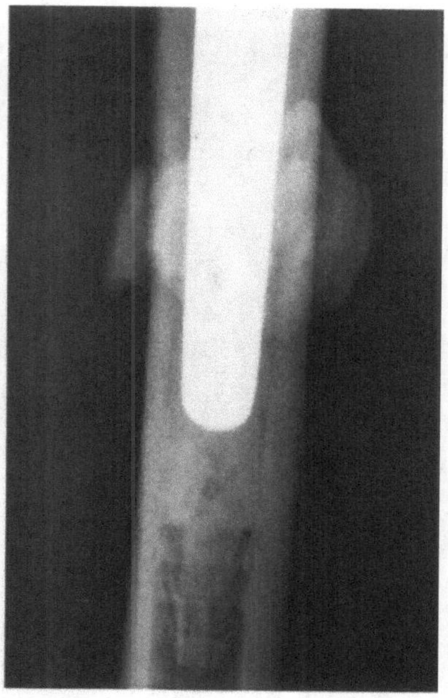

Fig. 14.6. Thigh pain due to cement leakage from the shaft. G.R., female, 73 years (O. 1187). Case 10. During a revision procedure, the removed titanium stem showed obvious corrosion. A drill biopsy was performed to collect a 5 mm diameter sample of cortical bone at the level of the corrosion. Cement leaked from the resulting hole during cementation and formed a mantle over three quarters of the shaft circumference. Initial non-specific pain developed into localised pain

14.4.5 Scar Pain

Occasionally a patient may experience his scar as particularly painful. One female patient with a complex range of symptoms was so bothered by her pain that we decided to perform a scar revision (see also Case 13).

14.4.6 Pain After Vascular and Nerve Injuries

■ **Neurogenic Pain After Major Nerve Paresis.** While the motor deficit predominates in a nerve paresis caused by implantation of a prosthesis, the patient may suffer pronounced pain that drags on for months (see also Chap. 10.5)

■ **Neurogenic Pain of the De-efferent Type After a Chronic Ischaemic Syndrome.** If an acute ischaemia associated with restricted flow in a major vessel, e.g.

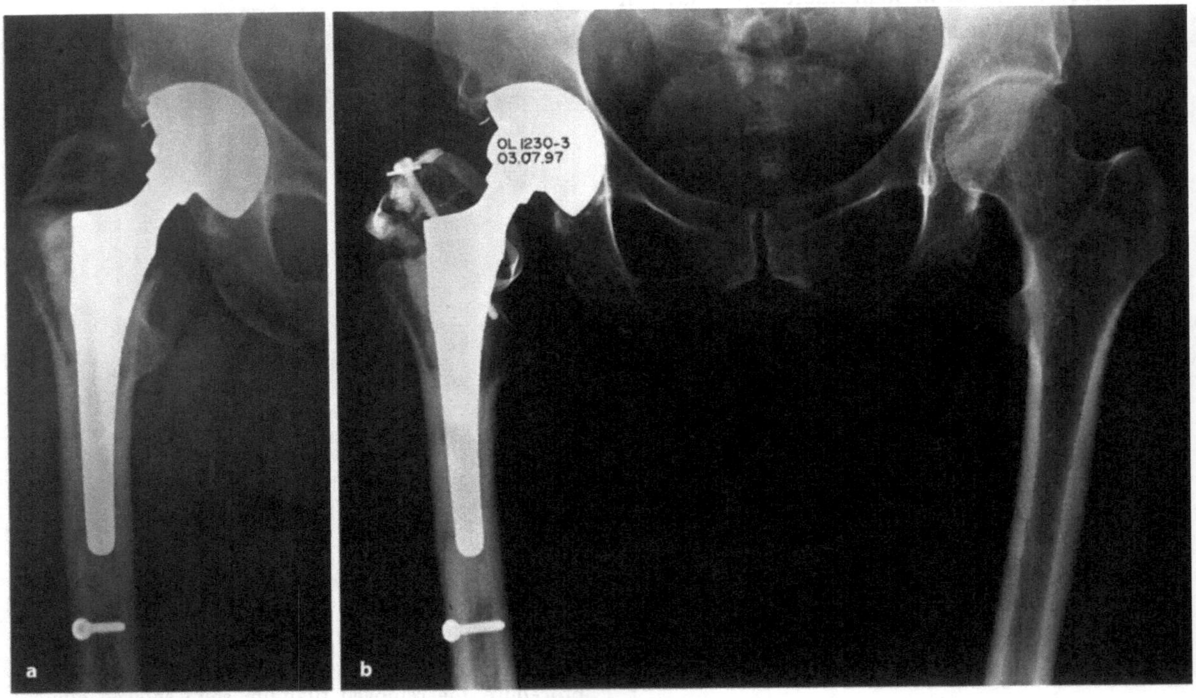

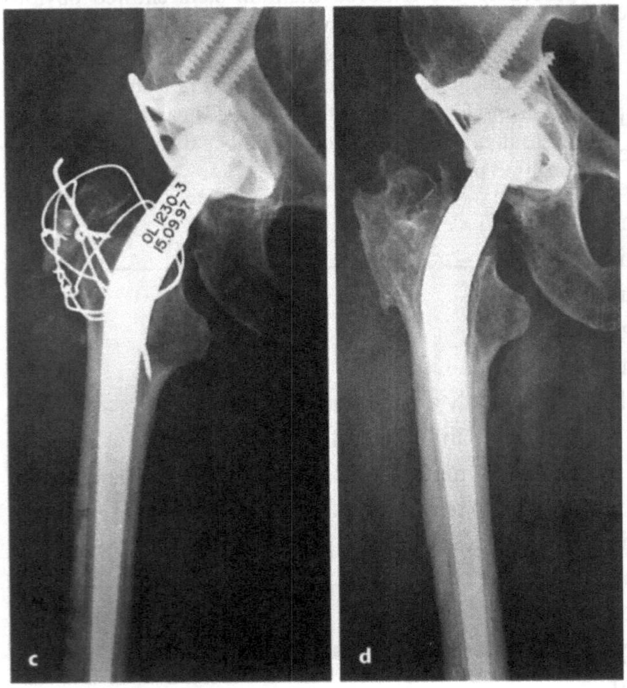

Fig. 14.7a–d. Trochanteric nonunion, cup loosening, "low-grade infection" and narrow spinal canal. F.S., female (O. 14200). Case 11

a A PCA prosthesis was implanted in this patient with known hip and back pain. An oversized stem inserted by mistake had to be removed immediately – since it was cemented – and replaced by a smaller implant. Nevertheless, the stem was still slightly too long and a trochanteric fracture occurred postoperatively

b Because of persistent pain in the trochanteric area, an attempt was made to stabilise the trochanteric nonunion with titanium bands. Six months later the nonunion was still present (*picture*). A seam is also apparent above the cup, which has migrated towards the lesser pelvis. The back pain was clearly aggravated by the Trendelenburg limp. The patient was only able to lie on her back and walk with two sticks

c Cup and stem replacement with shortening and trochanteric fixation (similar to Fig. 8.10). An infection with coagulase-negative staphylococci was treated for 3 months with Ciproxin (ciprofloxacin, 2 × 750 mg/day) and Rimactane (rifampicin, 2 × 450 mg/day). After the nonunion had healed, the narrow spinal canal was corrected with spondylodesis of L4/S1

d Two and a half years later, removal of metal from the greater trochanter. Only limited improvement. Furthermore, two sticks were required for walking longer distances, a situation that did not change even after additional decompression of L3/L4 and metal removal from L4/S1. The patient considered arranging treatment for the rhizarthrosis that had been activated by the use of sticks and underwent total hip replacement for increasing coxarthrosis on the other side. There was a question as to which treatments would be paid for by the insurance company responsible for the first operation the common femoral artery, is not rectified in the short term, the ischaemia may nevertheless recover. However, the residual pain can be severe enough to necessitate amputation in some cases (see also Chap. 13).

14.4.7 Back Problems

As soon as a total hip replacement is indicated, the spine must be included in the corresponding investigations. Hips that are stiffened in a flexion contracture can contribute significantly to the development of low back pain. Such pain may therefore disappear after one-stage replacement of both hips, primarily because of the elimination of the extension deficit. However, if the back problems are predominantly neurogenic in origin, e.g. root compression due to a tight spinal canal or cramped intervertebral foramina, a total hip replacement is unlikely to be helpful in relieving the pain. Quite the opposite, in fact, since the corresponding symptoms would be exacerbated by the increased activity postoperatively. If the spine was not investigated prior to the hip operation, a corresponding examination must be performed in all cases of residual pain.

■ *Case 11.* A female patient experienced an exacerbation of existing hip and back pain as a result of complications following a total hip replacement (Fig. 14.7).

14.4.8 Polymyalgia rheumatica

Polymyalgia is a condition that affects elderly patients, though its aetiology is not fully understood. It is characterised by non-specific joint pain (back of the neck, shoulder, upper arms, buttocks, thighs [1]), often accompanied by a raised C-reactive protein level [4], and possibly by temporal arteritis. Morning stiffness lasting for more than 1 h is another feature. Polymyalgia responds well and quickly to treatment with small doses of cortisone.

■ *Case 12.* A 66-year-old patient (S.C., male, O. 2378) was free of local symptoms 6 weeks after a total hip replacement, but was complaining of back pain. After 2.5 months, he was complaining of increasing muscle pain on exertion in the shoulders and chest. His erythrocyte sedimentation rate was 92 in the first hour. The consulted rheumatologist initiated trial therapy with cortisone (20 mg/day), whereupon the patient's symptoms disappeared at a stroke. Today, 15 years later, he is completely free of symptoms, in respect of both his hip and polymyalgia, on a cortisone dosage of 2.5 mg/day.

14.5 Complex Clinical Pictures

In exceptional cases, an enormous variety of problems and pain types can combine to become strangely, and fatally, linked in a single patient. Apparently unrelated problems can concatenate or plague the patient at the same time, hardly giving him any rest. While some patients may gradually improve, others can become permanently burdened by the same, or new, pains. Fortunately, only a few patients are involved. Always remaining available to such patients is worthwhile, not because this offers constant opportunities for suggesting this or that operation, but so that the patient can be helped repeatedly through discussion or some simple measure. It is also important occasionally to refer such patients to a colleague in the same, or a different, discipline, who may view the problem with different eyes and thus come up with a different diagnosis.

■ *Case 13.* Residual pain in the trochanter area despite numerous attempts at treatment (Fig. 14.8.).

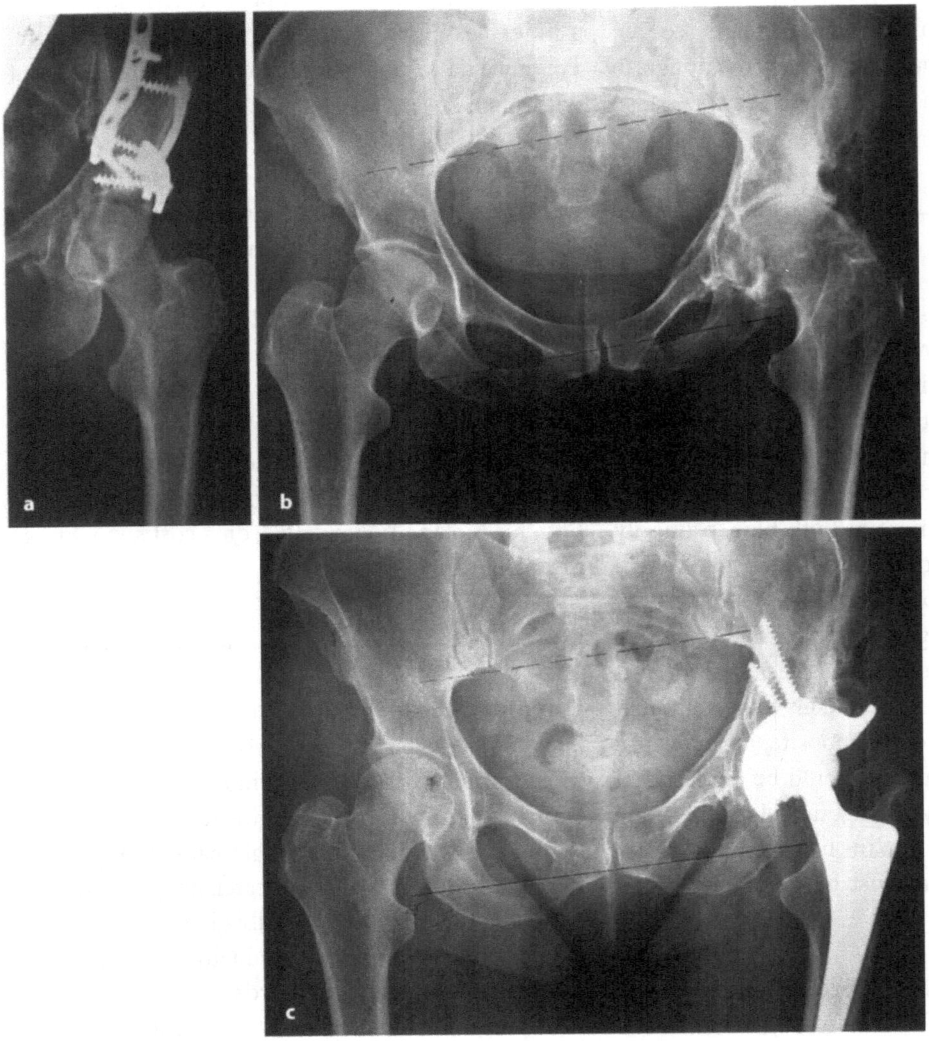

Fig. 14.8a–c. B.B., female (O. 10803). Case 13
a Not very satisfactory internal fixation of a left-sided acetabular fracture at 20 years of age. Although the patient had a slight permanent limp with an adduction contracture, she was still capable of walking flat out for 6 h or more up to the age of 42. The patient suffers from asthma
b Distinct increase in pain at age 45. Functional leg shortening of 1.5 cm with persisting adduction contracture and extension deficit of 10°
c While the prosthesis shows good integration 1 year after a total hip replacement, the patient still had an adduction contracture. Constant pain dorsal to the greater trochanter prevented any form of physical activity beyond what was absolutely necessary. The following were attempted: infiltrations, gait training, scar revision and tractopexy, pain therapy, a wide variety of analgesics, psychotherapy, all without actual success. Three years after the total hip replacement the patient was still suffering from the same pain despite consulting numerous specialists.

References

1. Bird HA, Esselinckx W, Dixon AS, Mowat AG, Wood PNH (1979) An evaluation of criteria for polymyalgia rheumatica. Ann Rheum Dis 38: 434–439
2. Maurer TB, Ochsner P, Schwarzer G, Schumacher M (2001) Increased loosening of cemented straight stem prosthesis made from titanium alloys. An analysis and comparison with prostheses made of cobalt-chromium-nickel alloy. Int Orthop (SICOT) 25: 77–80
3. Petersilge WJ, D'Lima DD, Walker RH, Colwell CWJr (1997) Prospective study of 100 consecutive Harris-Galante porous total hip arthroplasties. J Arthroplasty 2: 185–193
4. Vaith P, Hänsch GM, Peter HH (1988) C-reactive protein-mediated complement activation in polymyalgia rheumatica and other systemic inflammatory diseases. Rheumatol Int 8: 71–80
5. Willert HG, Brobäck LG, Buchhorn GH, Jensen PH, Köster G, Lang I, Ochsner PE, Schenk R (1996) Crevice corrosion of cemented titanium alloy stems in total hip replacements. Clin Orthop 333: 51–73

CHAPTER 15

Revision Rates Due to Aseptic Loosening After Primary and Revision Procedures

PETER E. OCHSNER, ULF RIEDE, MARTIN LÜEM,
THOMAS MAURER, RENATO SOMMACAL

This chapter presents a general analysis of our patient population in respect of revisions and re-revisions due to aseptic loosening. The results after primary implantation were most negatively affected by the use of a cemented titanium stem. The straight-stem prosthesis in its cobalt-chromium variant remains the most successful femoral implant used by us to date. A randomised study comparing this implant with the Virtec stem did not reveal any difference over a 5-year period. The results are slightly less favourable for the corresponding SL stem. Among the acetabular components, the cemented polyethylene cup, acetabular reinforcement ring and SL cup fared best in the primary procedures, while the acetabular reinforcement ring and antiprotrusio cage proved effective in revisions. For stem revisions, the cemented technique with a standard stem has proved most effective, while the uncemented SL revision prosthesis is recommended for situations with large defects. The analysis revealed that early revisions, though rare, were particularly unfavourable in a patient population with high mortality.

The presented data are primarily suitable for internal cross-comparisons, since any comparison with external data, for example data from the Swedish hip register, can be problematic.

The revision rates among our patients and the various implants used by us were analysed in respect of aseptic loosening. The implants were compared and rated, taking into account the respective indication. Comparison of our graph curves with those of other publications is only permissible if the preconditions of the investigations are identical, or at least similar.

The quality of life of the implant recipients is not examined in this book, since this aspect has been, and is being, addressed in separate studies, for example in relation to the SL revision stem [1], the straight stem and the SL titanium and cobalt-chrome alloy prostheses [8] and the antiprotrusio cage [9].

15.1 Definitions

■ **Revision Due to Aseptic Loosening.** A revision is defined as any operative procedure in which at least the cup or the stem is completely replaced as a result of an aseptic problem, generally loosening. The replacement of minor individual components, e.g. cup inlays or stem heads, is not counted as a revision.

■ **Reoperation.** A reoperation refers to any procedure in which neither the stem nor the cup is completely replaced. A reoperation can involve a revision of a haematoma, infection, fracture or trochanter without a change of component, or the removal of periarticular ossification. These reoperations are enumerated and addressed in earlier chapters.

15.2 Plotting of Curves

The data presented in the graph curves are based on (see also Chap. 1):

- Personal follow-ups with radiographs (standard follow-ups after 1, 2, 5, 10, 15 years and additional individually determined interim follow-ups)
- Follow-ups using questionnaires completed by the patient at home

All patients living abroad are able to be included in the survival curve evaluations in terms of the aforementioned four groups.

Included without exception are all primary operations and all aseptic revisions. In view of the relatively modest numbers involved, additional subdivision according to sex, age group and preoperative diagnosis is only useful in statistical terms for fairly large groups. The age distribution and average ages are, however, shown on all curves. Septic revisions are analysed in Chap. 5.

We use the Kaplan-Meier curve. One disadvantage of this type of curve is that the death of a patient is evaluated in exactly the same way as a patient lost to follow-up for other reasons. This gives disproportionate weighting to a prosthesis revision at a late stage, as can be seen from the comparison between Fig. 15.9 and Fig. 15.12. This error can be corrected to a certain extent by analysis of the "competing risk" [7]. In the method used by us, mortality and revision are evaluated competitively (see also Sect. 15.5.6).

■ **Curve Presentation.** The presented graph curves are intended to give as transparent an insight as possible (see legends to Figs. 15.1, 15.2).

■ **Special Factors Influencing the Results.** *Revisions* are always recorded immediately in our statistics. By contrast, patients not undergoing a revision appear in the statistics only when they are examined after the specified interval between each follow-up appointment, which ranges from 1 to 5 years. The delay in integrating the positive results suggests that the results for the non-definitive section of the curves will tend to be slightly better for the subsequent years.

Comparison with the Swedish register: An annual link with the central national hip register enables Swedish researchers to record which patients are still living and which have died [5]. The maximum delay in recording positive results is thus one year.

Problem patients are recorded at an early stage, thanks to systematic follow-ups and additional interim follow-ups in cases of doubtful findings. Since revisions are implemented at a correspondingly early stage, the surgery is often less time-consuming and the period of suffering for the patient is shorter. The waiting lists are only 2–3 months long. This follow-up and revision policy tends to produce higher revision rates.

Comparison with the Swedish Register: The patients are not given regular follow-up appointments, and a revision is usually performed only if the patient spontaneously visits the doctor because of problems, a revision is considered urgent and the patient actually undergoes surgery after a period on the waiting list.

Our patient population includes a surprising excess of male patients, with 55% undergoing primary operations and 63% revision procedures (see also Chap. 2). Since all statistical analyses indicate that revisions are, on average, performed earlier for men than for women, this fact has an adverse impact on our results.

The number of cases presented here are comparatively low. The dominant negative event in our patients is the failure rate for cemented titanium stems [6, 8]. As explained below, this event also affects the survival curves for the other components. By contrast, the numerous stem revisions enabled us to check many stable acetabular implants in situ.

In view of the foregoing, it follows that the curves presented here are of value primarily for internal comparisons, and that caution is indicated in any comparison with curves presented by other authors, including those based on the Swedish hip register. The curves are more useful the more one knows about the detailed underlying factors.

15.3 Analysis of Revisions After Primary Operations

15.3.1 Overview

The total population of patients receiving primary implants during the period 1984–2000 was subdivided into one group with and one without a cemented titanium stem. This distinction was made because the revision rate after the primary implantation of cemented titanium stems was much higher than that for the other strategies [6]. The cemented titanium stems were used only between July 1987 and November 1993 (Fig. 1.2, Chap. 2).

■ **Hip Prostheses Without a Cemented Titanium Stem.** The curve profile is characterised by a gradual increase in revision rates over time (Fig. 15.1). Thus, prostheses were completely or partly replaced in 3.2%, 5.8% and 7.6% of cases, respectively, in the first, second and third 5-year periods. Overall acetabular components appear to be more susceptible to revision than femoral ones, with nine stem and 15 cup revisions.

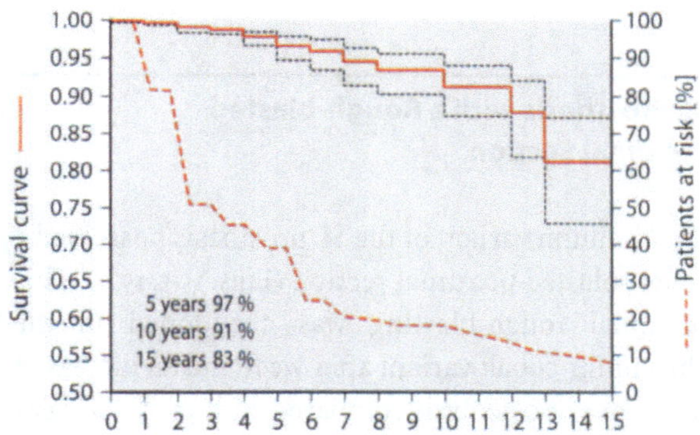

Fig. 15.1. All primary total prostheses without cemented titanium stems. n=1006; 890 patients (1984–2000), female: 45.1%, average age: 67.6 years (SD: 10.7 years). 21 revisions (five stem, 11 cup and four total prosthesis revisions). Comments on the curve: The survival curve processes the events (revisions) in annual increments. The *finely-dotted lines* represent the 95% confidence interval. The survival figures are stated for each 5-year period. The number of patients "at risk" on which the curve is based at the respective point is additionally shown by a *roughly-dotted curve* (*right-hand scale;* see also comment on the curve for Fig. 15.2)

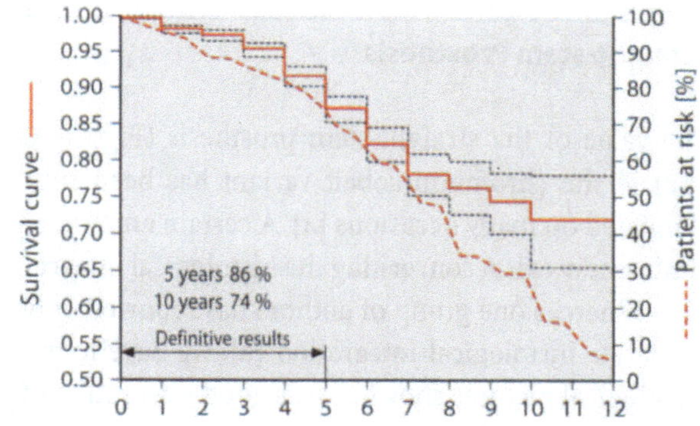

Fig. 15.2. All primary total prostheses with cemented titanium stems. n=564; 506 patients (1987–1993), female: 45.2%, average age: 68 years (SD: 10.1 years). 104 revisions (80 stem, four cup and 20 total prosthesis revisions). Comment on the curve: for implants which, as in this case, are only used for a defined period, the section in which no further changes in the curve are expected (i.e. all patients have already been followed up) is labelled "Definitive results"

■ **Hip Prostheses with a Cemented Titanium Stem.** The revision rate during the first 5 years was almost as high (Fig. 15.2) as that in the first 15 years in the group receiving other stems (Fig. 15.1). However, the revision rate did decline gradually over time. Thus, in the first 5-year period 13.9% of prostheses required complete or partial revision, compared with 12% in the second 5-year period. Nevertheless, it is unlikely that the curves will intercept at a later date. The revisions involved primarily the stem.

15.3.2 Femoral Components

The straight-stem, SL and Virtec prostheses – all cemented – were used as routine implants (Fig. 2.9a, Sect. 3.3.2). Adequate data are available for the first two types in the titanium and cobalt-chromium versions. The Virtec prosthesis, however, has been in routine use only since 1996 (Fig. 2.8). As regards the other implants, either the numbers involved are too small or the types used are not sufficiently comparable to allow a survival curve to be drawn up.

Straight-stem Prosthesis

The value of the straight-stem prosthesis (Figs. 15.3, 15.4) in the chromium-cobalt variant has been substantiated on many occasions [4]. A certain amount of controversy exists concerning the histological integration. Whereas one group of authors has reported only moderate histological integration [2], we have found histological pictures showing very good integration of cement and prosthesis in our own patients over an average period of 10 years (Fig. 3.4c,d). The two variants, "standard" and "lateralising", are evaluated together.

■ **Chromium-Cobalt Variant.** The chromium-cobalt prosthesis shows excellent long-term behaviour (Fig. 15.3). The increase in the revision rate over time is very gradual, and the curve remains favourable.

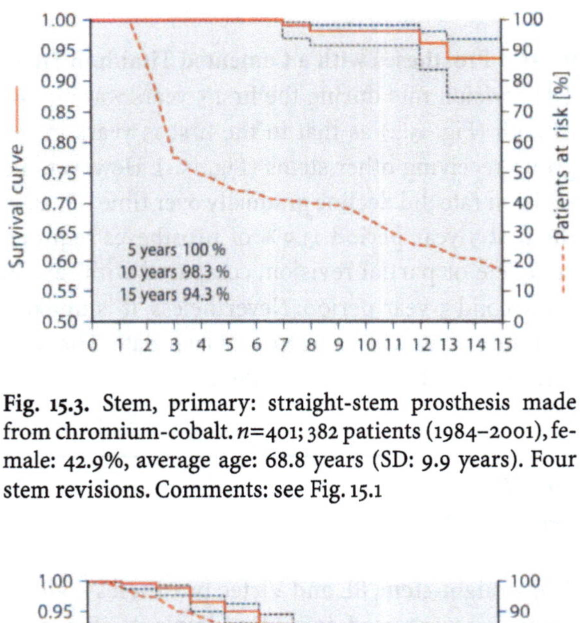

Fig. 15.3. Stem, primary: straight-stem prosthesis made from chromium-cobalt. n=401; 382 patients (1984–2001), female: 42.9%, average age: 68.8 years (SD: 9.9 years). Four stem revisions. Comments: see Fig. 15.1

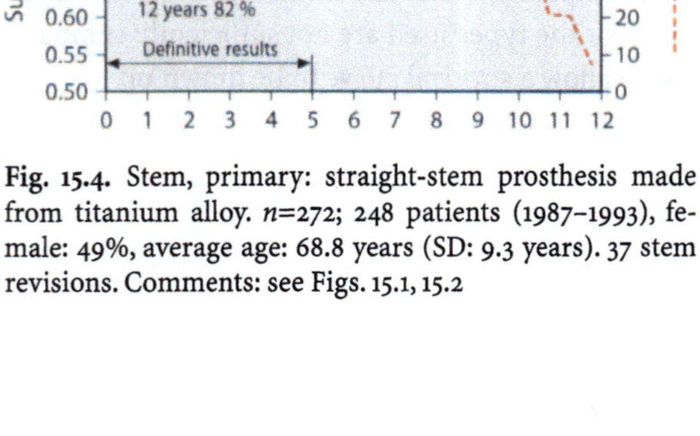

Fig. 15.4. Stem, primary: straight-stem prosthesis made from titanium alloy. n=272; 248 patients (1987–1993), female: 49%, average age: 68.8 years (SD: 9.3 years). 37 stem revisions. Comments: see Figs. 15.1, 15.2

This positive result is all the more remarkable given the very high proportion of male patients (57%) compared with other studies. Male populations are associated with a poorer survival rate, on average, than female groups. The early implants were fitted with a 32-mm head made from cobalt-chromium or ceramic. Compared with the currently used 28-mm heads, the larger heads produced increased wear, with a consequent increase in granulation tissue and associated loosening (Fig. 3.4d).

■ **Titanium Variant.** The revision rate for the titanium variant during the first 5 years is already higher than that noted during the first 15 years for the chromium-cobalt variant (Fig. 15.4). The high revision rates for the first 5 years are already definitively confirmed, while the subsequent flattening of the curve may change slightly. The results are on a similar scale to those for uncemented PCA prostheses [5]. The underlying reasons are not fully understood. The observed corrosion [11] is presumably just an early stage of loosening. A prime suspect is the much greater elasticity of the titanium alloy, which probably leads to early fatiguing of the cement [6]. This view is supported by the more frequent cases of loosening observed among men who perform strenuous physical work and those with small prosthesis sizes. This prosthesis was withdrawn in 1993.

SL Prosthesis with a Rough-blasted Proximal Section

The titanium variant of the SL prosthesis possessed a rough-blasted proximal section (Figs. 15.5, 15.6). This proximal rough-blasting was abandoned in the chromium-cobalt variant after we found an increased incidence of osteolysis compared with the fine-blasted straight-stem prosthesis. The currently marketed version is fine-blasted over its whole surface, though this variant was not used in our hospital.

■ **Chromium-Cobalt Variant.** The survival curve for this prosthesis is definitive for the first 5 years (Fig. 15.5). Because of increased rates of osteolysis, we have abandoned the use of this implant in favour of the previously used straight-stem prosthesis. Today, 5 years after this decision was made, the revision rate is acceptable but nevertheless higher than that for the

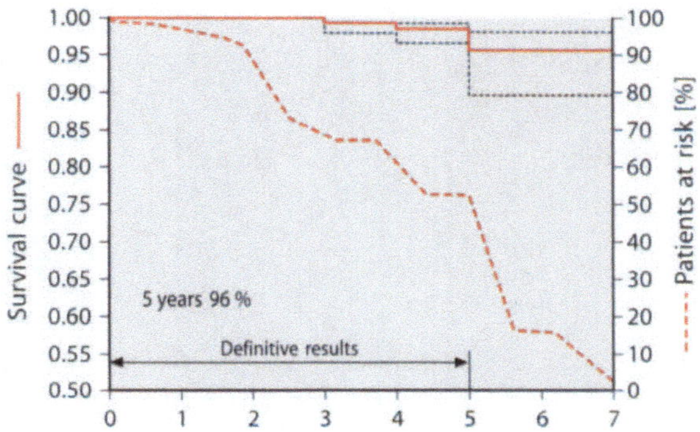

Fig. 15.5. Stem, primary: SL stem made from chromium-cobalt, rough-blasted proximally. n=255; 235 patients (1993–1996), female: 38.3%, average age: 66.7 years (SD: 11.0 years). Three stem revisions. Comments: see Figs. 15.1, 15.2

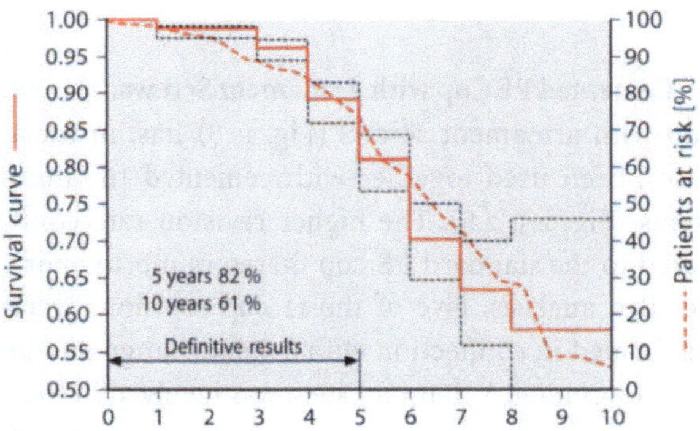

Fig. 15.6. Stem, primary: SL stem made from titanium alloy, rough-blasted proximally. n=233; 217 patients (1990–1993), female: 37.3%, average age: 69.1 years (SD: 9.5 years). 56 stem revisions. Comments: see Figs. 15.1, 15.2

traditional straight-stem prosthesis (Fig. 15.3). The number of osteolyses has also continued to increase [8]. The consequences of our decision to abandon the rough-blasting for the SL stem are not known because of the lack of any comparison group.

▪ **Titanium Variant.** This prosthesis is responsible for the poorest series in our patient population (Fig. 15.6). The revision rate for this stem in the first 10 years was some 20 times higher than that for the cobalt-chromium straight-stem prosthesis, and twice as high as that for the titanium straight-stem prosthesis. Fortunately, the revision rate curve seems to show signs of flattening out over the past 2 years. It is not clear which of the differences in shape and surface compared with the straight-stem prosthesis are most important, i.e. the absence of a central groove (prevention of varus tilting), the proximal rough-blasting (poorer integration with the cement in practice) or the absence of a cement abutment collar (stabilisation against subsidence). However, in view of the much poorer results observed for the two titanium variants, the greater elasticity of the titanium in combination with cement should be viewed as a particularly negative factor [6].

Virtec Prosthesis

This straight-stem variant, which is oval in cross-section in contrast with the traditional straight stem (Figs. 2.9a, 3.4c) has been used since July 1996 in parallel with the straight-stem prosthesis on a randomised basis. During the first 4.5 years of the ongoing study, no stem in either group has had to be replaced because of aseptic loosening. The annually checked clinical results have not yet revealed any differences between the two prostheses, and it is still too early to draw any definitive conclusions.

CDH Prosthesis

The CDH prosthesis is an implant reserved for difficult cases, for which it is particularly suited, given its small dimensions, oval cross-section and narrow CCD angle (Figs. 2.9a, 3.8, 7.4). The profiles recorded for this prosthesis in our own patients are fairly short on average, since patients with correspondingly difficult management problems are being referred to us in greater numbers only with our increasing experience. The total number of 79 primary implants was also distributed across three alloys (cobalt-chromium, titanium and steel; Fig. 1.2) In view of its small size, the titanium version of this implant was particularly affected by the high elasticity (Fig. 6.3). Instead of our own data, we would refer readers to the study on the patient population of M.E. Müller [3].

15.3.3 Acetabular Components

If cemented titanium stems are disregarded, revision operations after primary implantations were more likely to be indicated because of cup rather than stem loosening. As a routine acetabular implant, the polyethylene cup was used initially, followed by the polyethylene cup with armament screws and, subsequently, the uncemented SL cup in its first and second variants (Figs. 2.5, 2.6). For situations involving a poor acetabular bone stock, we implanted the acetabular reinforcement ring from the outset and, occasionally, the antiprotrusio cage in drastic cases (see also Sect. 3.3.1).

Polyethylene Cups

■ **Cemented Polyethylene Cup.** The cemented polyethylene (PE) cup (Fig. 15.7) was almost invariably combined with a chromium-cobalt cemented straight stem. The sex distribution and average age were closely matched in these two groups. A comparison of the two (Fig. 15.3) reveals similarly shaped curves, but with a sharper drop for the PE cup, i.e. a slightly higher revision rate. Because of the small numbers involved, the confidence intervals overlap. A detailed analysis of the X-ray series gives the impression, as yet not scientifically verified, that the loosening tendency is reduced if a thick cement layer is applied cranial to the PE cup rather than a thin, or barely visible, layer. All five revised PE cups show a seam, three of which show linear wear of over 2 mm. Since wear promotes loosening via granulation tissue, an improvement in the outcome for cemented PE cups can be expected merely by the use of a more favourable pairing.

In view of the positive 10-year results, we have started implanting the cemented PE cup again in patients from 75 years of age.

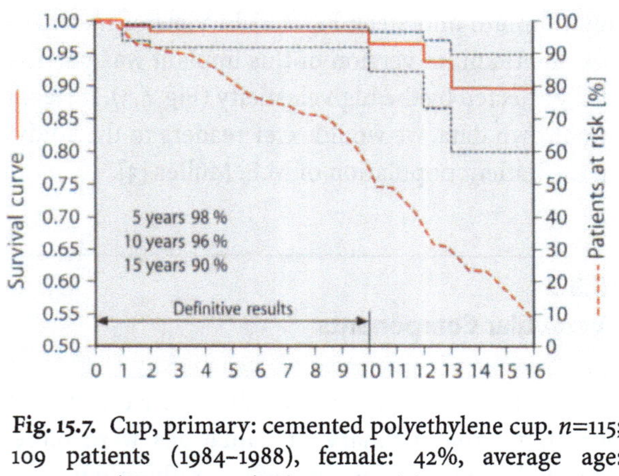

Fig. 15.7. Cup, primary: cemented polyethylene cup. n=115; 109 patients (1984–1988), female: 42%, average age: 67.3 years (SD: 9.7 years). Five cup revisions. Comments: see Figs. 15.1, 15.2

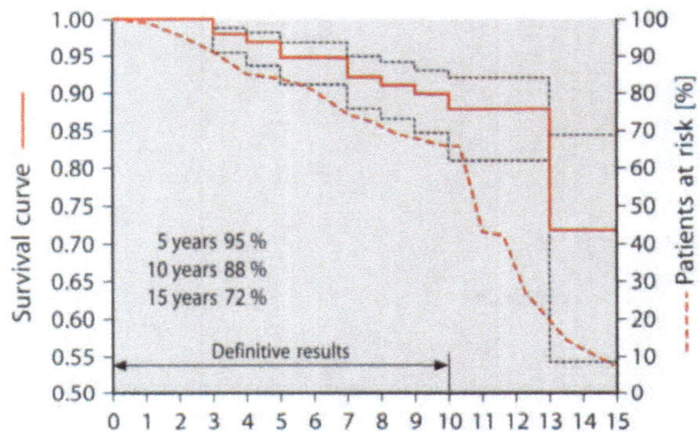

Fig. 15.8. Cup, primary: cemented polyethylene cup with armament screws. n=111; 103 patients (1984–1989), female: 42%, average age: 68.4 years (SD: 9.4 years). 12 cup revisions. Five revisions were performed secondary to a stem revision indicated as a result of stem loosening, in four cases involving a cemented titanium stem. Comments: see Figs. 15.1, 15.2

■ **Cemented PE Cup with Armament Screws.** The PE cup with armament screws (Fig. 15.8) has, in most cases, been used together with cemented titanium stems (Fig. 2.5, 2.8). The higher revision rate compared to the standard PE cup therefore merits more detailed analysis. Five of the 12 cup revisions were performed in connection with a stem change due to stem loosening. A titanium stem was involved in four cases. In some cases, the cup was changed because of discernible cup wear rather than any loosening. It is unlikely that a cup revision procedure would have been performed in these five cases if the stem had remained firm. However, even after these five cases are deducted, the results are worse than those for the cemented PE cup without armament screws.

Acetabular Reinforcement Ring According to M.E. Müller

We have used the acetabular reinforcement ring (Fig. 15.9) since 1984 primarily in patients with a small acetabulum and a defective bone stock (see also section 3.3.1, Fig. 2.5). The results have been excellent. This is our only patient group with a predominance of females, which probably explains why the results were slightly better than expected. Up to the 10-year follow-up point, they are probably better than those for the cemented PE cup. A comparative statement for the period up to 15 years is not yet possible because of the inadequate numbers of monitored patients. With a total of just two revisions, we have not been able to

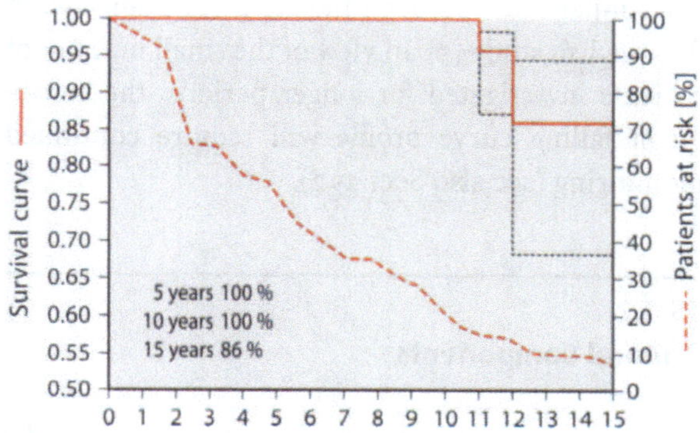

Fig. 15.9. Cup, primary: acetabular reinforcement ring according to M.E. Müller. n=286; 260 patients (1984–2000), female 63%, average age: 66 years (SD: 12 years). Two cup revisions. Comments: see Fig. 15.1

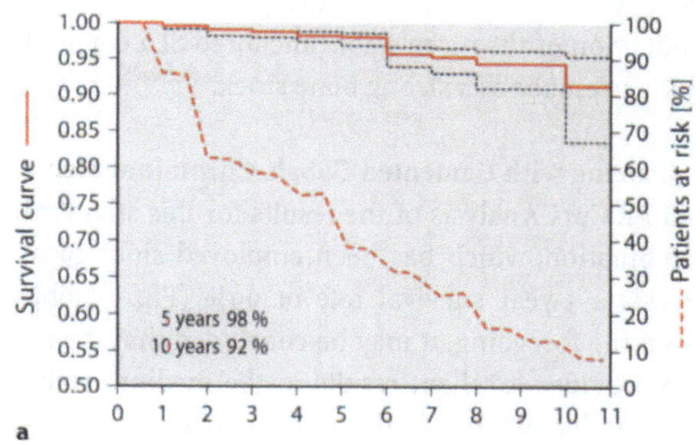

a

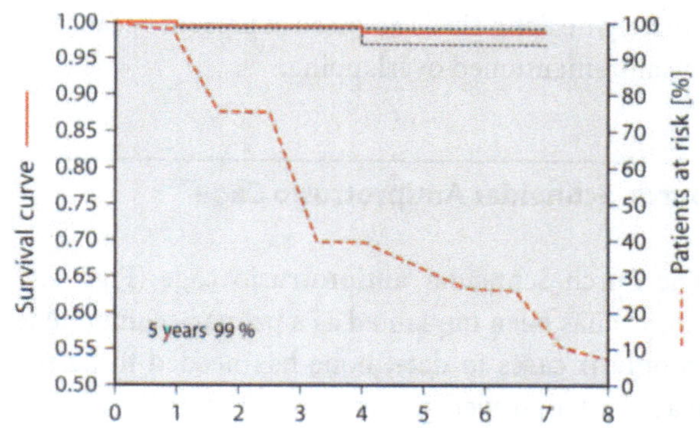

b

Fig. 15.10a,b. Cup, primary: SL cups 1 and 2
a Total patient population: n=1034; 883 patients (1989–2000), female: 41%, average age: 68 years (SD: 10 years). 20 cup revisions, including six on their own and 14 in connection with femoral revisions due to aseptic loosening of titanium stems. Comments: see Fig. 15.1
b Reduced patient population after the change to the cemented cobalt-chromium stem: n=567; 515 patients (1993–2000), female: 43%, average age: 69 years (SD: 9.4 years). Two cup revisions

determine any effect of the change in material from steel to titanium.

The comparison of the two curves (PE cup vs. acetabular reinforcement ring) is informative in providing a better understanding of the Kaplan-Meier curve. The numerical value for the PE cup, with a much smaller base population and five revisions after 15 years, is better than that for the acetabular reinforcement ring with more than twice as many implants and just two revisions. These two revisions were only performed after 10 and 11 years, respectively, at which point the comparison group was already very small. As a result, the survival curve for the acetabular reinforcement ring was much more greatly affected than the curve for the PE cup, which included a number of revisions performed at an early stage. This scenario is one of the reasons for introducing the "competing risk curve" [7] (see also Sect. 15.5.6).

SL Cup, Uncemented, Types 1 and 2

This cup is the most commonly used individual component in our patient population (Figs. 15.10a,b). Since the SL2 cup was introduced only in 1997, it will be assessed jointly with the SL1 cup in this review. The assessment is hampered by the combination with cemented titanium stems and pairing with Metasul joints (Fig. 15.10a).

■ **Combination with Cemented Titanium Stems.** Fourteen cups implanted during this period were subsequently revised concurrently with a loosened titanium stem. Whenever a lack of osteointegration was suspected, the cup was also changed, even if no clinical symptoms were present. Merely a new inlay was inserted only if clear osteointegration of the shells was present, as confirmed after removal of the inlay by inspection of all screws and the in-growth of bone into the medial slot of the cup. These hips were not counted as cup revisions. A few individual cups which, in retrospect, proved to be firmly anchored, were also forced out of their sockets by an abrupt tilting movement with the inserter as part of extended stability testing.

■ **Pairing with Metasul.** The SL cup was combined with the Metasul joint pairing in 111 (11%) of cases. This pairing resulted in four cup and three total prosthesis revisions. As soon as we became aware of this trend, we used the Metasul pairing only after the introduction of the more stably anchored SL2 cup and in the presence of a strong bone stock.

■ **Pairing with Cemented Cobalt-Chromium Stems and PE Cup.** Analysis of the results for this standard combination, which has been employed since 1993, reveals a 5-year survival rate of 99% (Fig. 15.10b). From the foregoing, it may be concluded that the SL cup provides excellent results in the medium term, but that the outcome in the long term cannot, unfortunately, be definitively assessed at present because of the aforementioned overlapping.

Burch-Schneider Antiprotrusio Cage

The Burch-Schneider antiprotrusio cage (Figs. 2.5, 2.6, 3.1) has been implanted as a primary component in only 11 cases to date; none has needed to be replaced after an average of 5.5 (0–14) years.

15.4 Analysis of the Re-revisions After Revision Operations

15.4.1 Overview

The graph in Fig. 15.11 includes all patients undergoing a first revision. After 10 years, 82% have managed without the need for a re-revision. These figures are of a similar order of magnitude to those published in the Swedish study [5]. In view of the small number of patients investigated for longer periods, the subsequent falling curve profile will require continued monitoring (see also Sect. 15.2).

15.4.2 Femoral Components

The revision rate for stems is far more crucial to the overall curve (Fig. 15.11) than that for cups. Consequently, the trend for revisions is precisely the opposite of that for primary prostheses.

■ **Uncemented SL Revision Stem.** With a survival rate of 92%, the SL revision stem (Fig. 15.12) achieved good 5- and 10-year results. The revisions were, without exception, indicated because of early loosening, which resulted in a poor outcome in the very first year. One patient sought to avoid a recommended revision simply by waiting. The 10-year revision rate of 8% therefore relates precisely to 8% of all patients receiving this prosthesis, since all patients actually experienced the risk event in time (see also Sect. 15.5.6). However, given the bone defects and the often poor initial situation, the clinical results and patient satisfaction are amazingly good [1].

■ **Cemented Stems.** Following a cemented stem revision (Fig. 15.13), 97% of the implants survived without subsequent replacement for 5 years and 89% for 10 years. An analysis of the mortality curve for the

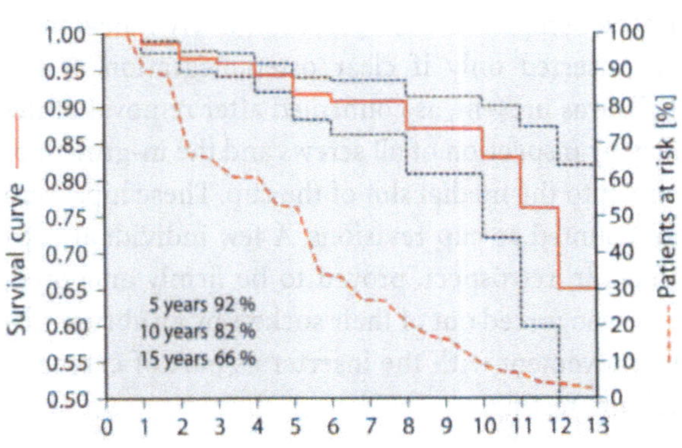

Fig. 15.11. All first revisions indicated as a result of aseptic loosening. n=381; 328 patients (1984–2000), female: 37%, average age: 70.3 years (SD: 9.8 years). 21 re-revisions (13 stem, one cup and seven revisions of both components). Comments see Fig. 15.1

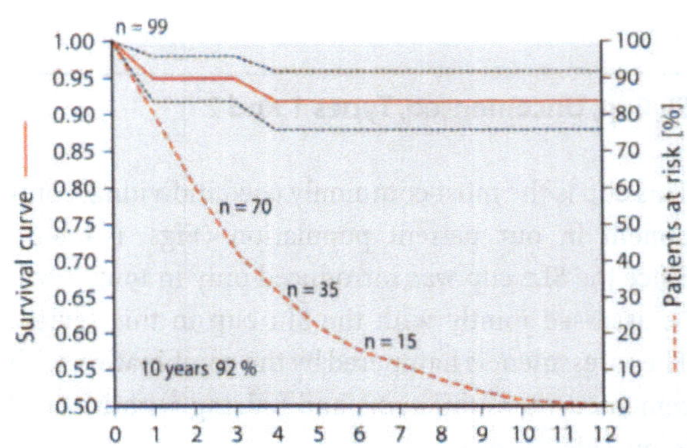

Fig. 15.12. Stem revisions: uncemented SL revision stem (Wagner), including first and multiple revisions. n=99; 85 patients (1988–1999), female: 44%, average age: 71 years (SD: 10.7 years). Six stem revisions. Comments see Fig. 15.1

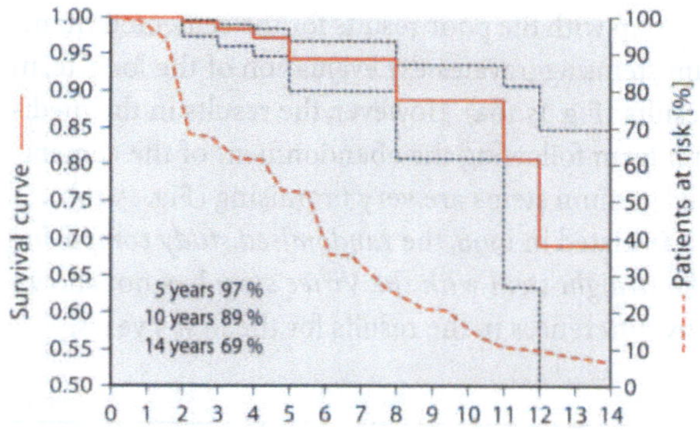

Fig. 15.13. First revisions of the stem: cemented stems. n=221; 209 patients (1984–2000), female 28%, average age: 70.3 years (SD: 10 years). Nine stem revisions. Comments: see Fig. 15.1

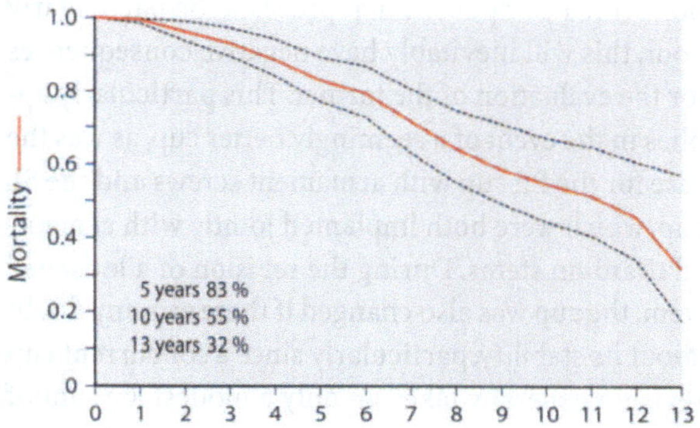

Fig. 15.14. Mortality curve of patients from Fig. 15.13, same patient population. Comment: This curve has a different scale and has been smoothed

same group of patients reveals 5- and 10-year survival rates of 83% and just 55%, respectively, while only 32% of the patients were still alive after 13 years (Fig. 15.14). As a result of the substantial mortality, very few patients were still being followed up after 10 years, and the corresponding survival data are therefore very unreliable.

15.4.3 Acetabular Components

■ **Acetabular Reinforcement Ring According to M.E. Müller.** The acetabular reinforcement ring (Fig. 15.15) is our preferred implant for acetabular revisions, being used in 59% of cases. It is used in situations with obvious defects, albeit not in the most serious cases (Figs. 2.7, 3.1d). The survival rates of 98% after 5 years and 91% after 10 years are statistically reliable, given

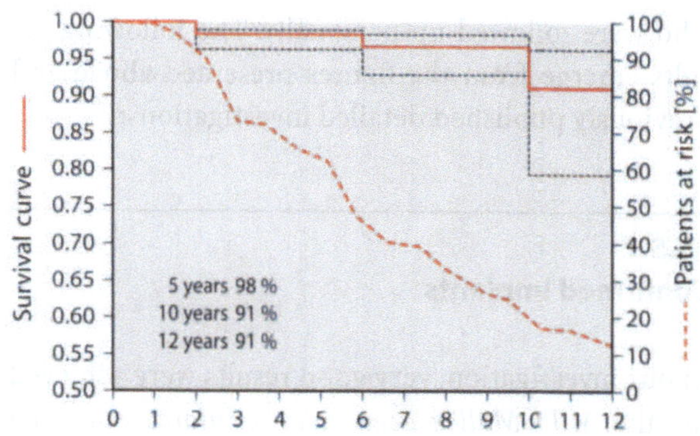

Fig. 15.15. Cup revisions: acetabular reinforcement ring according to M.E. Müller. n=203; 192 patients (1984–2000), female: 43%, average age: 72 years (SD: 10.4 years). Three cup revisions. Comments: see Sect. 15.1

the substantial numbers involved. The results were achieved primarily with titanium shells, while only about one sixth of the implants were manufactured from steel. The effect of rough-blasting, which was introduced in 1998, is not yet discernible (Fig. 13.10).

■ **Burch-Schneider Antiprotrusio Cage.** Of the 66 revisions performed to date, on average 5 (1–15) years ago (Figs. 2.6, 2.7, 3.1e), not a single component has had to be replaced because of aseptic loosening, while just one required replacement due to loosening in association with a fistulating late infection [9]. This implant is used in seriously defective situations and is also one of our most successful. Good results after an average period of 12 (8–21) years have likewise been reported for those patients who were originally operated on by Burch, who was one of the developers and is also our adviser [10].

■ **Other Acetabular Implants.** The other, much more rarely inserted, implants (cemented PE cups, SL cups) were used only if no defective situation was present. These are neither amenable to statistical analysis nor representative of the normal revision situation.

15.5 Conclusions

This study offers the advantage of a closed patient series in a single hospital. A crucial factor is the comparison between the curves for the revision/survival rates and the functional results. This is possible in our case thanks to the large proportion of patients who were followed up personally. The following results emerge from the figures presented above and previously published detailed investigations:

15.5.1 Confirmed Implants

In our investigation, very good results were achieved for the *M.E. Müller acetabular reinforcement ring* (Figs. 15.9, 15.15) and the *Burch-Schneider antiprotrusio cage,* when used both as primary implants and in revision procedures. When combined with the corresponding surgical techniques, these two components remain firmly anchored and provide good primary stability (Sect. 3.3.1).

15.5.2 Abandoned Implants

All of the cemented titanium stems (straight stem, SL and CDH) (Figs. 15.4, 15.6) led to poor results, and all three were therefore abandoned. In view of less favourable results in a direct comparison, the *SL stem made from a cobalt-chromium alloy with a rough-blasted proximal section* (Fig. 15.5) was abandoned in favour of the classical straight stem (Fig. 15.3), while the *cemented PE cup with armament screws* (Fig. 15.8) was abandoned in favour of the same cup without armament screws (Fig. 15.7).

15.5.3 Re-introduced Implants

On the basis of the long-term results, the classical *straight stem prosthesis made from a cobalt-chromium alloy* (Fig. 15.3) was re-introduced as a standard prosthesis, while the *cemented PE cup* (Fig. 15.7) with improved cementation technique was re-introduced as an alternative option for elderly patients.

15.5.4 Decisions Still Outstanding

No definitive assessment can yet be made concerning the *SL cup in its first and second variants,* since the overlap with the poor results for the cemented titanium stems aggravates the evaluation of the long-term results (Fig. 15.10a). However, the results in the medium term following the abandonment of the cemented titanium stems are very promising (Fig. 15.10b).

Initiated in 1996, the *randomised study comparing the straight stem with the Virtec stem* has not shown any differences in the results for the first 5 years.

15.5.5 Difficulty of Evaluating a Single Component as a Counterpart to a Poorer Component

If a better implant is tested concurrently in combination with a component that proves to be particularly poor, this will inevitably have negative consequences for the evaluation of the former. This particularly applies in the event of a seemingly better cup, as was the case for the PE cup with armament screws and the SL cup, which were both implanted jointly with cemented titanium stems. During the revision of a loosened stem, the cup was also changed if there was any doubt about its stability, particularly since a concurrent cup revision generally takes up only a modest amount of additional time. As a result, the revision rate for cups was increased out of consideration for the patient's safety (Fig. 15.8, 15.10). In contrast with cups, stems are less likely to be replaced concurrently with a loosened cup if the former appear to be firm, since the corresponding procedure takes much longer and thus increases the associated operation risk for the patient.

15.5.6 Comparative Evaluation of the Kaplan-Meier and Competing-Risk Curves

A *revision performed shortly after implantation* affects the probability for the whole patient population (Fig. 15.12). The total number of revisions is therefore relatively high, and the clock for the time of revision already starts ticking shortly after the primary operation. As a result, the likelihood of a re-revision is greatly increased. Moreover, patients requiring a revision after just 1 or 2 years are almost always dissatisfied. The Kaplan-Meier curve, however, is relatively little affected by this scenario (Fig. 15.12).

Mortality increases in line with the age at implantation. In our revision patients, the mortality after 10 years was already as high as 41% (Fig. 15.14). A revision 10 years or more after implantation in a group associated with high mortality involves only a small proportion of operated patients, since a significant percentage of the patients have died without a revision (Fig. 15.13). It should be borne in mind that a patient is generally satisfied if further revision is required only after several years have elapsed. However, the Kaplan-Meier curve falls much more sharply compared with an early revision, since a late revision concerns only a relatively small group (Fig. 15.13). This is offset, at least in part, by the recently introduced "competing-risk curve" [7] (Figs. 15.16, 15.17), in which the death of a patient is assessed as a competing event in relation to revision. The resulting 10-year failure rate of 8% calculated for uncemented SL revision stems is correspondingly higher than the 6% figure calculated for cemented stem revisions. Having subjected the significance of the "competing-risk curve" to an in-depth analysis, we believe that it should generally replace the Kaplan-Meier curve in the evaluation of operation results in cases where the death of the patient is not itself checked as a comparative criterion.

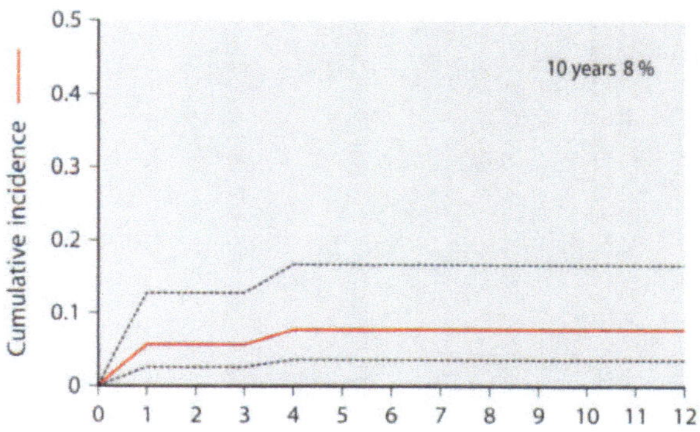

Fig. 15.16. "Competing-risk curve" for stem revisions with the uncemented SL revision stem (Wagner, illustrations. Same numerical bases as for Fig. 15.12). Comment: Since this curve counts the events (revisions), the percentages correspond to the number of revised prostheses. They complement those in the Kaplan-Meier curves.

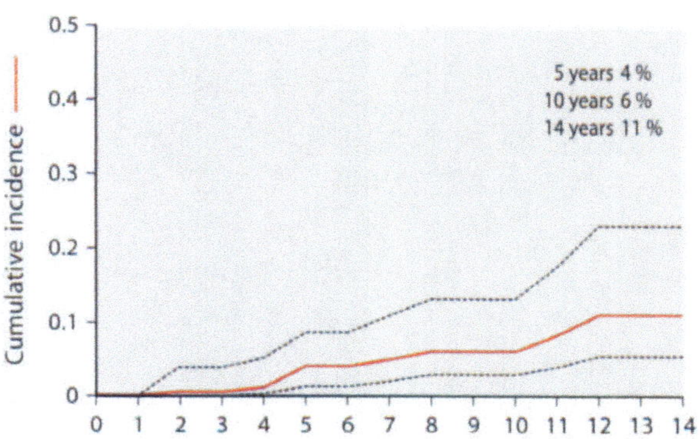

Fig. 15.17. "Competing-risk curve" for first revisions with cemented stems. Same numerical bases as for Fig. 15.13. Comment: see Fig. 15.16. (We should like to thank Mr. G. Schwarzer of the Institute for Medical Biometrics and Medical Informatics at Freiburg University for calculating and preparing Figs. 15.14, 15.16 and 15.17)

15.5.7 Assessment of the Generous Revision Policy

We take the view that regular patient check-ups after 1, 2, 5, 10 and 15 years, supplemented by any interim control required in the event of abnormal findings, can help disclose any problems in a timely manner. This enables us to perform a revision at a time when the patient has not yet suffered for very long from the effects of his problem prosthesis. As a result, the patient requiring a revision feels well looked after. This can also be confirmed numerically. Of the 479 revision procedures performed by us, 29.2% concerned patients who had undergone the primary hip replacement in our department. Only 11 (12%) of these patients preferred to go elsewhere for their revision operation.

A new study revealed almost identical clinical results 10 years after the primary implantation of a cemented titanium prosthesis both for those of our patients who had not required a revision and those who had undergone a revision in the interim.

References

1. Bircher HP, Riede U, Lüem M, Ochsner PE (2001) Der Wert der SL-Revisionsprothese nach Wagner zur Überbrückung großer Femurdefekte. Technik und Resultate. Orthopäde 30: 294–303
2. Draenert K, Draenert Y, Garde U, Ulrich CH (1999) Manual of cementing technique. Springer, Berlin
3. Gill TS, Sledge JB, Müller ME (1998) Total hip arthroplasty with the use of an acetabular reinforcement ring in patients who have congenital dysplasia of the hip. J Bone Joint Surg [Am] 80: 969–979

4. Lützner J, Ochsner PE (2000) Langzeitergebnisse mit der Orginal M.-E. Müller-Geradschaftprothese aus CoNiCrMo-Schmiedelegierung (Protasul-10). Orthop Praxis 36: 416–421
5. Malchau H, Herberts P (1998) Prognosis of total hip replacement. The national hip arthroplasty registry. University of Göteborg, Sweden
6. Maurer TB, Ochsner PE, Schwarzer G, Schumacher M (2001) Increased loosening of cemented straight stem prostheses made from titanium alloys. An analysis and comparison with prostheses made of cobalt-chromium-nickel-alloy. Int Orthop (SICOT) 25: 77–80
7. Schwarzer G, Schumacher M, Maurer TB, Ochsner PE (2001) Statistical analysis of failure times in total joint replacement. J Clin Epidemiol 54: 997–1003
8. Schweizer A, Riede U, Ochsner PE (2002) Comparative five-year results of two cemented straight stem models produced in two different alloys (cobalt-chromium and titanium). (submitted)
9. Van Koeveringe AJ, Ochsner PE (2002) Revision arthroplasty using Burch-Schneider antiprotrusio cage. Internat Orthop (in press)
10. Wachtl SW, Jung M, Jakob RP, Gauthier E (2000) The Burch-Schneider antiprotrusio cage in acetabular revision surgery. A mean follow-up of 12 years. J Arthroplasty 15: 959–963
11. Willert HG, Brobäck LG, Buchhorn GH, Jensen PH, Köster G, Lang I, Ochsner PE, Schenk R (1996) Crevice corrosion of cemented titanium alloy stems in total hip replacements. Clin Orthop 333: 51–73

Chapter 16

Preoperative Briefing

Peter E. Ochsner

The preoperative briefing primarily includes information about the benefits of the operation, alternative options, the treatment schedule, risks and costs. In orthopaedic surgery, the purpose of the briefing is to provide the patient with sufficient information to enable him to make his own decision about the need for an operation. The level of detail must be adapted to the patient, the planned procedure and the possible complications. Before the briefing, the doctor should acquaint himself with the personality and problems of the patient. Ideally, the briefing should be given before the patient is admitted to hospital. If the briefing is not provided by the operator himself, then the operator should at least be personally introduced to the patient. A record of the conversation in the patient's case notes or on a specially designed form provides important evidence of the briefing.

In addition to general complications, a total hip replacement can often be followed by limping, leg length discrepancies and haematomas. Particularly serious complications include the rare fatalities, nerve injuries and problems such as infections or recurrent dislocation that necessitate further operations. Aseptic loosening of the prosthesis is the most likely complication in the medium- to long-term.

16.1 Purpose and Content of the Briefing

In 1991, the Swiss Federal Court issued the following ruling on the subject of *briefing*: "The patient should be sufficiently informed of the procedure or treatment to enable him to provide his consent in full knowledge of the situation. However, the briefing should not induce a state of anxiety that would be detrimental to the patient's health." These two sentences are well balanced and serve as a guideline for the statements in this chapter. While the process of informed consent has become a legal obligation, certain limits have also been set.

A few general guidelines should be observed during a briefing session in order to ensure that nothing important is forgotten:

- What kind of specific *benefit* can our patient expect after an operation? What will this benefit be like if the result of the operation is only modest?
- What *alternatives* are available?
- What is included in the *treatment schedule*?
- What particularly common and particularly dangerous *risks* are involved? What do these mean for our patient should they arise?
- What *costs* can the patient expect as a result of the treatment?

16.1.1 Benefit to Be Expected for the Patient

The patient is entitled to have the expected benefit explained to him in realistic terms. The briefing must include the current health status of the patient. Orthopaedic patients, in particular, often suffer from other illnesses that can prevent them gaining the full benefit from the operation. The outcome in the event of only moderately successful treatment should also be addressed. The probability of success should be mentioned, particularly for more common procedures. Information about one's own results takes precedence over references to the literature. If one's own experience with the proposed method is limited, then the patient has a right to be informed of this fact.

16.1.2 Alternatives

The more far-reaching the proposed treatment, the more important it is to discuss the alternatives and provide a comparison of their results and risks. Not infrequently, a patient will decide to postpone a total hip replacement after being informed of the wavelike profile for hip pain in osteoarthritis or after being advised to try a course of physiotherapy.

16.1.3 Treatment Schedule

The patient has a right to be informed of the treatment schedule. The duration of hospital stay and the planned treatment, but also the expected adverse effects, are important not only to the patient but also to his family, since numerous arrangements will have to be made for the period after discharge from hospital. The relatives must be prepared for a period during which the patient will be dependent on others. Plans frequently have to be made in respect of holiday arrangements, the booking of outpatient nursing care after discharge from hospital, or of an in-patient health cure or stay in a rehabilitation clinic. The period of unfitness for work can have a considerable impact on the patient's future depending on the individual situation. A detailed briefing will enable the patient to discuss and coordinate the situation with his employer.

16.1.4 Risks

Openness and sensitivity are required when explaining the risks of a treatment. The likelihood of a complication and the commonest and most dangerous complications must be presented in one form or another, so that the patient is in a position to form his own clear judgement of the situation. As established in the aforementioned Federal Court decision, the doctor has to decide in each individual case how much detail to provide about complications. The patient's personality, in particular, needs to be taken into account. Anxious and self-confident patients, those with numerous illnesses and those who are perfectly fit cannot just be lumped together.

16.1.5 Costs

If the patient has to pay a part of the treatment costs himself, the question of costs will need to be broached. A cost estimate will be most helpful to the patient in enabling him to clarify the financial situation with his insurer.

Ultimately, the patient is responsible for weighing up all the above information, while the doctor provides assistance as required. According to another judgement of the Swiss Federal Court, issued in 1999: "The briefing is an exchange between doctor and patient, requiring the involvement of both parties."

16.2 General Conditions of the Briefing Discussion

16.2.1 Clarification of the Patient's Environment by the Doctor

One of the fundamental tasks of the doctor during the briefing process is to obtain as accurate a picture as possible of the patient and his circumstances. In orthopaedics, a knowledge of the condition to be treated and its consequences is not sufficient, of itself, as a basis for decision-making. Additional information about other people living with the patient, the patient's accommodation and occupational situation, hobbies, general lifestyle, on the one hand, and about the patient's general health, on the other, will provide the necessary background for an adequate consultation.

Patients can come to the orthopaedic surgeon with very differing objectives:

- The patient comes with the firm conviction that an operation is necessary.
- The patient's own doctor/friends had said that he needed treatment.
- The patient comes with a description of his complaint and is seeking preliminary advice.
- The patient is surprised by a medical opinion to the effect that an operation is necessary.

The doctor's skill consists in reliably identifying the aforementioned related factors and steering the conversation in the direction that is most appropriate *for the patient* on the basis of the described situation.

The briefing discussion provides a suitable opportunity, together with the patient, for addressing the material problems arising from a treatment, and for sounding out the patient's personal situation and the possibility of cooperation. The aim of a successful briefing is for the patient, in partnership with his doctor, to be able to come through the treatment period and – what is more difficult – to overcome any complications. Thus, the significance of this discussion is obvious. If a sufficient basis of trust cannot be built up, it may be appropriate to advise the patient to seek a second opinion or to hand over his management to another doctor.

16.2.2 Time of Briefing

From the timing standpoint, the briefing will be useful if it helps the patient determine the therapeutic strategy that is right for him. It is therefore sensible to arrange the briefing at an early stage. In our experience, the briefing discussion is best incorporated in a preliminary outpatient consultation during which the details of the procedure are also outlined. If the patient is given a written record of the discussion (Fig. 16.1), he will then have the opportunity to review his situation at leisure and, if necessary, cancel any further appointments. By appearing for operation, the patient further confirms his willingness to undergo surgery.

In cases of direct referrals for operation, an outpatient briefing procedure is not possible, and the patients can only be briefed on admission to hospital. To a certain extent, the briefing discussion is coloured by the impending operation that has already been arranged. It is difficult for a patient who is already in hospital to revise his decision to undergo surgery. Although this does occur, most of the patients concerned are subsequently advised against surgery by the relevant doctors.

In emergency situations, the briefing schedule presented above does not apply. Nevertheless, the doctors are still obliged to obtain the patient's informed consent. Even in these cases, a decision should only be made under pressure of time if so dictated by the prevailing medical need.

16.2.3 The Briefing Doctor

The advantage associated with an orthopaedic surgeon working in a private clinic compared to a public hospital is that the investigations, operation and follow-up are performed by one and the same individual. He even conducts the briefing discussion. Management of the patient is simplified, even if complications arise, since he is already familiar with the facts of the case.

In orthopaedic departments of public hospitals, the greater the number of doctors working together, the more difficult it is to achieve an effective briefing.

In a briefing during the preliminary outpatient consultation, the discussion is generally conducted by a *Facharzt* (specialised orthopaedic surgeon) and often by the operator. If the examining surgeon is a registrar, he is generally assisted by a fully trained specialist. If the patient is only briefed on admission to hospital, the doctor concerned is often a registrar. In the case of elective procedures, it is particularly important that the patient should still have the opportunity to talk personally with the scheduled operator. This contact not only serves as an occasion for briefing, but also primarily for reassuring the patient, who is then able to gain his own impression of the operator and his efforts in relation to the impending operation.

16.3 Legal Aspects of Briefing

16.3.1 Right to Briefing

The obligation to provide a briefing is based on the patient's right to physical integrity. Any treatment performed without the patient's consent is legally tantamount to the infliction of bodily harm. Before the patient can provide his binding consent, a corresponding explanation/briefing is essential, since this enables the patient to give his informed consent (German: *Einverständnis*, French: *choix éclairé*) on the basis of his own understanding. The duty to provide a briefing can also be derived from the law of contract. Viewed in terms of private law, the patient and doctor enter into a contractual relationship concerning an order for treatment, even though this is not specified in writing. The commissioned doctor therefore has a duty to inform the contracting patient about the subject matter of the order [4].

16.3.2 Scope

The scope of the briefing discussion can be defined in terms of time or content. Although the demands of lawyers as representatives of plaintiff patients will probably always exceed the perceptions of the doctors, the situation merits a brief analysis.

Very little of a binding nature can be specified about the length of the discussion. For some patients a basis of trust is created simply by a careful examination and a binding medical history. In such cases, the subsequent briefing discussion will not be very long. If the patient asks for time to think things over after a comprehensive briefing, then the briefing at the next consultation might perhaps be much more extensive. Considerable patience on both sides is often required in cases where patients are asking us to rectify remaining complications.

Radical differences of opinion exist concerning the extent of the briefing in respect of possible complications. Everyone agrees that common complications, but also rarer complications with serious consequences, should be mentioned. Unfortunately, the reports of successes in medical publications far outweigh the reports of complications. It is not easy therefore to provide realistic figures for the complications to be expected. This book aims to make a contribution in this respect.

16.3.3 Record Keeping

Even after a comprehensive briefing, both the patient and doctor forget many of the discussion points. When complications occur and the patient asks whether he had actually been informed of the possibility of their occurrence, mere oral confirmation by the doctor is often inadequate. Written documentation is particularly important in the case of a legal dispute, where the judge ultimately decides on the credibility of both parties' statements. Such hearings generally take place years after the event. Since the burden of proof concerning the briefing rests with the doctor, he will inevitably have to provide documentary evidence. The following options are possible:

- A record of the briefing discussion in the patient's case notes
- The signature confirming the patient's declaration of authorisation
- The completion of a (partially prepared) record accompanied by the patient's signature

LIESTAL CANTONAL HOSPITAL

Printer

ADMISSION REGISTRATION
ORTHOPAEDIC DEPARTMENT

Duration of operation ....

Ortho. **number** ....

Hospitalisation ....

Cost carrier ....

Type of treatment :
O 1. CL O 2. CL O 3. CL
O Hotel surcharge

Admission postop. inpatient O
day before O
..... days before O

Street :

Place :

For office use :

When : ....

Date of admission	Time	summoned

Specit : ill O
accident O
septic O

Telephone home: work :

Diagnosis

General ICD10 code

Autologous blood donations:
O 1 units O 2 units
O 3 units O 4 units

Long-term anticoagulation
O yes O no

Allergies :

Hb[1) ....gr%

Scheduled O **Operation** O **Cons. Therapy** O **Investigation**

O right
O left
O bilat.

Responsible Operator :

Follow-up treatment O outpatient
O spa treatment
O inpatient rehabilitation [2)]

To start O 6 weeks postoperatively
O immediately after discharge from hospital (LCH)

Additionally required files LCH
O Case notes (inpt./outpt.) and orthopaedic/traumatology x-rays before 1993
years ....
O Case notes from other departments in the hospital (name, year)
....
O X-rays from other hospitals

Files to be ordered from other hospitals by the secretariat (place, year) ....

Orthopaedic operating team for operation O order O prepare
....

Order sent to GP O for chest O ECG O ....

Investigations on admission O Normal laboratory O Chest O ECG
O Spec. laboratory:............... O Consultation: ....
O X-Rays: ....

Comments / special remarks

Date : Admitting doctor :

O Please tick as applicable

a

1) Only determine before donation if the Hb is suspected to be less than 11 g%
2) Indicate only for genuine disability / more complex rehabilitation problems

Form. 3772/95

Fig. 16.1a,b. Admission and briefing form used at our hospital
a Compilation of all the essential details for patient admission

Patient briefing conducted on: ....

by: ....

Scheduled operation: ....

....

....

Printer

Less recommended alternatives: ....

....

Patient was briefed on the possible occurrence of

- O Wound-healing problems, haematoma
- O Infection
- O Delayed bone healing
- O Implant loosening
- O Implant dislocation
- O Leg length discrepancy
- O Thrombosis, embolism
- O Neuroparalysis (e.g. .... nerve)
- O Circulatory problem (e.g. anterior tibial tendon syndrome)
- O ....
- O ....

Patient can expect:

- O Full functional performance
- O Functional improvement
- O Freedom from limping not certain
- O Improved mobility
- O Freedom from pain
- O Reduced pain
- O ....
- O ....

Approximate duration of treatment:

1. Duration of in-patient treatment approx. .... weeks
2. Full weight-bearing after approx. .... weeks
3. Total duration of treatment approx. .... weeks/months
4. ....
5. ....

Bone bank:

Do you agree that any bone necessarily removed at operation may, if not used for your own operation, be used for the benefit of other patients?

We would draw your attention to the fact that, for this purpose, a blood test for AIDS and hepatitis will need to be performed at the 6-month check-up.

O yes O no

The use of the following new implants/materials is scheduled for the operation:

- O Forked plate
- O New implant materials ....
- O Bone cement ....
- O Bone from the bone bank for ....
- O Other ....

Duration of briefing: ....

A copy is handed to the patient

Signature of patient: ....

b

Fig. 16.1b. Reverse side for recording the patient briefing

The *record in the patient's case notes* is currently the procedure most commonly used. However, since this is often incomplete and is done without the patient's knowledge, it only offers limited value as evidence and is susceptible to attack by the patient.

The *signature on a prepared declaration of authorisation* is a solution that we doctors have copied from the lawyers. But the lawyers consider the small print and preformulated explanations to be unacceptable, since there is no guarantee that the patient has actually understood the written text. This arrangement is more valuable if the patient not only signs the form, but also confirms that the written text has been explained to him orally in comprehensible terms.

The *completion of a (partially prepared) record accompanied by the patient's signature* offers the possibility of adaptation to the patient's individual case. It can be drawn up concurrently with the oral briefing, which takes up most of the time. The record is available at the end of the discussion for subsequent perusal and a copy can be given to the patient to take home (Fig. 16.1).

None of the above-mentioned solutions is entirely satisfactory. On the other hand, no one – at least no one in the European community – is demanding comprehensive written individual agreements. In view of the prevailing explosion in costs, we probably need to be careful about formulating any radical rulings. We orthopaedic surgeons are, however, in an exposed position. The Swiss Orthopaedic Association has therefore issued the following recommendations concerning content [1]:

- Diagnosis
- Course of the illness/accident with/without treatment
- Scheduled operation (approximate timetable, period of unfitness for work)
- Any necessary extensions to the operation
- Alternative treatments
- General complications that can occur after any operation
- Potential complications of the scheduled procedure
- Specific aspects
- Duration of the discussion, any witnesses
- Confirmation, signed and dated by the patient, to the effect that the listed points have been discussed comprehensively and in understandable terms, and that the patient's questions have also been answered

Foreign-speaking patients represent a particular problem. If the doctor is able to converse fluently in the patient's language, he can make a record of the briefing, minus an accompanying signature but including a reference to the circumstances of the discussion, and file this with the patient's case notes. If a detailed discussion with the patient is not possible, an interpreter should be engaged to translate the necessary explanations for the patient.

16.4 Specific Briefing Before a Total Hip Replacement

16.4.1 Complications of a General Nature

Two especially important complications in a total hip replacement are bleeding, which can lead to infections, and thromboses in major veins with the consequent potential for pulmonary emboli. Since the operation is an intermediate to major procedure, serious pre-existing conditions that adversely affect the patient's health pose an additional risk. Specific mention should be made of the possibility of a fat embolus in the lung, which is more likely to occur after procedures involving the femoral medullary canal [2]. Precautionary measures are detailed in Chap. 3.

16.4.2 Local Complications

The most important local complication after the implantation of a hip prosthesis is aseptic loosening of the implant (see also Chap. 15). The frequency of this complication is presented graphically in the form of survival curves (Figs. 15.1–15.17). These are not very comprehensible to the average patient and will require appropriate explanation. An overview of the other local complications is provided in Figs. 2.11 and 2.12, while further details can be found in the corresponding chapters. Leg length discrepancies, limping and haematomas are the commonest complications.

16.4.3 Specific Problems in Revision Operations

Thanks to modern surgical, anaesthetic and transfusion techniques, the risk of dying after a revision operation has been drastically reduced. Nevertheless, it should not be forgotten that patients scheduled for revisions are, on average, older and frailer (Figs. 2.2, 2.3), are more likely to suffer from illnesses that increase the surgical risk and to undergo a more major procedure, than patients awaiting primary operations. As regards the probability of the individual complications, leg length discrepancies, limping and postoperative haematomas are more likely to occur after revisions than after primary procedures. By contrast, neurological complications and periprosthetic fractures tended to occur less frequently in our patients (Figs. 2.11, 2.12).

16.4.4 Effect of Complications on Quality of Life

Patients cope with the various complications in very different ways. A particularly tragic event occurring in association with a total hip replacement is a fatality, whether due to an embolus, acute heart failure or a local vascular complication. Despite the explanations proffered during the briefing discussion, the patient does not expect to die from an elective orthopaedic procedure.

Patients generally find it very difficult to cope with neurological deficits triggered by the operation. An unsteady gait that only improves very slowly over 1 or 2 years represents a serious burden, and it is difficult to provide an accurate prediction about the extent of the recovery. Nor is there any known treatment that will noticeably improve the condition. The victim has to wait patiently to see how the situation develops (see also Chap. 11).

The next complications to be noted are those that lead to further surgical procedures after a brief period, such as early or delayed infections, dislocation tendency requiring revision, trochanteric nonunions or loosening in the first few postoperative years.

Chronic pain is another cause for dissatisfaction among patients, particularly since alleviation of pain is usually the main objective of the operation in the first place.

A limp, the need for sticks, restricted movement, leg length discrepancy and even a subsequent fracture occurring around the prosthesis generally affect quality of life only to a limited extent, or only in isolated individuals. Such complications are often based on a pre-existing condition that could not be rectified or could only be partially rectified. However, this fact does not exempt the orthopaedic surgeon from the obligation to carry out a meticulous pre- and postoperative examination in order to get to the root of the specific underlying causes.

References

1. Bereiter H (1996) Empfehlungen für die Patientenaufklärung. Bulletin der Schweizerischen Gesellschaft für Orthopädie 63: 18–23
2. Hirschnitz C, Ochsner PE (1996) Die klinische Relevanz von Fettembolien. Unfallchirurg 22: 57–73
3. Kuhn HP (2000) Operationsaufklärung – eine Optimierungsaufgabe. Schweizerische Ärztezeitung 34: 1838–1851
4. Ramer P, Rennhard J (1998) Patientenrecht. Beobachter-Buchverlag, Zurich

Subject Index

Page numbers in **bold** indicate exact definition of term

Sources of figures:

Figs. 3.2, 3.3:
Kindly made available by Centerpulse AG, Winterthur

Figs. 13.2, 13.4, 13.5, 13.6:
Original figures kindly provided by Prof. B. Nachbur; originally published in references numbered 13 and 14 in Chap. 13 above.

All other figures were produced specifically for this book at the Orthopedic department of the Kantonsspital Liestal. The Figs. 11.2, 11.3, 11.4, 11.5, 11.8. were produced in cooperation with the Cantonal Institute for Pathology at Liestal (Prof. W. Wegmann), and the Figs. 13.7, 13.8, 13.10 were produced in cooperation with the Institute for Anatomy of the University of Zürich (Prof. P. Groscurth).

MIX
Papier aus verantwortungsvollen Quellen
Paper from responsible sources
FSC® C105338

If you have any concerns about our products,
you can contact us on
ProductSafety@springernature.com

In case Publisher is established outside the EU,
the EU authorized representative is:
Springer Nature Customer Service Center GmbH
Europaplatz 3, 69115 Heidelberg, Germany

Printed by Libri Plureos GmbH
in Hamburg, Germany